Praise for
Population-Based Public Health Clinical Manual: The Henry Street Model for Nurses

"Population-focused nursing is a challenging concept, and this uniquely readable volume answers the need for a practical guide for new public health nurses and students. Each chapter explores nursing competencies developed by the Henry Street Consortium, providing real-life dialogue on issues commonly encountered by public health nurses. Topics such as evidence-based practice, effective communication, and leadership are welcome additions to the basic content on health systems, epidemiology, and other traditional public health themes. The authors capture the excitement and fears of new PHNs as they embark on their new public health career."

–Linda Spencer, PhD, RN
Coordinator, Public Health Nursing Leadership Program
Nell Hodgson Woodruff School of Nursing
Emory University

"This is a great resource for public health nursing education. It is comprehensive and filled with traditional and current applications for PHN practice. The format of the book has great utility, as it blends pertinent content with practice-based insights and strategies."

–Jean Bell-Calvin, MS, PHCNS-BC
Nursing Center Director
University of Wisconsin, Milwaukee
Silver Spring Community Nursing Center

Population-Based Public Health Clinical Manual

The Henry Street Model for Nurses

Marjorie A. Schaffer, PhD, MS, RN, PHN
Carolyn M. Garcia, PhD, MPH, RN, PHN
Patricia M. Schoon, MPH, RN, PHN

Sigma Theta Tau International
Honor Society of Nursing®

The Honor Society of Nursing, Sigma Theta Tau International, the only international honor society worldwide, is a global community of nurse leaders with members who live in 86 countries and belong to 469 chapters. Through this network, members lead in using knowledge, scholarship, service, and learning to improve the health of the world's people.

Sigma Theta Tau International
550 West North Street
Indianapolis, IN 46202

To order additional books, buy in bulk, or order for corporate use, contact Nursing Knowledge International at 888.NKI.4YOU (888.654.4968/US and Canada) or +1.317.634.8171 (outside US and Canada).

To request a review copy for course adoption, e-mail solutions@nursingknowledge.org or call 888.NKI.4YOU (888.654.4968/US and Canada) or +1.317.917.4983 (outside US and Canada).

To request author information, or for speaker or other media requests, contact Rachael McLaughlin of the Honor Society of Nursing, Sigma Theta Tau International at 888.634.7575 (US and Canada) or +1.317.634.8171 (outside US and Canada).

Print ISBN: 978-1-930538-97-9
ePub and .Mobi ebook ISBN: 978-1-935476-36-8
PDF ebook ISBN: 978-1-935476-37-5

Library of Congress Cataloging-in-Publication Data

Schaffer, Marjorie.
  Population-based public health clinical manual : the Henry Street model for nurses / authors, Marjorie A. Schaffer, Carolyn M. Garcia, Patricia M. Schoon.
    p. ; cm.
  Includes bibliographical references.
  ISBN 978-1-930538-97-9 -- ISBN 978-1-935476-36-8 (ePub and Mobi ebook) -- ISBN 978-1-935476-37-5 (PDF ebook)
  1. Henry Street Consortium. 2. Public health nursing. 3. Competency-based education. I. Garcia, Carolyn M. II. Schoon, Patricia M. III. Sigma Theta Tau International. IV. Title.
  [DNLM: 1. Henry Street Consortium. 2. Public Health Nursing. 3. Competency-Based Education. 4. Models, Educational. WY 108]
  RT97.S33 2011
  610.73'4--dc22
                    2011007032

First Printing, 2011

Publisher: Renee Wilmeth

Acquisitions Editors: Cynthia Saver, MS, RN, & Janet Boivin, RN

Editorial Coordinator: Paula Jeffers

Cover Designer: Katy Bodenmiller

Interior Design and Page Composition: Rebecca Batchelor

Principal Editor: Carla Hall

Development Editor/Project Editor: Billy Fields

Copy Editor: Kevin Kent

Proofreader: Barbara Bennett

Indexer: Johnna Van Hoose Dinse

Dedication

We dedicate this book to the public health nurses and educators who work together to create effective and meaningful learning experiences for nursing students. Your commitment and passion will live on in the public health nursing workforce of the future.

Acknowledgements

We wish to thank our colleagues in the Henry Street Consortium who generously shared their knowledge, experiences, and examples of the essence of public health nursing. The vision of Linda Olson Keller and Sue Strohschein for developing the public health nursing workforce of the future led to a federal Division of Nursing grant obtained by the Minnesota Department of Health. The "Linking Public Health Nursing Practice and Education to Promote Population Health" grant provided support for the development of the Henry Street Consortium. As a result of this support, public health nurses and nursing educators collaborated to develop the Henry Street Consortium competencies.

We wish to thank colleagues and recent graduates who reviewed chapters. Cecilia Erickson, Rebecca Hovarter, Renee Kumpula, Jessica Mallinger, Sarah Powell, and Sharon Cross provided helpful feedback for clarifying and revising our work. Megan Dohm, Kathy Fabro, and Arit Unanaowo searched and evaluated the literature for supporting several of the competencies. The colleges, universities, and health departments and agencies represented by Henry Street Consortium members are listed below.

Public Health Agencies
Anoka County Community Health & Environmental Services Department
Carver County Public Health Department
Chisago County Public Health Division of Health and Human Services
City of Bloomington Division of Public Health
Dakota County Public Health Department
Hennepin County Human Services & Public Health Department
Isanti County Public Health
Kanabec County Public Health
Metropolitan Area School Nurses
Minnesota Department of Health
Minnesota Visiting Nurse Agency
Saint Paul-Ramsey County Public Health
Scott County Public Health
Sherburne County Public Health Department
Washington County Department of Public Health & Environment
Wright County Human Services Agency

Colleges and Universities
Augsburg College
Bethel University
St. Catherine University
Crown College
Globe University & Minnesota School of Business
Metropolitan State University
Saint Mary's University of Minnesota
University of Minnesota

About the Authors

Marjorie A. Schaffer, PhD, MS, RN, PHN, is a professor of nursing at Bethel University in St. Paul, Minnesota. In 2010, Schaffer received the University Professor Award from Bethel University in honor of her scholarly work. A founding member of the Henry Street Consortium, she has taught public health nursing for more than 25 years. She has traveled to Norway as a Fulbright Scholar and Fulbright Specialist, most recently to consult on public health nursing education in Norway. She recently served as president of Chi-at-Large Chapter of the Honor Society of Nursing, Sigma Theta Tau International. She has coauthored articles on the Public Health Intervention Wheel and Henry Street Consortium. Schaffer has written more than 40 articles and book chapters and coauthored *Being Present: A Nurse's Resource for End-of-Life Communication*, also published by Sigma Theta Tau International.

Carolyn M. Garcia, PhD, MPH, RN, PHN, is assistant professor in the School of Nursing at the University of Minnesota and holds an adjunct faculty appointment in the School of Public Health. Her program of research is focused on adolescent mental health promotion and employs community-based participatory methods to develop, implement, and evaluate school-based, family-centric interventions for youths and their families. She has worked as a public health nurse for more than 15 years in settings ranging from teen clinics and detention centers to refugee camps in Rwanda and post-9/11 Red Cross disaster relief centers in Washington, DC. She teaches courses on public health nursing and qualitative research methods and advises undergraduate and graduate students' programs in nursing and public health. She currently serves on the professional advisory committee for the Minnesota Visiting Nurse Agency and recently served as president of Zeta Chapter of the Honor Society of Nursing, Sigma Theta Tau International.

Patricia M. Schoon, MPH, RN, PHN, is an adjunct associate professor at St. Mary's University of Minnesota and a clinical instructor for the University of Wisconsin, Oshkosh. She is a founding member of the Henry Street Consortium and has taught nursing and public health for more than 35 years. She received the Minnesota Nurses Association Nurse Educator Award in 2005 for her work on Nurses Day on the Hill and has developed an online political advocacy tool kit. She was president of Chi-at-Large Chapter and faculty advisor for Zeta Chapter of the Honor Society of Nursing, Sigma Theta Tau International. Schoon has developed innovative programs in the community, including a foot-care clinic for the homeless and a faith-based program for older adults. She has coauthored articles on the Henry Street Consortium and is the author of a chapter, *Population-Based Health Care Practice,* in a nursing leadership textbook.

Contributing Authors

Maureen A. Alms, BSN, PHN (Chapters 4, 9, 12, 13), is a public health nurse consultant with the Minnesota Department of Health (MDH). She provides consultation and technical assistance regarding public health practice to promote and maintain a strong public health infrastructure. Prior to working at MDH, she was a PHN team leader for Mental Health in Goodhue County.

Christine C. Andres, BSN, PHN (Chapters 9, 11, 12), is the family health supervisor at Kanabec County Public Health in Mora, Minnesota. She is actively involved in efforts to protect and promote the health of the residents of Kanabec County. She is a preceptor for nursing students and involved in training and development for PHNs in Kanabec County.

Linda J. W. Anderson, DNP, RN, PHN (Chapter 8), is an assistant professor of nursing at Bethel University in St. Paul, Minnesota. She teaches public health nursing theory and clinical in both the pre-professional and degree completion programs. Her current research interests include investigation of the public health nursing practice of faith community nurses and the development of faith community nurses as public health nursing preceptors for RN-to-BSN degree completion students.

Joyce Bredesen, MSN, RN, PHN (Chapter 5), is an assistant professor of nursing at Metropolitan State University in St. Paul, Minnesota. She teaches public health nursing theory and clinical in both the pre-licensure and degree completion programs. Her current doctoral project focuses on implications for clinical practice within the community setting for the homeless population. Other research interests include utilization of women's health care during pregnancy for underserved populations.

Bonnie Brueshoff, MSN, RN, PHN (Chapters 6, 13), is the public health director for the Dakota County Public Health Department in West St. Paul and Apple Valley, Minnesota. She manages and provides leadership for a staff of 150 with a budget of $14.5 million. Brueshoff has spent the majority of her 31 years in nursing in public health, focusing on prevention and early intervention programs, with an emphasis on maternal child health. She was a Robert Wood Johnson Executive Nurse Fellow from 2006 to 2009.

Sharon L. Cross, MSPH (Chapter 3), is the PHN supervisor for the Saint Paul-Ramsey County Public Health Teen Parent Program. Prior to working with the health department, she was a University of Minnesota School of Nursing senior teaching specialist and collaborated with colleagues on development of the PHN Competency Instrument to assess student learning. She has more than 30 years of experience in public health nursing.

Carol Flaten, DNP, RN, PHN (Chapter 7), is a clinical assistant professor at the University of Minnesota School of Nursing. Her public health nursing experience has included health promotion programs for families and for refugees, as well as tuberculosis prevention and control in foreign-born populations. Flaten's doctoral project examined quality improvement theory and implementation of a systems approach to improve the number of public health nursing visits to antepartum teens. She received the DNP Student, First Place Poster Award from the Midwest Nursing Research Society in 2010.

Patricia A. Henton, MPH, PHN (Chapter 11), is the community and family health unit supervisor at Chisago County Public Health Division of Chisago County Health and Human Services. She facilitates learning experiences of nursing students at Chisago County Public Health.

Karen Jorgensen-Royce, MSN, RN, PHN (Chapter 11), is a public health supervisor at Wright County Human Services, Buffalo, Minnesota. She supervises public health nurses who work with children with special needs, adults with disabilities, and elders. She assists in emergency preparedness and plans and coordinates the nursing student clinical experiences in Wright County.

Rose Jost, MEd, PHN (Chapters 5, 8), is the family health program manager for the City of Bloomington, Division of Public Health, Bloomington, Minnesota. She manages intensive home visiting services to high-risk families, health consultation for child care providers, health promotion education activities, school health services, and care of children with special health needs. She has a special interest in nursing education and maintains strong linkages with several university nursing education programs.

Noreen Kleinfehn-Wald, MA, PHN (Chapters 3, 4, 10), is the team leader for disease prevention and control for Scott County Public Health in Shakopee, Minnesota. She has 29 years of experience in public health in two Minnesota counties, inner-city settings, and in east Africa. She has primary responsibility for communicable disease investigation and management, immunization services, and has a special interest in public health data analysis.

Victoria Kyarsgaard, MS, RNC, PHN (Chapters 10, 13), is an assistant professor with 35 years of nursing experience in leadership, education, community health nursing, and maternal and child health. She teaches older-adult, maternal-child, community health, and leadership courses in both the undergraduate and degree completion programs. Her current research interests are developing cultural awareness in undergraduate nursing students and effective strategies for online nursing education.

Cheryl H. Lanigan, MN, PHN (Chapters 3, 9), is the director of quality improvement and analysis for family health at Minnesota Visiting Nurse Agency in Hennepin County, Minnesota. She coordinates nursing and resident experiences at MVNA and manages the MVNA Interpreter Program.

Karen G. Lindberg, MPH, PHN (Chapter 4), is the maternal-child health (MCH) program coordinator for Dakota County Public Health Department in Apple Valley, Minnesota. She mentors nursing students and public health nurses, coordinates MCH policy and program development, and provides training and consultation to state and local groups in the area of parent-child interaction and infant mental health.

Karen S. Martin, MSN, RN, FAAN (Chapter 3), is based in Omaha, Nebraska, and has been a health care consultant in private practice since 1993. She works with diverse providers, educators, and computer software companies nationally and globally. While employed at the Visiting Nurse Association of Omaha (1978–1993), she was the principal investigator of Omaha System research. She has been a visiting scholar and speaker in 20 countries and served as the chair of numerous conferences. She is the author of 70 editorials and more than 100 articles, chapters, and books combined.

Pamela Nelson, MS, RN, PHN (Chapter 12), is an assistant professor of nursing at Bethel University. Her areas of expertise include public health nursing and psychiatric/mental health nursing. She has completed research on the use of student portfolios to assess public health nursing competency development for baccalaureate and RN degree completion students.

Table of Contents

Foreword

The story of the Henry Street Consortium is about a group of public health nurses (PHNs) who overcame their differences to establish a powerful and influential collaboration. The Consortium comprises faculty representing schools that teach public health nursing, PHNs from local health departments providing clinical sites for nursing students, and a state health department PHN consultant.

The Consortium started with 13 health departments and five schools of nursing but has since expanded its membership. This partnership is unique not only because of the number of partners but also because of the nature of the collaboration—between health departments rural and urban, large and small, as well as between schools of nursing that normally compete for students and clinical sites. Though the Henry Street Consortium originated as part of a Minnesota Department of Health-Health Resources and Services Administration (HRSA) grant in 2001, this collaboration long ago earned its independence and set its own path.

The Consortium's name, of course, is taken from Lillian Wald's Henry Street Settlement—the birthplace of public health nursing in America. The beginning months of the Henry Street Consortium were challenging. Staff members from local health departments were intimidated by the credentials of the academic faculty, and the academic faculty members were hesitant to share their materials with faculty from other schools. The group worked hard to find common ground and sought a name with universal appeal. Henry Street was a good choice, not only because it gave everyone a common identity, but also because Lillian Wald was an ideal role model for the work that the Henry Street Consortium wanted to accomplish. The Consortium was committed to improving the health of its communities by redesigning the clinical experiences of public health nursing students.

The Henry Street Consortium proposed a bold goal—to prepare PHNs with the population-based competencies necessary for entry into public health nursing practice. Why did the Consortium develop new competencies when there were, in fact, numerous competencies? After reviewing existing competencies, Consortium members found that most competencies were written for expert PHNs. They wanted competencies appropriate for senior nursing students or new graduates. They wanted competencies that more clearly defined population-based practice. Henry Street Consortium members also wanted competencies that measured not only the distinctive skills and knowledge but also the characteristics and values that serve as the foundation of public health nursing practice. As Consortium members from academia and practice carefully listened to and learned from each other, they decided to develop a set of measurable, population-based public health nursing competencies for entry-level nurses that measured skills, knowledge, characteristics, and values. After much hard work, dozens of meetings, and endless drafts, they produced a set of competencies for novice-level senior nursing students or new graduates that is used by education and practice alike.

The Henry Street Consortium's commitment to public health nursing continues with this book. The Consortium's members have written an engaging book that embodies the mind, body, heart, and soul of public health nursing practice. It is written by PHNs who teach students in the clinical setting in conjunction with PHNs who precept students in their health departments. Many of these authors are nurses who would not normally, in the course of their work, write a book. That is one of the countless reasons that I am so taken with this book. It is delightfully grounded in real-life practice and full of concrete, practical examples and case studies. The student stories at the end of the book are a priceless gift. The authors leave a legacy of excellence in practice for future generations of the public health nurse workforce.

I hold a deep and abiding respect for the members of the Henry Street Consortium. It is a privilege to have been one of the original founders of the Consortium. The last chapter of this book concludes with a list of "personal characteristics that contribute to effective public health nursing practice." Many of these characteristics, in fact, exemplify the members of the Henry Street Consortium. The quality and depth of this book exemplify their creativity, humor, persistence, courage, and hard work. This book was an extraordinary undertaking by an extraordinary group of PHNs. Enjoy and use this book well.

–Linda Olson Keller, DNP, APHN-BC, RN, FAAN
Clinical Associate Professor, University of Minnesota School of Nursing
Chair of the Quad Council of Public Health Nursing Organizations
Robert Wood Johnson Executive Nurse Fellow, 2001 cohort

Introduction

Wouldn't it be great if you could easily download an application to your phone or computer that would give you all the tools you need to become a great public health nurse? One wonders how Lillian Wald, founder of public health nursing, would have used the technology that is at our fingertips when she walked the streets of New York City, caring for and living alongside the families in crowded tenements. Technological advances such as smart phone applications (apps) have dramatically increased our access to knowledge, data, and each other. However, though advances in technology might offer new ways to learn about and connect to things, information, and people, technology has limitations as to what it can provide. Similarly, other resources such as textbooks, journal articles, and even nursing faculty have limitations as well.

Developing competencies (i.e., skills, abilities, knowledge) that will help you become a great public health nurse takes more than mere access to or internalization of information and experiences from other people. The tools are important, but more important is the individual[md]the hands, heart, and mind that are using the tools to care and positively influence. Lillian Wald used what was available to her, and when something wasn't readily available, she fought to gain access. She was driven by something deep and profound. She was grounded in the lived experiences of those she was working to serve. She acted with purpose that might have begun with caring but was fueled by the relationships she established with the sick, the impoverished, and the needy.

Nursing, especially public health nursing, can be very overwhelming. The needs of individuals, families, and communities can appear insurmountable. Skills can feel awkward or too complex for any one person to manage, and oftentimes they are! The idea for this book originated from a shared recognition by public health nursing faculty, agency staff, and preceptors that public health nursing courses and clinical experiences are difficult for students and faculty alike. It is well established that clinical faculty struggle with finding enough enriching experiences for students. Often, one student is placed in a school-based experience, another student is placed with a local public health agency, and yet another might be placed in a correctional setting. On the one hand, the diversity in settings and opportunities facilitates opportunities for students to learn from one another as they share and reflect. However, this diversity also yields a challenge for faculty related to ensuring that all students are learning about and growing in all the core competencies. It can also be confusing for students who have difficulty adapting clinical learning expectations to diverse settings and who might or might not have a nursing instructor or public health nursing preceptor with them during all their clinical experiences.

The Henry Street Consortium (HSC), a group of public health nursing faculty from diverse schools of nursing and local public health nurses employed in health departments, schools, parish settings, and nonprofit community agencies, had been meeting regularly since 2003 to support positive, rich learning experiences for public health nursing students. The HSC developed a set of entry-level public health nursing competencies that all participants agreed to use in developing curriculum and clinical learning experiences. The HSC competencies are informed by key public health and public health nursing standards and guidelines, including the Quad Council core competencies, the Scope and Standards of Public Health Nursing, and Essential Public Health Services (see Appendix D at the end of the book). Companion documents include clinical guidelines and a menu of potential learning activities based on the competencies and recognized public health nursing interventions (MDH, 2001). What was missing, however, was a manual, or guide, for students and faculty to use in developing the skills necessary for effective entry-level public health nursing practice. We wanted a manual that would speak to students in an understandable, meaningful way and that would also address student concerns about practicing nursing in the complex and often unorganized world of the community. We needed to prepare future public health nurses for population-based practice. We hoped to motivate students to excel in their public health nursing clinical experiences and to engage in activities that facilitate learning and, in direct care, the health promotion of diverse individuals, families, communities, and populations. We sought to encourage students to think, think, think—to use their minds to grapple with moral and ethical dilemmas and complex health needs, disparities, and inequities.

For the Student Nurse:

- You have chosen a career as a nurse, and some of you might become public health nurses. This clinical manual was developed to be a tool you can use as you develop competencies and experience what it means to be a public health nurse.

- The knowledge and skills you acquire in your public health nursing course will enhance your effectiveness as a nurse, regardless of your employment setting. This manual will help you identify the public health principles that guide care for individuals, families, communities, populations, and systems. You will recognize and gain appreciation for public health's promotion of health and well-being and the prevention of disease and illness. And, you will become aware of public health nursing's overarching commitment to addressing health disparities and inequities with strategies that improve the well-being of individuals, families, communities, and systems.

- This manual will guide you in learning what public health nurses are, what they do, and what makes a public health nurse effective. It will guide you through the critical, or core, competencies you need to develop.

For the New Public Health Nurse:

- This manual provides an opportunity to orient yourself to the core competencies you are expected to demonstrate as a new public health nurse.

- As part of an orientation process, the manual will offer opportunities for reflection on a range of issues, challenges, and ethical dilemmas you will likely experience in one way or another during the initial months and first year of employment.

- Competencies such as assessment, collaboration, communication, and leadership are abilities all new public health nurses should possess; this manual offers you the opportunity to work through some of these broader competencies using public health nursing case studies and evidence from the literature.

- Additional competencies focus on developing critical relational nursing abilities, such as establishing caring relationships, demonstrating nonjudgmental acceptance of others, commitment to social justice principles, and holistically undertaking the nursing process of assessment, planning, intervention development, implementation, and evaluation.

- The collaboration of practicing public health nurses and public health nursing faculty to develop this manual contributes to high relevance of examples, practical application, and discussion of each competency.

For Public Health Nursing Faculty/Preceptors:

- This manual is a tool that can ensure your students are equally exposed to core competencies and a foundational level of knowledge with respect to public health nursing. For example, the initial chapters lay a critical foundation for public health nursing, and the subsequent chapters are individually devoted to a core competency. To help address this common difficulty of ensuring that all students receive the same foundational knowledge and skill development, regardless of clinical setting, clinical faculty might choose to assign a particular competency chapter to all students to ensure common ground. Another faculty might decide instead to assign different competencies to different students, depending on the scope of their individual clinical experience.

Organization of the Manual

This manual begins with a description of foundational public health nursing concepts. Then, each subsequent chapter is devoted to one core competency and organized according to the key competency characteristics. The elements of each competency chapter are outlined below.

Chapter Element	Description of the Element
Case study	A new case study is woven throughout each chapter to provide the reader with real-life scenarios experienced by student nurses or new public health nurses that address principles and challenges that are relevant to the core competency.
Notebook	The notebook is a table at the start of each competency chapter that states the competency, its components, and useful definitions of key chapter concepts.
Evidence Examples	Evidence examples provide the reader with summaries of research studies and other evidence-based practice sources that are relevant to the competency. These also offer a sense of the level of evidence available for each competency.
Activities	Each chapter has activities interwoven throughout the text, offering an opportunity for readers to reflect and engage in key ideas that are being presented.
Ethical Considerations	The ethical considerations section of each competency chapter applies ethical principles to a common dilemma that public health nurses might face. Three ethical frameworks are used: rule ethics (principles), virtue ethics (character), and feminist ethics (reducing oppression).
Learning Examples	The learning examples are additional examples of effective use of the competency in real practice that the reader can access as desired (i.e., additional articles, web-based resources).

Chapter Element	Description of the Element
Reflective Practice	The reflective practice section provides a conclusion to the case study with additional questions for the reader to consider.
Key Points	The key points section summarizes the main ideas of each chapter.
Think, Explore, Do	These opportunities are available for the reader as ideas for continued learning application of each competency. The course faculty might explore these opportunities and incorporate some into clinical assignments. For example, we might suggest a health education project or a social marketing activity to learn about and experience the core competency.

In summary, this manual appreciates public health nursing tradition and encourages adoption of innovative, future-thinking practice. Lillian Wald, the founder of public health nursing, was not bound by the traditions or limitations of nursing practice in her era. She challenged, questioned, and acted. She perpetuated change and demanded attention be given to the public health needs of children, families, and communities. She used every available asset and resource to combat poverty and disease, and when a resource didn't exist, she created one. She used evidence of the realities and challenges to inform solutions and strategies.

Today's public health nurse should do no less. Today's public health nurse has a growing base of evidence upon which to advocate for the health of those being served—evidence that ranges from a child's story to the results of a randomized controlled trial. We hope this manual promotes greater appreciation of what is expected from public health nurses and what makes an effective public health nurse. We hope the emphasis on evidence-based practice facilitates greater efforts by public health nurses to document effectiveness while continuing to appreciate, not minimize, the value of diverse sources of evidence. Your path toward becoming an effective nurse starts with you. It starts with your interest and determination to embrace what it means to be a nurse and, for some of you, a public health nurse. A commitment to figuring out nursing, or public health nursing, will take you on a journey that teaches, models, informs, changes, and challenges.

How can you not grow when faced with so many opportunities? Well, you can choose to ignore, deny, or reject what is being offered. Some nurses are hesitant to adopt emerging intervention ideas or practices that deepen, challenge, or conflict with the way things have always been done. Other nurses critically embrace new ways of thinking, acting, and evaluating. And still others advance the discipline of nursing by continually questioning, examining, and reflecting on what nursing is, what it isn't, and how it is practiced. We encourage you to become a nurse able to critique, willing to challenge, ready to adopt or reject, and eager to curiously and creatively problem-solve. With a commitment to becoming this type of nurse, you will have the tools you need. These internally driven tools, along with externally available resources (e.g., faculty, experiences, readings, this book), will contribute to your development into a successful and competent nurse. Finally, we hope this book finds its way into the tools that are within each of you—open hands, open hearts, and open minds—tools that will never be replaced by a downloaded application.

FOUNDATIONAL CONCEPTS FOR PUBLIC HEALTH NURSING PRACTICE

INTRODUCTION TO PUBLIC HEALTH NURSING PRACTICE

1

By Patricia M. Schoon

with Marjorie A. Schaffer and Carolyn M. Garcia

Key Terms

Community

Core functions of public health

Cornerstones of public health

Essential services of public health

Family

Health determinants

Health status

Key components of public health nursing

Levels of practice

Levels of prevention

Population

Population-based

Populations of interest

Populations at risk

Protective factors

Public health nursing

Risk factors

Scope of practice

Standards of practice

System

Practicing Nursing Where We All Live

Abby will soon be starting her public health nursing clinical and is struggling with the idea of practicing nursing outside the hospital. She was at lunch with two of her classmates, Alberto and Sia. "I can't imagine myself out in someone's home, or in a school, or in a community center or public health agency. How will I be respected without scrubs or my uniform? Is it really true that one of the most important skills in public health is listening and sometimes that is all that you do? I feel like I should be doing something."

Alberto responded, "My friend, Zack, had public health last semester. He said that it bothered him a lot at first that he had to listen and not tell his family what to do. He wanted to do more than listen—take a blood pressure or something. But after a while, he started to get comfortable. He said he really worked on his communication skills and got an A for therapeutic listening."

Sia commented, "I worry about all of this too. I was talking with Jen, a friend of mine who took public health last year. She said that on her first home visit, she went with her public health nursing preceptor. I hope our preceptors will do the same thing."

Abby said, "I am really worried about being out alone. I wonder what the neighborhood where my family lives will be like and if I will be safe."

Sia stated, "I already have my instructor's cell phone number on speed dial. We should get together with Jen and Zack and find out more about what they did to feel comfortable. I think they could give us some great advice."

Public Health Nursing

Public health nursing combines the theory and practice of nursing and the theory and practice of public health. Public health nursing, like nursing practice everywhere, involves the interaction of the nurse and patient or client; the health of the patient or client; the influence of the home, health care, and community environment; and the nursing care provided. One of the unique features of public health nursing is that the patient, or client as the patient is often called in public health, can be an individual or family, a group of people, or a whole community. The client could also be a system within the community (i.e., a school or church or community health or social service agency). Public health nurses (PHNs) work in homes, clinics, schools, jails, businesses, religious organizations, homeless shelters, camps, hospitals, visiting nurse associations, health departments, and on Indian reservations. Public health nursing is most often practiced in the community, but it can also be practiced in other settings such as hospitals or long-term care facilities. The following sidebar provides the formal definition of public health nursing practice.

> ### Public Health Nursing
>
> Public health nursing is the practice of promoting and protecting the health of populations using knowledge from nursing, social, and public health sciences. The practice is population-focused with the goals of promoting health and preventing disease and disability for all people through the creation of conditions in which people can be healthy (American Nurses Association [ANA], 2007, p. 5; American Public Health Association [APHA], 1996).

"I still don't understand how public health nursing is different from practicing nursing in a hospital setting" Albert sighed.

Sia responded, "What I remember from our public health theory class this morning is that taking care of people in their homes is different because we have to take into account the home environment and the community."

The core concepts from nursing that shape public health nursing include:

- Caring and compassion

- Holistic and relationship-centered practice

- Sensitivity to vulnerable populations

- Independent practice

The core concepts from public health that inform public health nursing include:

- Social justice

- Population focus

- Reliance on epidemiology

- Health promotion and prevention

- The greater good

- Long-term commitment to community (Keller, Strohschein, & Schaffer, in press)

Public health nursing care is provided to individuals, families, communities, and populations through a population-based lens. This lens enables nurses to view their clients within the context of the community in which the clients live. All aspects of the client's life are considered as the public health nurse carries out the nursing process: assessment, diagnosis, planning, intervention, and evaluation.

Key Components of Public Health Nursing

Public health nursing practice is shaped by several key components. You will find all but one of the following key components described in this chapter. The Public Health Intervention Wheel, a key component, is discussed thoroughly in Chapter 2.

- Scope and standards of public health nursing practice (ANA, 2007)

- Cornerstones of Public Health Nursing (Minnesota Department of Health, 2007)

- Health determinants (U.S. Department of Health and Human Services (USDHHS), 2000; USD-HHS, 2010)

- Levels of prevention (Stanhope & Lancaster, 2008)

- Public health nursing process (ANA, 2007; MDH 2001)

- Core functions and essential services of public health (Core Public Health Functions Steering Committee, 1995)

- Public Health Intervention Wheel (MDH, 2001)

Levels of Public Health Nursing Practice

Public health nursing is carried out at different levels within society; these levels of practice are: individual/family, community, and systems (MDH, 2001, pp. 4–5).

Individual/Family Level of Practice

Public health nurses (PHNs) work with individuals and families to promote health and reduce risks. The family is the essential unit of all communities and societies. A *family* is defined as two or more people who identify themselves as a family, share emotional bonds, and carry out the functions of a family (Clark, 2008; Friedman, Bowden, & Jones, 2003). Family functions include:

- Provision of emotional support and encouragement
- Socialization of children to roles and community expectations
- Reproduction of family members by birth or adoption
- Provision of economic support
- Provision of necessities such as food, shelter, and caregiving

PHNs work with individuals and families in many different community settings. Working with families in the community helps you understand the diverse socio-economic, cultural, and environmental factors that influence the level of health, wellness, and disease of individuals and families.

If you are working with an individual or family to help them adapt or change their values, health beliefs, or behaviors to improve their health status, then you are working at the individual/family level of practice.

Community Level of Practice

You initially identify the nature or characteristics of a *community* when you begin to work with vulnerable individuals, families, and groups. A community can refer to a:

- Group of people or population group
- Physical place and time in which the population lives and works
- Cultural group that has shared beliefs, values, institutions, and social systems (Dreher, Shapiro, & Asselin, 2006, p. 23)

If you are working with members of the community to help the community adapt or change its values, health beliefs, or behaviors in order to improve the health status of the community, then you are working at the community level of practice.

Systems Level of Practice

A *system* is an institution or organization that can be in one or more communities. Key systems include health care systems, public health systems, schools, churches, government agencies, non-profit organizations, and businesses. PHNs practice at the systems level when they work with providers and professionals such as teachers, social workers, nurses, doctors, government officials, and members of the business community working for different agencies.

If you are working with members of systems to help these systems adapt or change their values, health beliefs, or the way they conduct their business (behaviors) in order to help them improve their capacity to meet the health needs of those they serve, then you are working at the systems level of practice.

The Relationships Among Individuals/Families, Communities, and Systems

Individuals, families, and systems are best understood within the context of the community in which they live. Individuals and families interact with, and are acted upon by, their social and physical environment and the systems that influence their health. For example, families living in an inner city neighborhood might not have access to a grocery store that sells fresh fruits and vegetables nor the money for transportation to the store. The neighborhood characteristics influence family access to quality food and their nutritional well-being. Figure 1.1 shows an example of the interrelationships among families, communities, and systems.

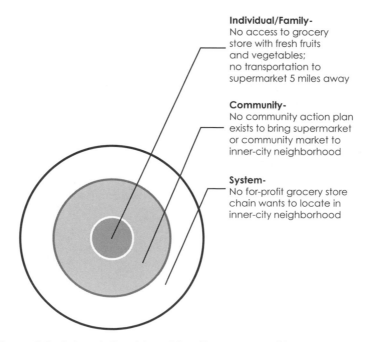

Individual/Family-
No access to grocery store with fresh fruits and vegetables; no transportation to supermarket 5 miles away

Community-
No community action plan exists to bring supermarket or community market to inner-city neighborhood

System-
No for-profit grocery store chain wants to locate in inner-city neighborhood

Figure 1.1 Interrelationships of families, communities, and systems

To make a difference for these families who live in this inner-city neighborhood, PHNs can:

- Work with families to see if they are eligible for food stamps or WIC (individual/family level)

- Work with a community action council to make them aware of the problem in the inner-city neighborhood and to inform them that they need to take action such as providing bus service from the neighborhood to a shopping center supermarket (community level)

- Help form a coalition of non-profit organizations and businesses to bring a cooperative store or other full-service grocery store to the neighborhood (systems level)

Table 1.1 summarizes the three levels of PHN practice and provides examples of how public health nursing is carried out at these levels.

Table 1.1   Levels of Public Health Nursing Practice

Individual/Family Level	Examples
Population-based, individual-focused practice changes knowledge, attitudes, beliefs, practices, and behaviors of individuals. This practice level is directed at individuals, alone or as part of a family, class, or group. Individuals receive services because they are identified as belonging to a population at-risk (MDH, 2001, p. 5).	• Home visiting to newborn and parents • Teaching hand washing to a first-grade class • Checking for presence of lead-based paint in a family home with preschool children • Developing a fall prevention plan for an elderly person living alone
Community Level	**Examples**
Population-based, community-focused practice changes community norms, community attitudes, community awareness, community practices, and community behaviors. They (PHNs) are directed toward entire populations within the community or occasionally toward target groups within those populations. Community-focused practice is measured in terms of what proportion of the population actually changes (MDH, 2001, p. 4).	• Writing a letter to the editor of local paper stressing the value of home visiting to parents of newborns • Creating a billboard about the hazards of lead-based paint • Holding community "town hall" meetings to make the community aware of safety hazards for elderly living alone

Systems Level	Examples
Population-based, systems-focused practice changes organizations, policies, laws, and power structures. The focus is not directly on individuals and communities but on the systems that impact health. Changing systems is often a more effective and long-lasting way to impact population health than requiring change from every single individual in a community (MDH, 2001, pp. 4–5).	• Meeting with legislators to advocate for reimbursement for home visiting with families of newborns • Developing a hand-washing program at an elementary school • Teaching local realtors how to recognize lead-based paint in a home • Developing a fall prevention protocol for nurses working with elderly in the community

Scope and Standards of Public Health Nursing Practice

All professional nurses have a *scope of practice* regardless of their clinical area of practice. A scope of practice refers to the boundaries of safe and ethical practice. A scope of practice is dependent on four components:

- Educational preparation
- Credentials
- State licensure law
- Clinical or employer role description

Professional nurses are also guided by *standards of practice*. These standards represent the professional guidelines developed by professional nursing organizations that specify how nurses carry out the nursing process in their clinical area of practice. One broadly accepted scope of practice and set of standards for public health nursing is the American Nurses Association (ANA) publication, *Public Health Nursing: Scope and Standards of Practice* (2007). Table 1.2 includes a listing of these standards.

Table 1.2 Standards of Public Health Nursing Practice and Professional Performance

Standards of Public Health Nursing Practice	
Standard 1. Assessment	The public health nurse collects comprehensive data pertinent to the health status of populations
Standard 2. Population Diagnosis and Priorities	The public health nurse analyzes the assessment data to determine the population diagnosis and priorities.
Standard 3.Outcomes Identification	The public health nurse identifies expected outcomes for a plan that is based on population diagnoses and priorities.

Standard 4. Planning	The public health nurse develops a plan that reflects best practices by identifying strategies, action plans, and alternatives to attain expected outcomes.
Standard 5. Implementation	The public health nurse implements the identified plan by partnering with others.
Standard 5A. Coordination	The public health nurse coordinates programs, services, and other activities to implement the identified plan.
Standard 5B. Health Education and Health Promotion	The public health nurse employs multiple strategies to promote health, prevent disease, and ensure a safe environment for populations.
Standard 5C. Consultation	The public health nurse provides consultation to various community groups and officials to facilitate the implementation of programs and services.
Standard 5D. Regulatory Activities	The public health nurse identifies, interprets, and implements public health laws, regulations, and policies.
Standard 6. Evaluation	The public health nurse evaluates the health status of the population.

Standards of Professional Performance

Standard 7. Quality of Practice	The public health nurse systematically enhances the quality and effectiveness of nursing practice.
Standard 8. Education	The public health nurse attains knowledge and competency that reflects current nursing and public health practice.
Standard 9. Professional Practice Evaluation	The public health nurse evaluates one's own nursing practice in relationship to professional practice standards and guidelines, relevant statutes, rules, and regulations.
Standard 10. Collegiality and Professional Relationships	The public health nurse establishes collegial partnerships while interacting with representatives of the population, organizations, and health and human services professionals, and contributes to the professional development of peers, students, colleagues, and others.
Standard 11. Collaboration	The public health nurse collaborates with representatives of the population, organizations, and health and human services professionals in providing for and promoting the health of the population.
Standard 12. Ethics	The public health nurse integrates ethical provisions in all areas of practice.
Standard 13. Research	The public health nurse integrates research findings into practice.

Standard 14. Resource Utilization	The public health nurse considers factors related to safety, effectiveness, cost, and impact of practice and on the population in the planning and delivery of nursing and public health programs, policies, and services.
Standard 15. Leadership	The public health nurse provides leadership in nursing and public health.
Standard 16. Advocacy	The public health nurse advocates to protect the health, safety, and rights of the population.

Source: American Nurses Association. (2007). Public Health Nursing: Scope and Standards of Practice. Silver Springs, MD; Author.

The definition of public health nursing presented earlier and the goals of public health nursing practice that follow help to define the professional scope of public health nursing practice. PHNs work to improve population health at the local, state, national, and international levels (ANA, 2007). Public health nursing goals are to promote and preserve the health of populations and the public, prevent disease and disability, and protect the health of the community as a whole. PHNs frequently partner with other health and social services professionals and community members to achieve these goals. Although PHNs are employed in many different settings, they always practice with a focus on the priority health needs of the community.

Population-Based Nursing Practice

Public health nursing practice is population-based because it starts by focusing on the population as a whole to determine the priority health needs of a community. "A *population* is defined as a collection of individuals who have one or more personal or environmental characteristics in common" (MDH, 2001, p. 2). PHNs in a variety of work settings can carry out population-based practice. To be population-based, public health nursing practice should meet five criteria:

- Focus on entire populations possessing similar health concerns or characteristics

- Be guided by an assessment of population health status that is determined through a community health assessment process

- Consider the broad determinants of health

- Consider all levels of prevention, with a preference for primary prevention

- Consider all levels of practice (individual/family, community, system) (MDH, 2001, p. 3–4; MDH, 2003)

ACTIVITY

Population-based health practice is often complex. Resolution of population-health problems generally requires multiple interventions, levels of prevention, and levels of practice. Read the following case study and respond to the questions.

How are the five criteria for population-based practice represented in the interpersonal violence case study?

What levels of prevention are involved?

What levels of practice are involved?

Case Study: Increase in Interpersonal Violence in the Community

The annual health report in Community A based on the biannual community health assessment documented an increase in interpersonal violence. The County Health Board establishes a goal to reduce this interpersonal violence. PHNs in a variety of work settings become involved in programs to achieve this health goal. PHNs working with families in their homes counsel families on how to prevent and report intra-familial abuse. School nurses work on anti-bullying campaigns with students, teachers, staff, and parent-teacher associations. Occupational health nurses start screening for increased worker stress and referral of stressed workers to employee assistance programs. PHNs participate in a media campaign to help increase the public's awareness of the seriousness of interpersonal violence and the need for more community intervention programs.

Populations in the Community

PHNs work with two types of populations in the community: *populations of interest* and *populations at risk* (MDH, 2001, p. 2). Table 1.3 defines these populations and provides examples of them.

Table 1.3   Populations Served by Public Health

	Population of Interest	**Population at Risk**
Definition	Population who is essentially healthy but could improve factors that promote or protect health	Population with a common identified risk factor or risk exposure that poses a threat to health
Examples	Families who live in urban areas with little opportunity for exercise because of lack of parks, playgrounds, or bike paths	Children who are not immunized for major childhood illnesses such as measles and chickenpox
	College students who have increased stress because of study needs and college debts and are looking for ways to reduce their stress level	Older members of a church congregation who live alone and are at risk for falls

Cornerstones of Public Health Nursing

The *Cornerstones of Public Health Nursing* (MDH, 2007) provide the foundation for population-based nursing practice (Schaffer et al., 2010). The Cornerstones, listed below, reflect the values and beliefs that guide public health nursing practice.

- Focuses on the health of entire populations

- Reflects community priorities and needs

- Establishes caring relationships with communities, systems, individuals, and families

- Is grounded in social justice, compassion, sensitivity to diversity, and respect for the worth of all people, especially the vulnerable

- Encompasses mental, physical, emotional, social, spiritual, and environmental aspects of health

- Promotes health through strategies driven by epidemiological evidence

- Collaborates with community resources to achieve those strategies, but can and will work alone if necessary

- Derives its authority for independent action from the Nurse Practice Act

  Source: Keller, Strohscheim, & Schaffer, in press; Minnesota Department of Health, Center for Public Health Nursing, 2007. Adapted from Original, 2004, by the Center for Public Health Nursing.

These Cornerstones are reflected in daily practice of PHNs when they:

- Organize their workload and schedule based on priority health needs of clients and community

- Take time to establish trust when visiting families in their homes

- Carry out holistic assessments of individuals and families within the context of culture, ethnicity, and communities

- Use evidence-based practice from nursing and public health sciences to select appropriate and effective interventions

- Collaborate with other members of the health care team

- Make critical decisions about the needs of their clients and the selection, implementation, and evaluation of interventions based on their professional knowledge and professional licensure

Abby is spending the day with her PHN preceptor. Her preceptor receives a referral to visit a family who just moved into the community and is homeless. The PHN knows that a health priority for her community and agency is to improve the health of homeless populations, particularly those in the population with young children. Recent data on the health needs of her county demonstrate that homeless families with young children have higher rates of malnutrition and developmental delays. Abby works with her PHN preceptor to modify her home-visiting plan for the day so that she can make an initial visit to this family at the local family homeless shelter. The family is Spanish-speaking and the PHN does not speak Spanish, so she arranges for an interpreter to accompany her on the visit to this family. The PHN has Abby call Social Services to see if the family's application for cash assistance and temporary housing in a family homeless shelter has been approved. The PHN has Abby gather information about local homeless shelters and food banks to take to the visit and has her get some bus passes for the family to use when they go to different agencies to apply for as-

sistance. After her busy day with her PHN preceptor, Abby discussed her visit to the homeless family with Alberto and Sia that evening. Their instructor has challenged them to identify the Cornerstones of Public Health Nursing found in their clinical visit that day.

Health Determinants

Public health nurses consider the multiple factors that determine the health of their clients. *Health determinants* are factors that influence the health of individuals, families, and populations. Health determinants can have a positive or negative influence on health.

- *Protective factors* are health determinants that protect one from illness and/or assist in improving health.

- *Risk factors* are health determinants that contribute to the potential for illness to occur or to a decrease in health or well-being.

Key health determinants include multiple interacting components. Biological, behavioral, and environmental factors interact and contribute to the health and illness of individuals, families, and populations (ANA, 2007; Marmot & Wilkinson, 1999; Public Health Agency of Canada, 2002; USDHHS, 2000; USDHHS, 2010; Zahner and Block, 2006).

Health Status

PHNs use the community assessment process and public health nursing process to determine the *health status* of individuals, families, communities, and populations. *Health status* refers to the level of health or illness and is the outcome of the interaction of the multiple health determinants. Health status indicators are used to measure health status. Health status indicators are frequently represented by statistical measures such as rates and percentages. Some common examples of population health status indicators are teen pregnancy rate, percent of low-birth-weight babies, neonatal mortality rate, percent of malnutrition in a group, and obesity rate. Rates and percentages of different population groups can be compared to determine similarities or differences in the health status of the different groups. Health status comparisons can also be applied at an individual level, such as identifying a child with malnutrition as having a lower level of health than a child who is not malnourished. Health status comparisons allow PHNs to determine their priorities for nursing care among individuals, families, communities, and populations. Figure 1.2 illustrates a health determinants model.

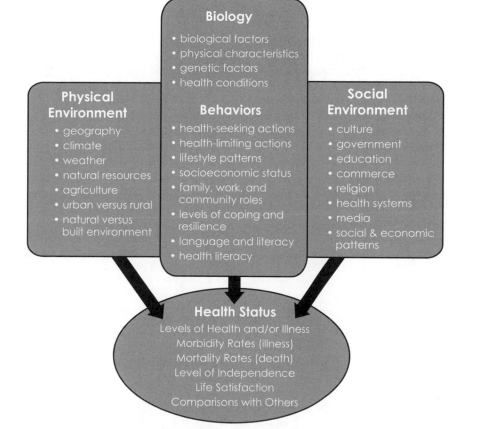

Figure 1.2   Health for individuals/families, communities, and populations

This health determinants framework is a comprehensive approach to assessing and intervening with clients in the community. In this model the social environment includes access to health care and health policy as aspects of health systems. PHNs can use it to organize and identify the complex contributors to the health status of specific individuals, families, and populations and to develop interventions to improve health. Health determinants, including protective and risk factors, exist at individual/family, community, and systems levels, so interventions should include elements that address factors in each level.

ACTIVITY

Review the following Health Determinants Analysis Case Study.

Identify the health status indicators for this community.

Identify health determinants that contribute to the health status of this community.

How would you modify the health determinants that negatively affect the health status of this community?

Case Study: Health Determinants Analysis

A community assessment in a small rural community determines that over one-third of the adult residents are overweight or obese. The assessment reveals 40% of the adults in this community report that they have high cholesterol and 30% report that they have high blood pressure. The majority of adults admit to eating out at fast-food restaurants at least five times a week. This community contains many fast-food restaurants, and the most common foods sold in them are high in fat, sodium, sugar, and calories. This community has few outdoor recreational sites, such as bike and walking paths, and the county board has voted down increasing tax levies to provide those paths. The local hospital does provide evening and weekend health education classes on modifying diet and exercise to lead a healthier life.

Levels of Prevention

The *levels of prevention* comprise a health intervention framework applied to the stages of health and disease for individuals and groups (Stanhope & Lancaster, 2008). The levels of prevention illustrated in Figure 1.3 help to determine appropriate activities and goals for an intervention.

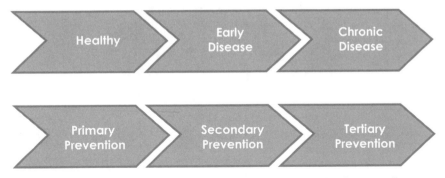

Figure 1.3 Stages of health and disease and levels of prevention

The major focus of many public health nursing activities is primary prevention. However PHNs provide care at all levels of prevention. In contrast, within the hospital setting, the focus of most nursing care is on ill patients and their family members. In the hospital setting, nurses more often provide secondary and tertiary prevention care but certainly might provide some primary prevention. The definition of each level of prevention follows.

Definitions of Levels of Prevention

Primary prevention both promotes health and protects against threats to health. It is designed to keep problems from occurring in the first place. It promotes resiliency and protective factors or reduces susceptibility and exposure to risk factors. Primary prevention occurs before a problem develops. It targets essentially well populations.

Secondary prevention detects and treats problems in their early stages. It keeps problems from causing serious or long-term effects or from affecting others. It identifies risks or hazards and modifies, removes, or treats them before a problem becomes more serious. Secondary prevention is implemented after a problem has begun, but before signs and symptoms appear. It targets populations that have risk factors in common.

Tertiary prevention limits further negative effects from a problem and aims to keep existing problems from getting worse. Tertiary prevention is implemented after a disease or injury has occurred. It alleviates the effects of disease and injury and restores individuals to optimal level of functioning. It targets populations who have experienced disease or injury.

MDH, 2000, p. 14

Three Core Public Health Functions and Ten Essential Services of Public Health

PHNs and other public health professionals who work for governmental public health agencies have a scope of practice that is unique based on identified *core public health functions* and the *essential services of public health* (Institute of Medicine (IOM), 1988). The three core functions follow.

- **Assessment**—Community assessment of population health needs by monitoring and investigating levels of population health and illness

- **Policy Development**—Development of health policies, goals, plans, and interventions to meet priority community health needs

- **Assurance**—Measurement of outcomes of health policies, goals, plans, and interventions and the competency and adequacy of public health professionals to determine that priority health needs of a community have been met in an efficient, effective, and timely manner

Public health departments, as official government agencies, and the public health professionals who work for them must comply with the health mandates, laws, and regulations at local, state, and federal levels. The public health agencies and staff are accountable to the communities they serve. The Ten Essential Services of Public Health (Core Public Health Functions Steering Committee, 1995) have been identified as those that need to be carried out by PHNs and other public health professionals to maintain the health of a community and its diverse populations. The Ten Essential Services with examples are outlined in Table 1.4.

Table 1.4   Ten Essential Services of Public Health

Essential Service	Examples
1. Monitor Health	• Carry out community assessment to determine levels of health and illness in community and populations
2. Diagnose and Investigate	• Check lead levels of preschool children, infants, and toddlers at risk for lead poisoning
	• Diabetic screening in Native American community

3. Inform, Educate, and Empower	• Teach first-time parents how to care for their new baby • Provide car seat education to new parents
4. Mobilize Community Partnerships	• Develop a network of community services for community-dwelling elderly
5. Develop Policies	• Work with county board members to develop a policy for playground safety in local communities
6. Enforce Laws	• Report suspected child abuse or neglect • Monitor compliance with immunization laws for school children
7. Link to/Provide Care	• PHNs and Emergency Department staff develop a referral and follow-up system for homebound elderly who visit the Emergency Department and then return home
8. Assure Competent Workforce	• Update public health nursing staff on H1N1 Virus • Teach rural PHNs how to do well-water testing
9. Evaluate	• Carry out evaluation studies to determine effectiveness of public health nursing programs such as home visiting to new families
10. System Management & Research	• Determine needs for public health services and service gaps in community • Provide data to justify how tax dollars improve the public's health

Source: Core Public Health Functions Steering Committee, 1995

PHNs employed by governmental agencies must meet the basic health needs of the community by providing the core functions and essential services necessary to maintain population health. Figure 1.4 demonstrates the relationship between the core functions and the essential services (Core Public Health Functions Steering Committee, 1995; USDHHS, 2010).

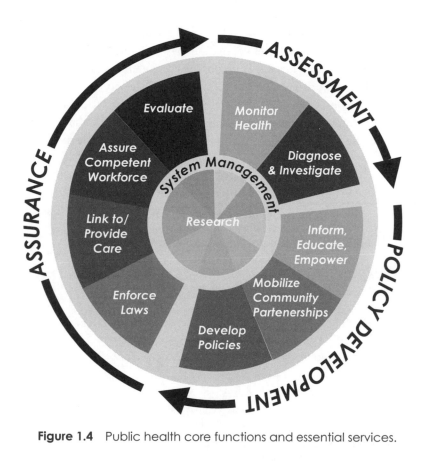

Figure 1.4   Public health core functions and essential services.

Essential Public Health Services Work Group of the Core Public Health Functions Steering Committee Membership: American Public Health Association; Association of Schools of Public Health; Association of State and Territorial Health Officials; Centers for Disease Control and Prevention; Environmental Council of the States; Food and Drug Administration; Health Resources and Services Administration; Indian Health Service; Institute of Medicine; National Academy of Sciences; National Association of County and City Health Officials; National Association of State Alcohol and Drug Abuse Directors; National Association of State Mental Health Program Directors; National Institutes of Health; Office of the Assistant Secretary for Health; Public Health Foundation; Substance Abuse and Mental Health Services Administration; U.S. Public Health Service Agency for Health Care Policy and Research, Fall, 1994.

Entry-Level Population-Based Public Health Nursing Competencies

Graduates of baccalaureate nursing programs are prepared for entry-level public health nursing practice. The Henry Street Consortium (2003) identified 11 entry-level competencies that are consistent with the national benchmark Quad Council Competencies developed in 2003 (Abrams, 2004; Quad Council, 2004) and that identify competencies from the novice to the expert levels of public health nursing practice. However, the Henry Street Consortium competencies focus only on entry-level practice and were developed specifically for baccalaureate nursing students and novice nurses entering public health nursing. The Henry Street Consortium Entry-Level Population-Based Public Health Nursing Competencies are listed in Figure 1.5. A more comprehensive listing of the competencies (see Appendix C) outlines the relationship between the Cornerstones and the Henry Street Consortium competencies, lists the behaviors that demonstrate the competencies, and includes examples of how to achieve these competencies. A comparison of the Henry Street Competencies with other professional standards and competencies is presented in Appendix D. The Henry Street Consortium competencies provide the organizing framework for this manual.

ENTRY-LEVEL POPULATION-BASED
PUBLIC HEALTH NURSING COMPETENCIES
For the New Graduate Or Novice Public Health Nurse

1. Applies the public health nursing process to communities, systems, individuals, and families

2. Utilizes basic epidemiological principles (the incidence, distribution, and control of disease in a population) in public health nursing practice

3. Utilizes collaboration to achieve public health goals

4. Works within the responsibility and authority of the governmental public health system

5. Practices public health nursing within the auspices of the Nurse Practice Act

6. Effectively communicates with communities, systems, individuals, families, and colleagues

7. Establishes and maintains caring relationships with communities, systems, individuals, and families

8. Shows evidence of commitment to social justice, the greater good, and the public health principles

9. Demonstrates nonjudgmental and unconditional acceptance of people different from self

10. Incorporates mental, physical, emotional, social, spiritual, and environmental aspects of health into assessment, planning, implementation, and evaluation

11. Demonstrates leadership in public health nursing with communities, systems, individuals and families

---

Figure 1.5   Henry Street Consortium Entry-Level Competencies

Key Points

- Public health nursing combines the theory and practice of public health and nursing.
- The goal of public health is to improve the health of the public.
- The Cornerstones of Public Health explain the beliefs and values of public health nursing practice.
- PHNs work to improve population health at the local, state, national, and international levels of practice
- Public health nursing practice is population-based, focusing on entire populations including populations of interest and populations at risk.
- Public health nursing is guided by an assessment of the community and considers the broad determinants of health.
- Primary prevention is the focus of public health nursing, but PHNs also provide secondary and tertiary prevention interventions.
- PHNs work at all three levels of practice (individual/family, community, and systems).
- PHNs are guided by the three core functions and ten essential services.
- There are 11 entry-level public health nursing competencies that are consistent with other nationally known standards of public health nursing practice.

Exercises

Reflective Practice

1. Review the Health Determinants model presented in this chapter.

    a. Identify key health determinants in each category in the model that have influenced your health status.

      - Biology _____
      - Behaviors _____
      - Physical Environment _____
      - Social Environment _____

    b. Which health determinants can you modify to improve your health status?

    _____

    _____

    c. Which health determinants cannot be modified?

    _____

    _____

2. Refer back to the Case Study: Health Determinants Analysis. You are working with this community to modify its health determinants

   a. How would you carry out the Core Functions of Public Health?

   _____

   _____

   b. Which Essential Services of Public Health would you be providing?

   _____

   _____

   c. What level or levels of prevention would you be practicing?

   _____

   _____

   d. Which Entry-Level Population-Based Public Health Nursing Competencies would you be developing?

   _____

   _____

3. What are the three most important things that you learned about public health nursing from reading this chapter?

   _____

   _____

4. What nursing strengths and skills that you have already developed will help you in this public health nursing clinical?

   _____

   _____

Alberto asked, "Let's see if I have this straight. The Cornerstones of Public Health Nursing and the scope and standards of public health nursing tell us what public health nursing is and how it is practiced. The Henry Street Consortium Population-Based Public Health Nursing Competencies focus on what we should be learning and practicing in our public health clinical activities. Do I have that right?"

Abby and Sia responded, "Yes. You've got it!"

EVIDENCE-BASED PUBLIC HEALTH NURSING PRACTICE   2

By Patricia M. Schoon
with Carolyn M. Garcia and Marjorie A. Schaffer

Key Terms

Critical appraisal	Interdisciplinary	Public health nursing process
Evidence-based practice	Interdisciplinary teams	Public health interventions

Abby is talking with Jaime, an RN who has returned to school to get his baccalaureate nursing degree. She asked him, "How do you use the nursing process in your hospital work? Did you ever think you could use it for an entire unit of patients and not just the patients you are caring for?"

Jaime replied, "It still seems kind of strange to me. But I am a member of the Quality Improvement Team. We just finished an audit to look at the incidence of patient falls to see if our unit is meeting the goals set by the hospital to reduce the patient fall rate. Our patient fall rate is still higher than the goal set by the hospital. We decided that we need to hold an in-service on assessing patients for their fall risk and the different protocols we can use to reduce patient falls. So, I guess if we think of my unit as a community, we are using the nursing process at more than one level of practice."

Abby pondered, "I guess I can kind of see that you are using the nursing process to assess the fall rate for the entire unit. The idea of using the nursing process with a system still seems very strange to me."

Jaime thought about the idea of nursing at the systems level and finally said, "Maybe if I think of the nursing staff on my unit as part of the hospital system, then the Quality Improvement Team can assess what they know about fall risk and prevention and design a program just for our staff to improve their skills in that area. What do you think?"

Abby sighed, "I kind of understand how I can use nursing process to assess the health needs of individuals, families, and communities, but I can't think how I would assess the health status of a system. Do systems have a health status?"

Jaime responded, "We use the term health systems to refer to hospitals. Do you think we can we use the term systems to refer to community agencies?"

Abby mused, "If a system, like a public health agency, doesn't have enough money to provide the health services that the community needs, then I guess it wouldn't be very healthy."

Jaime said thoughtfully, "Maybe we need to look at community health needs and determine if specific community systems, like hospitals, schools, educational systems, and public health agencies, have the resources to meet the priority needs of their community. If they don't have the resources, then maybe we plan interventions to help them get the resources or services they need."

Making Decisions Based on Best Practices

The Public Health Nursing Process

The *public health nursing (PHN) process* integrates concepts of public health, community, and all three levels of PHN practice (i.e., individual, community, and systems) into the nursing process (i.e., assessment, diagnosis, planning, implementation, and evaluation) (Minnesota Department of Health [MDH], 2003). This application of the nursing process is reflected in the American Nurses Association *Public Health Nursing: Scope and Standards of Practice* (2007), as illustrated in Figure 2.1.

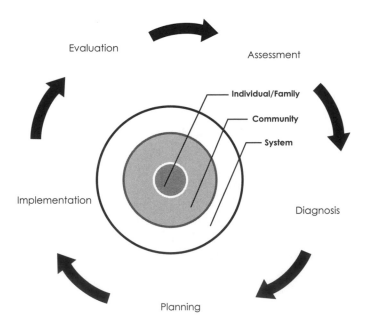

Figure 2.1   Nursing process at three levels of public health nursing practice

The nursing process applied to all three levels of practice will be discussed in subsequent chapters of this manual.

Interdisciplinary Practice

Public health nursing is *interdisciplinary* in that public health nurses (PHNs) often work with people in other professions to achieve public health goals. PHNs frequently work as part of *interdisciplinary teams*. Many of the interventions used by PHNs are also used by other professionals in the community. Each member of the team has a specific role and specific responsibilities that facilitate the implementation of coordinated and comprehensive interventions. Health team members can include nurses, social workers, physicians, epidemiologists, health educators, environmental health professionals, biostatisticians, and others. Other members of the team often include police and fire professionals, teachers, lawyers, child care professionals, governmental officials, and community members. See Chapter 5 for a more in-depth discussion of interdisciplinary collaboration.

Most educational preparation of different health professions occurs independently of each other or in "silos." This educational approach creates barriers that can interfere with the coordinated and collaborative efforts needed to improve population health. Duplication of services, gaps in services delivered, lack of understanding of the roles of different disciplines, and miscommunication can and does occur when professionals begin to work with each other after being "educated" separately (Institute of Medicine, (IOM), 2004). Whenever possible, public health nursing students should be given opportunities to work with other members of a community health team.

Competent interdisciplinary work depends on effective communicative ability across disciplines and team member cooperation. This cooperation requires members to be open to mutual listening and education to appreciate different ways of thinking (Gupta, 2006, 56).

> Abby commented, "My PHN preceptor told me that we are going to make a joint visit with the social worker to a family where a baby has Failure to Thrive. My preceptor is going to focus on assessing the health status of the baby, and the social worker is going to focus on the family support system and resources in the community for the mother. It will be interesting to see how they work together."
>
> Jaime responded, "I am going to an interdisciplinary child abuse team meeting with my preceptor. It is a county-wide team made up of police, social workers, lawyers, and public health nurses. It seems like my preceptor is always working with other people."
>
> Abby concurred, "It really does seem that PHNs work with lots of other disciplines. My preceptor says that is the best way to deal with community-wide health problems."

Public Health Intervention Wheel

Because PHN practice occurs at three levels, interventions must also be implemented at all three levels. *Public health interventions* are actions that PHNs take on behalf of individuals, families, systems, and communities to improve or protect their health status (MDH, 2001). A study of over 200 public health nurses from a variety of practice settings identified 17 population-based interventions specific to public health nursing that are found at all three levels of public health nursing practice: individual/family, community, and systems (Keller, Strohschein, Lia-Hoagberg, & Schaffer, 1998, 2004).

These interventions are organized in the *Public Health Intervention Wheel* illustrated in Figure 2.2. The Public Health Intervention Wheel is evidence-based and represents what PHNs do (Keller et al., 2004). PHNs often use more than one intervention at more than one level of practice (individual and family, community, or system) to influence the multiple health risks affecting individuals, families, and populations.

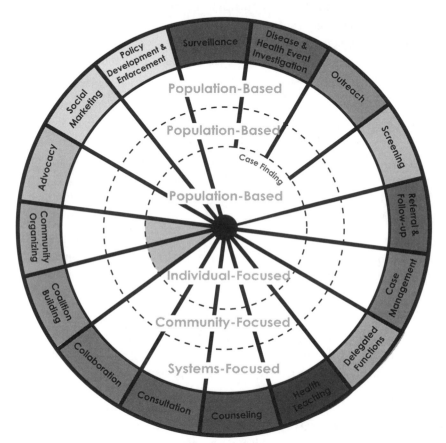

Figure 2.2   Public Health Intervention Wheel (MDH, 2001)

The intervention wheel has 17 interventions divided into 5 wedges with 3 to 5 interventions included in each wedge. Each group of wedges reflects a clustering of interventions that often occur together. A color version of the wheel that shows the wedges may be found at http://www.health.state.mn.us/divs/cfh/ophp/resources/docs/wheelbook2006.pdf. The three inner circles, called segments, represent the three levels of public health nursing practice (i.e., the individual/family segment, community segment, and systems segment). Most interventions are carried out at all three levels of practice. Sixteen of the interventions are independent nursing actions that can be practiced under your state Nurse Practice Act without a physician's orders. The seventeenth intervention, *delegated functions*, can include medical functions delegated by a medical professional or tasks or activities that the public health nurse delegates to another health staff member.

Definitions and examples of the 17 population-based public health interventions are outlined in Table 2.1. Interventions are organized within the five wedges on the Public Health Intervention Wheel designated by color of wedge after each intervention. The interventions described are all activities that nursing students can carry out.

Table 2.1   Public Health Nursing Interventions

PHN Intervention	Definition	Examples
Surveillance (pink wedge)	Surveillance describes and monitors health events through ongoing and systematic collection, analysis, and interpretation of health data for the purpose of planning, implementing, and evaluating public health interventions (MDH, 2001, p. 13).	• Investigate and report the incidence and prevalence of sexually transmitted infections in the local teen population (community level) • Work with a school nurse at an elementary school to develop a tracking program to identify the incidence and prevalence of student-on-student bullying before and after the implementation of an anti-bullying curriculum (systems level)
Disease and health event investigation (pink wedge)	Disease and other health event investigation systematically gathers and analyzes data regarding threats to the health of populations, ascertains the source of the threat, identifies cases and others at-risk, and determines control measures (p. 29).	• Identify and follow up on cases of sexually transmitted infection in a high school population to identify sources of infection and provide treatment (individual/family level) • Gather information about radon levels in your community and determine high-risk geographical areas (community level)
Outreach (pink wedge)	Outreach locates populations of interest or populations at risk and provides information about the nature of the concern, what can be done about it, and how services can be obtained (p. 41).	• Interview people at a family homeless shelter to determine who needs information about the location of local food shelves and WIC clinics (individual/family level) • Develop brochures for local grocery stores to hand out about nutritional needs for children and the location of local food shelves and WIC clinics (systems level)

PHN Intervention	Definition	Examples
Case finding (pink wedge)	Case finding locates individuals and families with identified risk factors and connects them to resources (p. 55).	• Identify new immigrants from southeast Asia who might be at risk for tuberculosis (TB) (individual/family level) • Give at-risk immigrants information on where to receive Mantoux (individual/family level)
Screening (pink wedge)	Screening identifies individuals with unrecognized health risk factors or asymptomatic disease conditions in populations (p. 63).	• Organize a blood pressure screening clinic at a community center (systems level) • Conduct blood pressure screening for African-American males (individual/family level)
Referral and follow-up (green wedge)	Referral and follow-up assists individuals, families, groups, organizations, and communities to utilize necessary resources to prevent or resolve problems or concerns (p. 79).	• Give an elderly person who is homebound information about how to contact a local Meals on Wheels program and then contact the individual a week later to see if he or she has successfully reached the Meals on Wheels program (individual/family level) • Work with Emergency Department (ED) nurses and home visiting nurses to develop and use a referral process for elderly individuals seen in the ED that need home health care services (systems level)
Case management (green wedge)	Case management optimizes self-care capabilities of individuals and families and the capacity of systems and communities to coordinate and provide services (p. 93).	• Work with parents of a newborn with Down's Syndrome to identify services in their community that they can use to help them (individual/family level) • Work with a PHN and school nurse to coordinate in-home and school health services for children with severe developmental delays (systems level)

PHN Intervention	Definition	Examples
Delegated functions (green wedge)	Delegated functions are direct care tasks a registered professional nurse carries out under the authority of a health care practitioner, as allowed by law. Delegated functions also include any direct care tasks a registered professional nurse entrusts to other appropriate personnel to perform (p. 113).	• Provide immunizations at a community flu clinic under standing orders from medical personnel (individual/family and systems levels) • Direct a peer counselor to work with a new diabetic to organize a grocery list and menu plans (individual/family level)
Health teaching (blue wedge)	Health teaching communicates facts, ideas, and skills that change knowledge, attitudes, values, beliefs, behaviors, and practices and skills of individuals, families, systems, and/or communities (p. 121).	• Teach a class for teen moms about how to care for new baby (individual/family level) • Develop a program on childcare for new moms at a local high school (systems level)
Counseling (blue wedge)	Counseling establishes an interpersonal relationship with a community, system, family, or individual intended to increase or enhance their capacity for self-care and coping. Counseling engages the community, system, family, or individual at an emotional level (p. 151).	• Provide support for parents who are coping with providing care for their dying child at home (individual/family level) • Provide crisis management services to a community that has just experienced a devastating tornado (community level)
Consultation (blue wedge)	Consultation seeks information and generates optional solutions to perceived problems or issues through interactive problem-solving with a community, system, family or individual. The community, system, family or individual selects and acts on the option best meeting the circumstances (p. 165).	• Help a recently divorced father who has custody of his two children to problem solve balancing parenting and work responsibilities (individual/family level) • Consult with a peer-counseling group for diabetes management to help them develop strategies for working with individuals with diabetes in their community (community level)

PHN Intervention	Definition	Examples
Collaboration (red wedge)	Collaboration commits two or more persons or organizations to achieving a common goal through enhancing the capacity of one or more of them to promote and protect health (p. 177).	• Partner with the nurse and social worker in an adolescent correction facility in developing a program to help inmates maintain contact with caring individuals in their family or friendship network (systems level) • Work with the county parks and playground department and local young parents group to develop a plan to provide more bike and walking paths for family use (community and systems level)
Coalition building (red wedge)	Coalition building promotes and develops alliances among organizations or constituencies for a common purpose. It builds linkages, solves problems, and/or enhances local leadership to address health concerns (p. 211).	• Establish a network of agencies to work together to develop a community disaster plan (systems level) • Develop an alliance between local environmental groups, waste management, and recycling organizations to improve community recycling (community level)
Community organizing (red wedge)	Community organizing helps community groups identify common problems or goals, mobilize resources, and develop and implement strategies for reaching the goals they collectively have set (p. 235).	• Organize a group of renters from several low-income housing developments to work together to improve the safety of their buildings (community level) • Help organize group of low-income housing services organization, community homeless shelters, and county human services to develop strategies to provide a more streamlined program for placing homeless people in affordable housing (systems level)
Advocacy (yellow wedge)	Advocacy pleads someone's cause or acts on someone's behalf, with a focus on developing the community, system, individual, or family's capacity to plead their own cause or act on their own behalf (p. 263).	• Help a client file an appeal for an insurance denial for home-care services when the client meets eligibility criteria stated in insurance policy (individual/family level) • Lobby legislators for support of community mental health programs (systems level)

PHN Intervention	Definition	Examples
Social marketing (yellow wedge)	Social marketing utilizes commercial marketing principles and technologies for programs designed to influence the knowledge, attitudes, values, beliefs, behaviors, and practices of the population of interest (p. 285).	• Create a video for teen parents on how to help their infants and toddlers meet developmental milestones (individual/family level) • Participate in a televised panel discussion about the effects of drug and alcohol use during pregnancy on the fetus (community level)
Policy development and enforcement (yellow wedge)	Policy development places health issues on decision-makers' agendas, acquires a plan of resolution, and determines needed resources. Policy development results in laws, rules and regulations, ordinances, and policies. Policy enforcement compels others to comply with the laws, rules, regulations, ordinances, and policies created in conjunction with policy development (p. 313).	• Participate on a county task force to revise county human services guidelines for mandating reporting of suspected child abuse or neglect (systems level) • Talk to a church group about the need to support a bill for community nutrition programs for children living in poverty (community level)

Source: Modified from MDH, 2001 by adding examples.

Notice the wedge that includes consultation, counseling, and health teaching. When public health nurses are working with a new mother and baby, they might use all three of these interventions to help the mother know how to best care for her new baby.

> *Jaime said, "I am going to a meeting with my PHN preceptor this afternoon about how the different county agencies and the school district are working together as a team to try to reduce smoking among high school students. I guess that would be an example of collaboration, but I am not sure what level of practice that would be."*
>
> *Abby pondered, "I think maybe the agencies and school district working together is at the systems level. If they used an intervention like social marketing to let teens know about the availability of a smoking cessation program at their school, then they would be practicing at the community level."*
>
> *Jaime responded, "Teens at risk for smoking are a population within the community and PHNs work with populations within the community. Well, if the team's goal is to change the smoking behaviors of high school students who are individuals and they used the interventions of health teaching I guess those actions would be at the individual/family level. This gets kind of confusing at times."*

ACTIVITY

Review the public health nursing interventions and examples in the Table 2.1.

What other interventions besides social marketing and health teaching could be used for the smoking cessation program in the high school? Choose two interventions.

What level of practice would you use with each intervention?

What members of the interdisciplinary team at the high school could carry out these interventions?

How might the PHN or school nurse work with these team members?

How might their roles and responsibilities be the same or different?

Public health nurses take a comprehensive approach in dealing with public health problems in the community. They use multiple interventions to achieve primary, secondary, and tertiary prevention goals at all three levels of practice and when possible, work with other members of the interdisciplinary team and members of the community. Table 2.2 demonstrates this comprehensive approach using lead poisoning as an example.

Table 2.2   Three Levels of PHN Practice & Three Levels of Prevention with Public Health Interventions

Level of Practice	Primary Prevention	Secondary Prevention	Tertiary Prevention
Individual/Family	**Health Teaching** • Teach parents of young children how to keep their children safe from lead poisoning	**Screening, Referral and Follow-up** • Screen individual children's lead levels • Refer to primary care provider for diagnosis and treatment	**Case Management and Collaboration** • Work with children who have long-term neurological deficits • Team might include a PHN, a PT, an OT, an SW, and an MD
Community	**Social Marketing and Outreach** • Staff a booth at county fair and hand out brochure on lead poisoning and children	**Screening, Referral and Follow-up** • Hold a lead-screening clinic at the county fair	**Case Management and Social Marketing** • Determine resources available for families with lead poisoning and create list of resources
Systems	**Health Teaching** • Provide education to pediatric clinic staff about lead poisoning risks in their client population	**Collaboration** • Coordinate services for referral, diagnosis, and follow-up with local pediatric clinics and schools	**Case Management and Collaboration** • Develop a case management protocol for working with a PHN, physical therapist, occupational therapist, social worker, and medical team

ACTIVITY

Read the following case study and answer the following questions.

Who do you think should be members of the task force for fall prevention?

Should interventions be aimed at individuals, communities, or systems?

What interventions would the task force be likely to use in developing and implementing the fall prevention program?

Case Study: Fall Prevention Program for the Elderly

Over the last year, the number of elderly seen in the Emergency Department at a local hospital for injuries related to falls increased by 50%. The hospital contacted the local Visiting Nurse Agency and asked them to join a task force to develop and implement a fall prevention program for elderly living in the community. The hospital wanted to reduce the number of elderly with fall injuries seen in their Emergency Department by 50% over the next year.

Evidence-Based Practice

Public health nursing practice seeks to be *evidence-based*, which means that the interventions used by PHNs are selected because they have been shown to work, to be effective. Evidence-based practice (Melnyk & Fineout-Overholt, 2005) is a problem-solving approach to clinical practice that includes the following:

- Systematic search for and critical appraisal of the most relevant evidence to answer a burning clinical question

- One's own clinical expertise

- Client preferences and values

Abby wondered about how PHNs knew what to do when they worked with their clients. She said, "The PHNs keep talking about evidence-based practice, but I am not sure exactly what that is."

Jaime reported, "Today my PHN preceptor and I made a home visit to an elderly woman who lives alone. We did a fall risk assessment and a home safety check. I asked the PHN how she selected the risk assessment and the home safety check tools. She told me that a committee of PHNs reviewed journal articles to find research reports on what assessment tools were effective for determining fall risks in older adults. They also looked at what home safety checks had been developed specifically for frail older adults living at home. Then they tried out the home safety check tools and picked the one that fit best with what their PHNs needed to know about the home environment. I think this is the way you do evidence-based practice, but I need to read more about it."

Abby commented, "One of the PHNs at my agency went to a fall prevention workshop given by an occupational therapist (OT) and a physical therapist (PT) at the local hospital. They taught the workshop participants how to screen older adults for fall risk and what type of interventions would help to reduce the fall risks, like using assistive devices, installing good lighting, removing slippery rugs, and wearing non-skid slippers. Do you think this information could be considered evidence-based? The OT and PT said they were reporting on what they had found worked best with their patients."

Jaime said, "I guess we could review the material on evidence-based practice in our textbooks and then talk more to our PHN preceptors."

"Good idea," said Abby. "Let's do it."

Using interventions known to be effective is important. PHNs are accountable to their clients (individuals/families, communities, and systems) and to the public to determine the effectiveness of an intervention and to justify the use of resources. Public health nurses have carried out research to demonstrate the effectiveness of many interventions provided to individuals, families, and communities. Though research for evidence-based practice might be limited in public health nursing, you should use it whenever it exists (Brownson, Baker, Leet, & Gillespie, 2002; Keller & Strohschein, 2009). Table 2.3 provides examples of interventions that have been found to be effective (Quad Council, 2007).

Table 2.3   Effectiveness of Selected Public Health Nursing Interventions

Individual/Family Level	
Intervention	**Results**
Health teaching	• Statistically significant increases in the prevention of scald burns (Corrarino, Walsh, & Nadel, 2001)
	• Improved vaccination rates for infants born to women chronically infected with hepatitis B virus (Corrarino, 2000)
Home visiting by PHNs or PHN-led interdisciplinary teams (Home visiting as an intervention includes the use of multiple interventions such as health teaching, counseling, and case management.)	• Reduced child maltreatment reports involving mothers identified as perpetrators of child maltreatment (Eckenrode et al., 2000)
	• 90% of pregnant women with substance abuse problems and not in treatment entered treatment, and 100% had full-term births (Corrarino et al., 2000)
	• Higher than average prenatal hemoglobin levels and higher rates of breast-feeding (Fetrick, Christensen, & Mitchell, 2003)
	• At-risk families showed significant reductions in postnatal depression screening scores and improvement in parental role (Armstrong, Fraser, Dadds, & Morris, 1999)
	• Significant increase in the use of primary care providers by indigent mothers as a regular source of sick care and better recall of health education information (Margolis et al., 1996)

Standardized home-visiting programs	• Long-term, sustained improvement in the lives of women and children (Izzo et al., 2005; Olds et al., 2004a; Olds et al., 2004b)
	• A program for building trusting relationships and coaching maternal-infant interaction resulted in improved maternal and child health (Kearney, York, & Deatrick, 2000; Olds et al., 2002)
Case management and teaching	• Interventions to parents of children with asthma resulted in statistically significant cost reduction for hospitalizations and emergency room visits (Corrarino & Little, 2006)
	• Case management, monitoring, and teaching to women covered by Medicaid who were at risk for delivering low birth weight infants, resulted in a low-weight birth rate that was less than that of commercial enrollees of the same insurer (Milbank Memorial Fund, 1998)
Community Level	
Surveillance	• PHN obtained critical surveillance information for emergency preparedness (Atkins, Williams, Silenas, & Edwards, 2005)
Coalition building	• PHN developed statewide and local community partnerships and coalitions for influencing policy development and organizational redesign (Padget, Bekemeirer, & Berkowitz, 2004)
Systems Level	
Health teaching	• PHN demonstrated the need for and developed, disseminated, and encouraged the use of head lice treatment guidelines among health care providers (Monsen & Keller, 2002)

Source: Excerpted from Quad Council, 2007

Before using an intervention, you need to look in the literature or consult with expert PHNs to identify specific interventions that can meet the unique needs and characteristics of your clients. Your own experiences as a nursing student can also be a guide as to what interventions you can carry out effectively. Nursing interventions should be both effective and efficient. Questions you can ask to determine effectiveness and efficiency are listed in Table 2.4.

- **Effective interventions** are those that fit the client's situation and preferences and result in the desired outcomes.

- **Efficient interventions** are those that take the least amount of resources and achieve desired outcomes in the shortest period of time.

Table 2.4   Analyzing Effectiveness and Efficiency of Interventions

Determining Intervention Effectiveness	Determining Intervention Efficiency
• Is the intervention culturally and developmentally congruent with the client's status and situation? • Is the intervention acceptable to the client? • Does the outcome of the intervention demonstrate improvement of the client's health status?	• What are the costs of the intervention (money, time, people involved, and other resources) for the PHN, the other members of the health team, the agencies involved, and the client? • Are the costs of implementing the intervention justified by the health benefits for the client and the community?

PHNs need to have effective and efficient methods for collecting and analyzing data on client problems, interventions, and client outcomes. The *Omaha System* is the premier management information system for public health nursing that meets this challenge by providing an organized data classification system that has been used extensively to demonstrate the effectiveness of interventions and provide credible evidence for best practices in public health nursing (Martin, 2005).

You can use several evidence-based practice models to help you in your search for credible evidence. The model we are using in this manual is based on the *Johns Hopkins Nursing Evidence-Based Practice Model and Guidelines* (Newhouse, Dearholt, Poe, Pugh, & White, 2007). The levels of evidence are illustrated in Figure 2.3. You will find examples from all levels of evidence in the remaining chapters of this manual. While the levels of evidence are presented in a hierarchical manner in Figure 2.3, this does not mean that lower levels of evidence should be discounted or that higher levels of evidence such as random controlled trials (RCTs) represent the "gold standard" in public health. It is important to thoughtfully consider and analyze information from all levels of evidence. For example, the use of qualitative research, particularly when studying culture and ethnicity, has led to significant understanding of how diverse populations and people view themselves and the world around them.

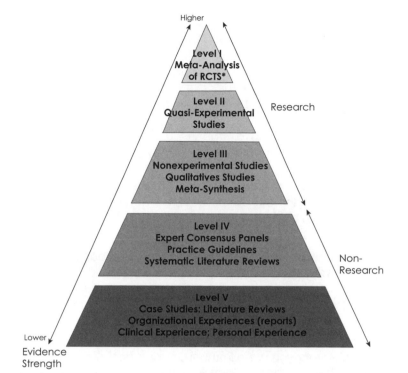

Figure 2.3 Levels of evidence: Adapted from Keller & Strohschein, 2009, as modified from Johns Hopkins Nursing Evidence-Based Practice Model and Guidelines (Newhouse et al., 2007)
*Randomized controlled trials or experimental research

You can find explanations of the levels of evidence with examples in Table 2.5.

Table 2.5   Levels of Evidence

Research Evidence

Level I: Research—Experimental (Randomized Controlled Trial)
Experimental studies have three distinct features:

1. **Randomization** of subjects by assignment to experimental or control group.

2. **Manipulation** of the subjects by introducing an experiment or treatment or independent variable (X) to the experimental group and observing the effect on the dependent variable, what you hope to change (Y)—for example, providing anti-smoking education to adolescents to determine the impact of education on smoking behaviors.

3. **Control** by introducing a comparison group that does not receive X and comparing the effects of the experiment on Y in both the experimental and control group. For example, what was the rate of smoking among adolescents who participated in an anti-smoking campaign versus the rate of smoking among adolescents who did not participate in an anti-smoking campaign? The researcher is looking for causality—does participation in an anti-smoking campaign cause a decrease in smoking among adolescents?

Example: The research reported here is part of the Nurse Family Partnership ongoing research and intervention program. The effect of prenatal and infancy nurse home visits on mothers' fertility and children's functioning 7 years after the program ended was studied using a randomized, controlled trial of 743 primarily black women enlisted in a public system of obstetric and pediatric care. The nurse home visiting program reduced women's rate of additional births, improved the stability of their partner relationships, facilitated children's academic adjustment to elementary school, and reduced childhood mortality from preventable causes (Olds et al., 2007).

Level II: Research—Quasi-Experimental

Quasi-experimental research uses scientific method like experimental research, but the distinct features vary somewhat.

- **No randomization** of the subjects, as to do so would be unethical. Subjects might be sorted into groups, but researchers do not control who is in each group. It would be unethical to withhold immunizations from children to see the effects on their health as the benefits of immunization and hazards of nonimmunization are known.

- **Some manipulation** in that subjects are placed in different groups based on their exposure to X (i.e., children who were vaccinated (X) versus children who were not) to study the impact of vaccination on child's health (Y). In other cases, only one group of subjects receives a pretest and post-test to determine the effects of intervention (X) on subjects' health (Y).

- **Some control** in that the researcher compares the effect of X on Y among different groups. So, what percent of children who were immunized for measles and mumps contracted the diseases compared to the percent of measles and mumps contracted among children who were not immunized?

Example: An educational program was designed to improve the nutrition of homeless children living in a family homeless shelter. Four nutritional courses were taught to 56 women by clinic nurses. Mothers scored higher on nutritional knowledge in post-test than they did in pretest; however, those mothers could make little change in the nutrition of their children because the cafeteria food did not change. The cafeteria food was heavily dependent on donations. This factor suggested that other interventions need to be implemented to improve nutritional status of homeless children living in homeless shelter (Yousey, Leake, Wdowik, & Janken, 2007)

Level III: Research—Non-Experimental (Descriptive, Qualitative)

These studies have no randomization, no manipulation, and little control.
- Non-Experimental Descriptive or Correlational Research (Quantitative)

- The purpose of descriptive research is to identify and describe characteristics of phenomena using quantifiable measures (for example, identifying the sleep habits and hours of sleep of parents who have a multiple birth).

- The purpose of correlational research is to compare the relationship between two or more variables (for example, comparing quantitatively the similarities and differences of hours of sleep among parents who have a multiple birth versus parents who have a single birth). If you discovered that fewer parental hours of sleep correlated with a multiple birth, that is useful information, but you could not infer that fewer hours of sleep were caused by the multiple birth.

Example: Disparities and trends in TB risk factors and treatment outcomes between correctional inmate and non-inmate populations were identified. Data from the national TB surveillance system from 1993to 2003 were analyzed. Findings demonstrated that inmates have a higher rate of TB than non-inmates and inmates were less likely to complete treatment (MacNeil, Lobato, & Moore, 2005).

Qualitative Research

The purpose of qualitative research is to develop an understanding of the meaning of life experiences. Patterns of behaviors, attitudes, beliefs, and values might be identified. This research might be carried out through observation (participating in or observing the life experiences of others), discussions or interviews, historical review of events and documents, or an analysis of a culture or subculture. The results are summarized and interpreted. For example, you might want to find out how a new immigrant group takes care of its ill family members. Observation and discussion might be the most effective methods to find out this information.

Example: A descriptive qualitative study was conducted to determine best practices in outreach. Ten public health nurses were interviewed. Strategies for effective outreach and barriers to effective outreach were identified. Knowledge of community resources, sharing information, and support of colleagues were identified as factors which increased effectiveness of outreach. Barriers were lack of knowledge related to resources, inconsistent awareness of importance of community assessment to identify resources, and incomplete understanding of intervention of outreach. Recommendations for improving the effectiveness of outreach were presented *(Tembreull & Schaffer, 2005)*.

Non-Research Evidence

Level IV: Clinical Practice Guidelines (CPGs) and Systematic Reviews
- **Clinical Practice Guidelines** are statements that include recommendations, strategies, and information that help health care professionals and patients make decisions about patient care. These guidelines are developed by groups of experts (for example, professional organizations and societies, government agencies, health care organizations, and other public and private organizations) who conduct a rigorous review of the scientific literature and research evidence.

Example: The Centers for Disease Control and Prevention (CDC) has published guidelines for immunizations for children and adults (www.cdc.gov).

- **Systematic Reviews** are evidence reports based on a broad search of the research literature and a critical appraisal of the research related to a specific clinical topic or question. The systematic review is different from a literature review which identifies research in a specific clinical area but does not critically appraise the research itself.

Example: Professional organizations publish systematic reviews of nursing research such as *The Cochrane Database of Systematic Reviews* published by the Cochrane Collaboration, and *Worldviews on Evidence-Based Nursing,* a peer-reviewed journal published by Sigma Theta Tau International (Newhouse et al., 2007).

Level V: Expert Opinion and Organizational Experience
Expert opinions are the written or verbal reports and advise of experts based on their extensive clinical expertise and experience. These written and verbal reports can be in the form of case studies; narrative literature reviews; advice and consultation from experts; quality improvement reports; financial data; program evaluations; practitioner experience and expertise; and patient experience. Journal articles, conference presentations and proceedings, webinars, and organizational websites, and online discussions are common communication methods for dissemination of expert opinion.

Example: The American Nurses Association (ANA), the American Public Health Association (APHA), the Association of Community Health Nurse Educators (ACHNE), and the Association of State and Territorial Health Officials (ASTHO) are professional organizations that provide ongoing written and oral expert advice in public health and public health nursing. These associations also develop and disseminate practice guidelines for nursing and public health.

PHNs need to be critical consumers of public health and nursing research. One of the most difficult skills is to know how to translate evidence from the literature or from consultation with experts into the context of one's professional nursing practice. The PET Process Model developed by Johns Hopkins helps the nurse to think through a clinical problem in an organized way (Newhouse et al., 2007). Figure 2.4 illustrates the PET process.

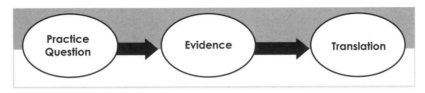

Figure 2.4   The Johns Hopkins Nursing Evidence-Based Practice Process PET (Practice Question, Evidence, and Translation)
(Newhouse et al., 2007, p. 202)

PRACTICE QUESTION

You should start by putting the clinical practice concern in the form of a question, such as, "What is the most effective way to improve the physical health of newborns during a home visit?"

One helpful way to frame your clinical practice question is to use the PICOT approach (Stillwell, Fineout-Overholt, Melnyk, & Williamson, 2010), which includes the following elements in the question:

- P Patient population

- I Intervention of interest

- C Comparison intervention of interest

- O Outcome(s) of interest

- T Time it takes the intervention to achieve outcomes

PICOT Question: Will pregnant adolescents (P) who receive weekly home visits from a public health nurse (I) as opposed to no home visits from a public health nurse (C) have improved birth outcomes (O) at the completion of the current pregnancy (T)?

ACTIVITY

Use evidence-based practice in your public health nursing clinical. You can start by creating your PICOT question.

What at-risk client (individual/family or population) are you working with most often in your public health nursing clinical?

- What is the primary health concern?

- What interventions are you using?

Complete a PICOT question to focus your study of the evidence.

- P   Patient population =

- I   Intervention of interest =

- C   Comparison intervention of interest =

- O   Outcome(s) of interest =

- T   Time it takes the intervention to achieve outcomes =

EVIDENCE OF BEST PRACTICES

After the PICOT question has been developed, you can start to look for the evidence of "best practices." Consider all five levels of evidence-based practice as you look for answers to your question.

Much of the evidence for effective public health nursing comes from Levels III, IV, and V of the evidence-based practice model. It is often not ethical, possible, or practical to randomly place people in an experimental or a control group, especially if placement in either group could possibly have a negative effect on an individual's health or well-being. An example of an unethical approach would be to do a study comparing the incidence of lung cancer of smokers and nonsmokers by assigning individuals randomly to the smoking and nonsmoking groups, thus causing harm to those placed in the smoking group. It is also unethical to withhold a treatment already known to be effective; for example, it would be inappropriate to conduct a study to determine the effectiveness of immunization for measles using a control group because the value of immunization for measles and the harm from non-immunization are well established.

For ethical, logistical, and financial reasons, quasi-experimental and nonexperimental studies are much more common than randomly controlled trials. Consequently, much of the evidence for public health nursing is from quasi- or nonexperimental studies. An increasing body of qualitative research in public health nursing exists. Understanding the context of the family, culture, and community; the meaning of events; and the impact of these factors on the clients' health behaviors and health status is often best discovered through use of qualitative research methods. Public health nurses also learn a great deal from their practice experiences and those of their colleagues. Case study examples can be found in the literature, shared at professional conferences, or reported on the Internet. These anecdotal reports are also part of the practice evidence of public health nursing.

When public health nurses are considering a new intervention or strategy, they can find it useful to conduct a *rapid critical appraisal of the literature* (Fineout-Overholt, Melnyk, Stillwell, & Williamson, 2010). A *critical appraisal of the literature* is a systematic process you can use to examine and synthesize the research data presented in an article or a group of articles. Generally, each article is examined, or reviewed, and then synthesized together. For each article you review, you want to ask a few questions to complete a rapid appraisal:

- What is the level of evidence of this study or report?

- If research, how well was the study conducted?

  - Was the purpose of the study clear?

  - Were the research questions stated?

  - Were the research methods explained and did they address the research questions?

  - Were the results of the research presented in an understandable manner?

  - Were ethical guidelines addressed?

  - Were the strengths and limitations of the research discussed?

  - Were the recommendations made based on the findings of the study?

  - How useful are the study outcomes and recommendations to your clinical practice?

Compare and contrast the studies and reports you have appraised. Select the best studies or reports with the most credible evidence that fit your clinical situation and address your specific question. Then develop a set of recommendations for action based on the evidence. This critical appraisal process was used effectively by public health nurses in a county health department to develop a set of guidelines for pediculosis management based on best practices (Monsen & Keller, 2002).

Evidence Example: Best Practice Evidence Leads to Pediculosis Management Guidelines.

Public health nurses in a county health department collaborated with epidemiologists, nursing students, and faculty to design and implement an effective population-based pediculosis management project. The focus of the project was the development of pediculosis treatment and prevention guidelines based on recognized best practices that were acceptable to both epidemiologists and practicing public health nurses. Guideline strategies had to meet two criteria: they had to be based on the life cycle of the louse, and they had to help reduce the barriers families experienced in lice prevention and control. Public health nurses disseminated these guidelines to community providers and reinforced their use through consultation and educational sessions. Two critical changes occurred as a result of the project. First, community providers significantly changed their recommendations for the treatment of pediculosis after nursing intervention. Second, public health nurses increased their population-based practice skills, continued to use those skills to address pediculosis, and extended those skills to additional population-based initiatives (Monsen & Keller, 2002, p. 201).

ACTIVITY

Use the PICOT question you have developed to focus your search for best practices in the literature.

Look for evidence of "best practices" for the intervention you selected.

- What electronic database or databases will you use?

- Carry out your literature search. Obtain help from the reference librarian if you are having difficulty with your keyword search.

- Select three to five journal articles that address your PICOT question about "best practice interventions." You may use articles that represent different levels of evidence. Make sure you select the articles that have the most credible evidence.

Carry out a rapid critical appraisal. Answer the following questions about each article you have selected:

- Who is the population being studied?

- What is the intervention being studied?

- What is the level of evidence of this study or report?

- If the article is a research study, how well was the study conducted?

- How useful are the study outcomes and/or report recommendations to your clinical practice?

Compare and contrast the studies you have appraised using your answers to the questions. For example, do the studies have similar or different results?

- Select the best studies or reports.

- Which articles have the most credible evidence that best fits your clinical situation and answers your specific question?

- Determine a course of action (interventions) based on the evidence.

TRANSLATION

Now you are ready to translate your best practice evidence into your own clinical practice. Make sure that your recommendations for action are appropriate and feasible for your client and specific clinical situation. Develop your nursing intervention plan based on your best practice evidence and recommendations, your own clinical experience, and client preferences and values. Then implement your plan and evaluate the outcomes of your interventions.

ACTIVITY

Evaluate the effectiveness of your actions or interventions.

Did your client(s) achieve the behavioral outcome?

Was your client satisfied with the outcome?

How did your intervention and client outcome compare with the evidence you found in the literature?

If your client did not achieve the behavioral outcome or the client's outcomes were inconsistent with best practice, review the best practice literature again. Look at all levels of evidence available. Consider consulting with a clinical expert.

If you follow through on these steps, you will be practicing nursing from an evidence-based practice framework. As a professional you will be accountable for your own nursing practice, so you need to be aware of and use best practices. You will find that we present many levels of evidence in this manual to provide justification for using specific interventions.

Jaime commented, "I think I am going to do my intervention paper on ways to reduce smoking in high school students. I have to start looking for evidence-based practice articles. I wonder how I should go about that."

Abby said, "I have been working with the college reference librarian to research my topic. She suggested that I use three databases: CINAHL, PubMed, and the Cochrane Database of Systematic Reviews. I have found a few good articles in each database."

Jaime responded, "Great! I will try those databases, too!"

Key Points

- The public health nursing process guides the actions of the PHN.
- PHNs work at all three levels of practice (individual/family, community, systems).
- Interdisciplinary teams are generally more effective and efficient in achieving public health goals.
- PHNs carry out 17 interventions unique to public health nursing; 16 of these interventions are practiced independently as part of professional nursing practice.
- PHNs frequently use multiple interventions concurrently to achieve public health goals.
- Public health nursing practice is evidence-based.
- There are six levels of evidence, and it is appropriate to use all of the levels of evidence.
- One way for PHNs to demonstrate accountability is to use an evidence-based approach in selecting, planning, implementing, and evaluating use of interventions.

Exercises

Reflective Practice

1. What do you think are the major differences between the nursing process and the public health nursing process?

   a. What will you do differently when using the public health nursing process?

   b. How will you prepare for this difference?

   _____

   _____

   _____

2. What other disciplines will you work with most often in your public health clinical?

   a. What additional information do you need to know about the other health disciplines?

   b. How will you find out the information that you need?

   _____

   _____

   _____

3. What public health nursing interventions have you used in previous clinical experiences?

   a. How will you carry out these interventions in your public health clinical?

   b. How will this be the same or different from what you have done before?

   _____

   _____

   _____

4. Have you used an evidence-based practice approach in other nursing clinical experiences?

   a. What have you learned in reading this chapter that you did not know before?

   b. How will your past experiences and your new knowledge help you practice evidence-based public health nursing?

   _____

   _____

   _____

ENTRY-LEVEL POPULATION-BASED PUBLIC HEALTH NURSING COMPETENCIES

II

COMPETENCY #1:
Applies the Public Health Nursing Process to Communities, Systems, Individuals, and Families

By Patricia M. Schoon
with Karen S. Martin, Sharon L. Cross,
Noreen Kleinfehn-Wald, and Cheryl H. Lanigan

Cherise and Zack were listening to Shannon, their public health nurse (PHN) preceptor, tell them about the clients they were about to visit for the first time. Shannon told them about the halfway home for young adults with emotional and behavioral disorders. This home has 25 residents, age 18–25, who live in congregate housing, sharing housekeeping, laundry, and cooking duties. The residents have been admitted from hospitals, chemical dependency treatment centers, local jails, homeless shelters, and from homes where family caretakers had become overwhelmed. Cherise was assigned to work with a young woman who had been admitted from a homeless shelter the previous weekend. Cherise asked, "How will I do a family assessment when I don't know anything about my client's family? She doesn't even live with them! Her family is still living at the homeless shelter."

Zack responded, "I am more concerned about the community assessment we have to do for the half-way house. Is a halfway house a community? I am confused."

Cherise said, "Well, I guess the first thing we do is go and visit with them. We need to get them to trust us if we are to help them."

CHERISE AND ZACK'S NOTEBOOK

Competency #1: Applies the public health nursing process to communities, systems, individuals, and families

- Identifies the population(s) for which the PHN is accountable

- Assesses the health status of communities, systems, individuals, and families

- In partnership with communities, systems, individuals, and families, develops a plan based on priorities (including nursing care plans for individuals/families)

- Implements the plan with communities, systems, individuals and families

- Evaluates—Measures outcomes of public health nursing interventions

---

Useful Definitions

Public Health Nursing Process: Integrates concepts of public health, community, and all three levels of PHN practice (i.e., individual, community, system) into the nursing process (i.e., assessment, diagnosis, planning, implementation, and evaluation) (Minnesota Department of Health, 2001).

Health Status Indicators: Measure the level of health or illness of an individual/family, community, or population, such as incidence or prevalence of disease, birth and death rates, level of independence, life satisfaction, and quality of life.

Health Determinants: Factors that influence the health of individuals, families, and populations. Health determinants can have a positive or negative influence on health.

Protective factors: Health determinants that protect one from illness and/or assist in improving health.

Risk factors: Health determinants that contribute to the potential for illness to occur or for a decrease in health or well-being.

Health Informatics: Public health informatics is defined as the application of information, computer science, and technology to public health practice, research, and learning (Centers for Disease Control and Prevention, 2010a).

Electronic Health Records (EHRs): "Longitudinal collection of clinical and demographic client-specific data that are stored in a computer readable format" (Martin, 2005, p. 461).

Community Assessment: The process of systematically collecting information about a community's structure, processes, and dynamics, its physical and social environment, its populations, and its level of health and wellness to determine its strengths, its resources, its populations of interest and populations at risk, its health needs, and its health priorities.

Family Assessment: The process of systematically collecting information about family structure, processes, and dynamics, their physical and social environment, and their level of health and illness to determine their strengths, resources, health needs, and health priorities.

Population: A group of people who share one or more characteristics such as geographic location, culture or ethnicity, age, sex or gender, developmental level, or health concern.

Priority Setting: Organizing health concerns by hazard level so that health risks that place individuals/families, communities, or populations at greater risk are dealt with first.

Partnership: A relationship between two or more individuals or organizations that is mutual, egalitarian, and goal-oriented.

Thinking and Doing Population Health—Nursing Process Leads the Way

Public health nurses work with individuals and families wherever they find them in the community and in whatever condition they find them. The priority for PHNs is health promotion and disease prevention, but PHNs also work with individuals and families who have chronic health conditions to help them achieve their health potential and, whenever possible, to manage their own lives and health care needs. Cherise and Zack's clinical is in a halfway house with young adults who have emotional and behavioral disorders and currently are unable to live by themselves or manage their own health care needs. They are going to need to discover their clients' potential for self-care and wellness to help them reach that potential. Instead of using a problem-based approach, they need to use a strengths-based approach as they carry out the public health nursing process. Because their clients live in the community, they need to find out as much as they can about the support systems and resources and also the resource gaps within the community.

Partnering with Individuals, Families, and Communities

PHNs need to understand the context of the lives of the people in the community in which they work. PHNs must know and understand the history, culture, and lifestyle of individuals, families, populations, and communities. For example, in a post-clinical seminar, students were discussing the stresses and crises of the families they were visiting. They stated that they did not understand how these families could function with so much stress. One of the students, a recent immigrant, said she thought these families were fairly well off—they had housing, food, and were safe in their homes. The country she emigrated from was in turmoil. She had seen family members murdered, their cattle slaughtered, homes burned, and people without food or clothing. These people, she thought, had stressful lives. The other students reflected on her comments. They came to realize that people view the world from their own experiences. Understanding and appreciating the lived experiences of people is important. Knowing about and understanding each other helps promote the opportunity for people to work together in a mutually respectful manner that can build on each other's strengths.

PHNs work in partnership with individuals, families, and communities. Partnerships are mutual relationships based on trust. PHNs establish trust with individuals, families, and communities by respecting their rights to make their own health decisions and by adapting nursing practice to fit the lived experiences and daily lives of those individuals, families, and communities. PHNs direct their efforts to meet the priority health needs identified by their clients. PHN practice includes the "3 Es":

- **Egalitarian (equal)** relationships with individuals, families, and communities

- **Enhancement** of individual, family, and community strengths, resilience, and resources

- **Empowerment** of individuals, families, and communities to advocate for and manage their own health care needs

Public Health Nursing Process

The public health nursing process builds on the basic nursing process of assessment, diagnosis, planning, implementation, and evaluation. Public health is interdisciplinary and inclusive by nature. At the community level, this means that the public health nursing process from start to finish is conducted within an interdisciplinary practice framework and involves partnering.

Data Collection, Data Management, and the Public Health Nursing Process

Data comprise the engine that drives the problem-solving process in nursing practice. Therefore, you need to have a system and process for data collection and management in place at the beginning of the nursing process. For this reason, we are discussing data before we discuss the components of the public health nursing process. Many public health and community agencies have electronic health records (EHRs) and automated health information systems (HIS). Though you will find more than one HIS in use, a system specifically created for public health nursing is useful as an example. The Omaha System, a standardized terminology initially developed for practitioners in the community, provides a problem-solving approach based on the nursing process (see Evidence Example). The Omaha System is the foundation of health information systems used by interdisciplinary team members at many health departments and other community provider sites. This HIS allows PHNs to collect and analyze data throughout the nursing process on individuals, families, and populations. The automated system facilitates aggregating data on individuals and families into larger data sets of populations so that patterns can be discerned within populations. This aggregation of data also allows PHNs to look at outcome data for specific programs and interventions. The Omaha System allows PHNs to collect their own evidence-based practice data.

Evidence Example: The Omaha System

The Omaha System was developed by the Visiting Nurse Association of Omaha (Nebraska) and seven test sites to enhance practice, documentation, and information management. Four federally funded research studies were conducted between 1975 and 1993. DeLanne Simmons, Chief Executive Officer, envisioned a computerized management information system that incorporated an integrated, valid, and reliable clinical information system focused on clients who received services, not on the practitioners who provided the services (Martin, 2005; Omaha System, 2010; Martin, Monsen, & Bowles, 2011).

The Omaha System enables health care providers to analyze and exchange client-centered coded data. It was designed to be relatively simple, hierarchical, multidimensional, and computer-compatible and to be used by interdisciplinary practitioners to guide their practice and document and communicate information about clients from admission to discharge. It exists in the public domain (no fee or license) and is intended for use across the continuum of care. It is based on a conceptual model depicted in Figure 3.1 that reflects the pivotal position of the individual, family, and community; the partnership with practitioners; and the value of the problem-solving approach. In other words, the Omaha System encourages critical thinking and operationalizes the nursing process. The problem-solving approach complements the strengths-based approach that focuses on building developmental assets and increasing the health of youth and communities (Martin, 2005; Omaha System, 2010).

The Omaha System consists of three components:

Problem Classification Scheme (client-centered assessment that engages individuals, families, and communities)—The Problem Classification Scheme is a hierarchy that includes domains; individual-, family-, and community-centered problems; modifiers; and signs/symptoms.

Intervention Scheme (plans, pathways, care activities, and service delivery terms to improve safety, quality, and effectiveness)—The Intervention Scheme is a hierarchy of interventions that includes categories, targets, and client-specific information.

Problem Rating Scale for Outcomes (evaluation that provides usable information for measuring and reporting client progress across time)—The Problem Rating Scale for Outcomes consists of knowledge, behavior, and symptom status concepts and Likert-type rating scales.

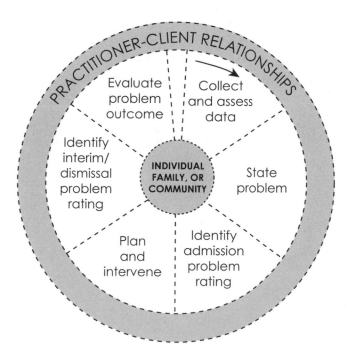

Figure 3.1 Omaha System model of the problem-solving process
Source: Martin, 2005, p. 7, used with permission

See the Evidence Example of an Omaha System case study.

Evidence Example: Omaha System Case Study

Anna K.: Older Woman who had a Chronic Cardiac Condition and Attended a Screening Clinic

Information Obtained during the First Visit/Encounter

Public health nurses at the Dakota County Public Health Department (Minnesota) developed health clinics for senior citizens. The clinics offered screening for health concerns, particularly hypertension, heart disease, and depression; accurate health information for prevention and treatment; and outreach and referral coordination for home care, equipment, medical assistance, and other community services. Because interaction time was limited, the nurses developed standardized protocols and forms based on the Omaha System to increase the efficiency and effectiveness of assessment, interventions, and documentation. When new clients visited the clinics, the nurses considered four problems, Communication with Community Resources, Mental health, Circulation, and Medication regimen. If those problems did not reflect clients' presenting data, the nurses selected and documented other pertinent problems, interventions, and outcome ratings.

When Anna K. came to the senior clinic for the first time, she reported that she had a history of dizziness and high blood pressure, but could not recall previous readings. When the nurse checked her vital signs, her blood pressure was 152/86 sitting and 154/82 standing; her pulse was 60 and regular. Her weight was 138 pounds, appropriate for her reported height. They talked about hypertension, blood pressure guidelines, the Circulation protocol, and Anna's data. The nurse suggested strategies to increase Anna's safety when she was dizzy. The nurse recorded Anna's vital signs on a health card, gave the card to her, and suggested that she have her blood pressure re-checked monthly and recorded on the card. She asked her to show the card to her doctor during future appointments.

Anna said she took two "heart" pills fairly regularly. She agreed to bring them with her when she returned to the Senior Clinic the following week so she and the nurse could discuss them. The nurse planned to use the Medication regimen protocol if appropriate, and record them on Anna's health card.

Application of the Omaha System

Domain: Physiological

PROBLEM: CIRCULATION (high priority problem)

Problem Classification Scheme

Modifiers: Individual and Actual

Signs/Symptoms of Actual:

- syncopal-fainting episodes/dizziness
- abnormal blood pressure reading

Intervention Scheme

Category: Teaching, Guidance, and Counseling

TARGETS AND CLIENT SPECIFIC INFORMATION:

- anatomy/physiology (circulatory system)
- mobility/transfers (avoid falls)
- signs/symptoms-physical (importance of vital signs, when to notify physician, dizziness)

Category: Case Management

TARGETS AND CLIENT SPECIFIC INFORMATION:

- continuity of care (show doctor her health card with monthly blood pressure checks)

Category: Surveillance

TARGETS AND CLIENT SPECIFIC INFORMATION:

- medical/dental care (schedule and go to appointments)
- signs/symptoms-physical (vital signs, circulatory status, weight, blood pressure)

Problem Rating Scale for Outcomes

Knowledge: 2-minimal knowledge (some information about normal/abnormal blood pressure readings but not impact on health; did not know previous readings)

Behavior: 4-usually appropriate behavior (usually took medications, has blood pressure checked periodically, seeks health care)

Status: 3-moderate symptoms (blood pressure exceeded expected range for non-diabetic client)

Elizabeth A. Vance, BSN,RN, PHN
Nurse Case Manager
Allina Home & Community Services
St. Paul, Minnesota

Carol A. Fish, MS, RN, PHN
Public Health Supervisor
Dakota County Public Health Department
West St. Paul, Minnesota

Source: Vance & Fish, 2010

Community and population data can be gathered from a variety of sources. Primary data is information you gather. Secondary data is information gathered by others. PHNs collect and use primary data when they aggregate their client data to look at program and service outcomes. PHNs also collect primary data through key informant interviews and focus groups (a small group of people gathered together to discuss a specific issue). PHNs access and use secondary data when they use health statistics data gathered by county, state, and national agencies such as the United States Department of Health and Human Services and state health departments.

Public Health Nursing Assessment

Public health nursing assessment is a systematic deliberative and holistic process of collecting data about a client (individual, family, community, or systems) that leads to an understanding of the client's health determinants, health status, and priority health concerns and needs. PHNs also need to carry out *strengths-based assessments* so that intervention plans for health concerns and problems are based on the clients' abilities to manage their own health care needs. *Strengths-based assessments* identify clients' abilities, resources, and resilience and examine health needs and problems.

Individual and Family Level of Practice

The family is the focus of care when PHNs work at the individual/family level of practice. The family is the primary unit of society and is responsible for carrying out the functions that allow family members to survive and thrive. The basic functions of the family are listed below.

- *Relational Support*—Meet the emotional, nurturing, and support needs of family members.

- *Socialization*—Instill attitudes and values; educate members to fulfill family and societal roles and responsibilities.

- *Reproduction*—Ensure survival of family and society through birth, adoption, and caregiving.

- *Economic*—Provide financial resources sufficient to meet family needs.

- *Provision of Basic Needs*—Provide for food, shelter, clothing, safety, communication and transportation, and health care.

    Adapted from Clark, 2008, p. 326

Family assessment is a holistic process in which all of the factors that influence a family's level of health and wellness are considered. You need to identify the health determinants (protective factors and risk factors) for individuals and families who have similar characteristics. For example, postpartum depression is one of the most common forms of depression and places new mothers and other family members at risk for harm. Knowing this, a PHN would include a postpartum depression screen as part of the assessment of a pregnant or postpartum client. If a mother is experiencing postpartum depression, an assessment of the children to determine their own health and safety would be appropriate. Families that live in poverty are more likely to have inadequate nutrition than families with adequate incomes, so a PHN would include a family nutritional assessment when working with poor families. The following outline presents the components of family assessment.

- Family Structure, Processes, and Dynamics

    - Family beliefs, values, and goals

    - Family members, relationships, roles, and responsibilities

    - Family development and life trajectory

    - Communication and decision-making patterns

- Cultural and lifestyle patterns including caregiving and caretaking
- Ability of the family to meet its basic needs
- Ability to nurture and support family members
- Family coping, strengths, resilience, flexibility, and ability to grow and change
- Home and Community
  - Living environment (home and community; physical and social components)
  - Links to community organizations and support systems (e.g., schools, faith-based communities, work, community organizations)
  - Community resources
- Health, Wellness, and Illness Patterns
  - Health behaviors, health risk factors, and protective factors
  - Existing health problems and health threats
  - Health literacy and cultural compatibility with existing health care services
  - Access to and use of health care services
  - Ability to manage family health care needs and resources
  - Unmet health care needs and family health priorities

Whether an individual lives alone or with others, the same family functions are relevant. If you are working with an individual who lives alone and has no known family or whose family lives elsewhere, you still need to use the same family assessment approach.

PHNs carry out assessment as part of the nursing process in a community setting such as a home, school, or clinic. Most of the information is gathered through observation and listening. When in the home setting, PHNs are guests of the family members and need to follow the family's lead in communications, timing, length and place of visit, and the roles of the nurse and family members. To assess the family, PHNs must first establish a trust relationship with family members based on mutual respect and understanding (McCann & Baker, 2001; Eriksson & Nilsson, 2008). Asking about personal family matters and health situations requires families to disclose information they generally do not share with strangers, so the development of a trust relationship needs to precede or occur simultaneously with the interviewing process. Andrew Gardner (2010) found that one way to engage clients and help them to feel comfortable was to start by being open and friendly; this seems obvious but can be challenging for student nurses learning to be professional, maintain boundaries, and create an environment conducive to effective nursing practice. An appropriate level of openness certainly can facilitate a connection and mutual understanding. This is sometimes a difficult balancing act as genuine friendship needs to occur within a professional context of the nurse-client relationship. The initial visit to a family is critical in establishing the nurse-client trust relationship (see Evidence Example).

Evidence Example: Public Health Nurses' Views of a Good First Meeting

Swedish researchers (Jansson, Petersson, & Uden, 2001) used focus groups to determine what public health nurses believed constituted a good first home visit with parents of newborns. A good first visit is considered key to developing an effective relationship with parents. Three criteria were identified:

Creating trust through good contact/reciprocal relationships, listening, being a guest and having an equal role with parents, and having time, privacy and peace and quiet

Creating a picture of the family's life situation by getting a holistic impression of family, seeing them in their home environment, getting a picture of what the clients are like, and taking in, consciously and unconsciously, the mood and a variety of information about the family

Creating a supportive climate by confirming and affirming parents feelings, abilities and responsibilities and increasing their responsibilities while providing a safety net

Source: Jansson, Petersson, & Uden, 2001

Cherise has been introduced to her client, Nicole, a 23-year-old homeless woman. Nicole is shy, talks to Cherise in monosyllables, and does not make eye contact. She responds to many questions by telling Cherise to ask her mother. Nicole's mother will be visiting this afternoon. Cherise decides to return to visit with Nicole and her mother.

ACTIVITY

If you were Cherise, how would you go about completing a family assessment with Nicole and her mother? Consider role-playing this interview with some of your classmates.

How would you establish a trust relationship with Nicole and her mother?

Where and how would you interview Nicole and her mother?

How would you provide for privacy and confidentiality?

What family information would you want to collect from Nicole and her mother?

The PHN continues the nursing process by moving into identification of the individual or family's health priorities and mutual goal-setting. After goals have been established, a plan of action is developed with the family. Unlike the acute care setting, working with families in the home and community setting often takes place over a longer period of time that might involve many visits. Home visiting and the nursing process are compared in Table 3.1. The orientation phase might take one to three visits on average. The working phase might take multiple visits that last months or possibly years.

Table 3.1 How the Nursing Process Occurs in Home Visits

Home Visiting Components	Nursing Process
Orientation Phase • Introduction • Determine purpose of visit and visit activities with client • Engage in social conversation • Assessment • Identify and state client's problems	**Assessment and Diagnosis** • Individual and family assessment • Strengths-based assessment—protective factors identified • Resources identified • Health risks and active health problems identified • Unmet health needs identified
Working Phase: Identification • Client asks questions and identifies nurse as someone who can help • Client identifies problems • Nurse provides health teaching, support and counseling, follow-up assessment, referral, and advocacy	**Planning and Implementation** • Mutual planning, priority setting, goal-setting • Primary interventions used are health teaching, counseling, referral and follow-up, and advocacy
Working Phase: Mutual Relationship • Client uses nurse as resource and accesses community resources • Nurse engages client in mutual problem-solving	**Implementation** • Primary interventions used are case management, health teaching, counseling, collaboration, and consultation
Resolution and Termination • Problems solved or ongoing but stable • Client becomes independent of nurse or continues to need support • Relationship ends when client no longer needs nurse or no longer participates in plan (moves or refuses participation in plan or visits)	**Evaluation** • Evaluation of outcomes: outcomes met, partially met, or not met • Replan—change in goals, outcomes, and/or interventions • New priorities or emerging problems identified and nursing process continues

Source: Adapted from McNaughton, 2005

PHNs carry equipment they need to complete assessments on individual family members. For example, common equipment used on maternal/child health visits includes baby scale, BP cuffs, stethoscopes, tape measures, disposable thermometers, developmental screening tools, growth grids, and thermometers for determining temperature of bath water.

PHNs often carry laptops and smartphones to access information and enter family data into EHRs during the home visit. Based on a federal mandate, all health providers including health departments are expected to have EHRs by 2014 (Martin, Monsen, & Bowles, 2011). PHNs use practice guidelines or clinical pathways that might be automated or paper-based. They use automated databases specific to individual client and family situations. For example, public health agencies have screening, assessment, and monitoring databases for newborns, infants, children, antepartum, postpartum, and family clients. PHNs collect admitting data on each client during their initial visits to their clients. They monitor and record health changes at each visit.

> *Cherise met with Nicole and her mother. She was able to complete a family assessment and also to determine Nicole's individual health problems. Nicole's mother stated that things had been going well until both she and her husband lost their jobs and their health insurance and Nicole went off her medications. She and her husband are looking for jobs. She said they are very determined to keep their family together. Nicole was not doing well in the homeless shelter, so the halfway house seemed like a good option until they find an apartment. Nicole's current health problems include lack of health insurance; lack of a mental health provider; no medications to control her mental health problems; and several broken teeth and visible dental caries. The homeless shelter has a health clinic; the halfway house had a social worker. Cherise, Nicole, and her mother decide that their priority is finding a mental health provider and a way to get medications for Nicole. Nicole cries when her mother leaves, stating, "I want to go with my mother. I am so lonely here."*

ACTIVITY

What are Nicole and her family's strengths or protective factors?

What are their risk factors?

If you were going to use the interventions of surveillance and case management in working with Nicole and her mother, what ongoing assessments would you carry out?

Community Level of Practice

PHNs assess communities to determine their level of health and wellness. The assessment is carried out in partnership with the community. Table 3.2 presents an overview of the public health nursing assessment process at the community level. Many geographic communities such as cities, counties, and states conduct a community assessment on a periodic basis, commonly every 2 years. They do this to monitor changing health conditions of the populations in their communities and to establish community priorities for health goals, funding, and actions. The governmental agencies conducting the assessment partner with other community organizations and members to ensure that the diversity of the community and all points of view are reflected in the assessment. PHNs are part of the team that collects and analyzes the community data. Table 3.2 outlines a process for completing a community assessment.

It is important to conduct a strengths-based assessment as part of the community assessment process. PHNs work to enhance community strengths so that communities can be as independent as possible in solving their own health care problems and managing their own health care needs. The following Evidence Example provides an example of how a strengths-based assessment facilitates community capacity building.

Evidence Example: Recognizing Strengths in a Rural Community

An ethnographic study identified the health care needs and strengths of a community with a large number of multicultural rural elders in a southwestern county in New Mexico (Averill, 2003, p. 449).

The following major health needs were identified:

- Escalating costs of prescriptions for elderly living on fixed incomes

- Limited access to primary health care, home care, specialty care, hospice, and emergency care

- Social isolation and loneliness due to living in an isolated area, abandonment by younger family members, and being unable to drive or leave home

The following major strengths were identified:

- Knowledge, experience, and traditions of a culturally and ethnically diverse community of elderly with rich traditions of healing, health, and family caring

- Core group of dedicated professional nurses in acute care, home care, hospice care, educational outreach, and public health

- Pre-existing community-based action group made up of diverse community planners, educators, advocates, healthcare providers, public school officials, and administrative and municipal representatives

Source: Averill, 2003

After they visited their clients in the halfway house, Cherise asked Shannon, "I have never heard of halfway homes for adults with emotional and behavioral disorders. Who thought to build a home for them?"

Shannon responded, "The public health department carries out a community assessment periodically to determine the priority health problems of the people living in the community. We want to know what the major health needs are and which needs are met and which are unmet. We also look at the assets or resources of the community to determine the community's capacity to manage its own health care needs and solve its own problems. Then we prioritize and decide what services to offer, what the funding should be, and how to allocate resources to our different programs. During the last community assessment process, we found out that 10% of adults in our community had chronic mental health problems and many are on medications to control their symptoms. Many of our public health nurses provide case management services in the home to try to keep our mental health clients stable and on their psychotropic medications. When we analyzed our caseloads, we found that we were not providing services to young adults with mental health problems."

The United States Department of Health and Human Services (USDHHS) conducts an assessment of the nation's health every 10 years. The report for the assessment conducted for the year 2000 was called Healthy People 2010 and the report for the assessment conducted for the year 2010 is called Healthy People 2020

(USDHHS, 2000, 2010.) The 2020 report outlines goals to be achieved between 2010 and 2020. Many states also conduct assessments of their population health every 10 years using the Healthy People guidelines.

The population data collected in public health includes population health status, health differences or health status gaps between populations (health disparities), and health determinants (causes of health and illness within the population). Health status data are considered the "vital signs" of the population and include the following:

- Mortality (death rates) data

- Morbidity (illness rates) data

- Health behaviors data (e.g., smoking, exercise, obesity, use of seat belts)

- Health and life satisfaction data (how satisfied one is with current health and lifestyle)

- Functional health data (ability to live independently and manage own health care needs)

These population "vital signs" are called global health status measures.

Table 3.2   PHN Assessment Process for Communities

Determine Assessment Target
• Identify community or population(s) to be assessed
Develop a Working Relationship with Community Partners
• Identify all potential partners
• Select and recruit interdisciplinary and community partners
• Engage as many community partners as possible
Planning
• Determine data needed to identify community strengths and health concerns or problems
• Identify methods for data collection
• Identify who will collect the data and when data will be collected
Data Collection
• Gather data on community's perception of their strengths, problems, and health influences
• Gather data on health determinants (protective factors and risk factors)
• Gather data on health status outcomes
• Gather data about the systems that influence the community's or population's health (social, economic, educational, political, and legal)
• Collate the assessment data

Data Analysis

- Collaborate with partners on data analysis
- Synthesize and summarize descriptive data for entire community and for diverse populations within the community.
- Consider using some of the data management tools found in Chapter 4. Identify the community strengths and resources (health determinant protective factors)
- Identify the factors that have negative impact on health (health determinant risk factors)
- Identify the community's health outcomes by health goal categories such as those found in Healthy People 2020 (www.healthypeople.gov)
- Compare the differences in protective factors, health risks, and outcomes among populations in the community
- Explore the relationships among identified risk and protective factors to determine populations and community level of wellness and capacity for managing their own health needs.
- Identify the major health concerns of the community based on data analysis and discussion with the community
- Identify the population(s) at greatest risk based on comparative analysis of different populations and community as a whole

Reporting

- Prepare reports (written, audiovisual, verbal presentations)
- Share data and conclusions with the community

Determining Health Priorities and Goals

- Determine community health priorities in partnership with the community
- Identify goals for each priority
- Identify the measurable health status outcomes for each priority
- Select populations at greatest risk in community for targeted interventions

Source: Modified from Minnesota Department of Health, 2003

For a comprehensive community assessment tool see Table 3.3.

Table 3.3 Community Assessment

Part 1: Determinants of Health

Section I. Biology

Unit of Analysis	*Data*
Geographic Area: Population by Census Track, Community, County, State, Country Population at Risk by Common Characteristic (i.e., ethnic, cultural or religious group, age or developmental stage, common health risk [potential or actual])	• Population at last census • Population density • Population changes last decade • Demographics: Age, race, gender • Physical characteristics • Genetic factors • Health conditions

Sources of Evidence:

Section 2. Behaviors

Socioeconomic Characteristics	• Employment (employed versus unemployed) • Income levels • Poverty level • Educational levels • Language literacy
Lifestyle Patterns	• Living arrangements (type of housing, people in household, relationship of people in household) • Homelessness • Family, work, and community roles • Religious affiliations or memberships • Patterns of social conformity or non-conformity (lawfulness, antisocial behaviors, lawlessness)
Health Behaviors	• Health-seeking actions • Health-limiting actions • Coping and resilience • Health literacy

Sources of Evidence:

Section 3. Physical Environment

Natural Environment

- Geography (terrain, climate, weather, natural resources)
- Air and water quality
- Recreation

Built Environment

- Urban versus rural, suburban
- Transportation (roads, bridges, public and private transportation services)
- Transportation access (ground, airports, waterways)
- Governmental and protective services (police, fire, emergency response)
- Public and handicapped access and accommodation
- Leading industries and worksites
- Educational facilities
- Shopping (food, clothing, other)
- Agriculture
- Water, sanitation, waste management, and recycling services
- Vector control (insects, rodents, large animals, ticks and fleas)
- Air and water quality or contamination control
- Housing stock (type, age, condition, availability)
- Recreational facilities
- Parks, playgrounds, athletic fields

Sources of Evidence:

Section 4. Social Environment

History of Community

- Pattern of settlement
- Immigration and migration patterns
- Key events

Culture and Ethnicity

- Diversity in community
- Festivals and celebrations

Political and Social Climate

- Conservative, liberal, independent, libertarian

Religious Institutions	• Denominations and membership • Calendar of holidays and events • Community and volunteer services
Commerce and Workplace	• Businesses, retail and shopping, banks, business community organizations • Workplace (worker organizations, unionization, workplace safety and hazards) • Distance from place of residence to workplace and commuting patterns
Education	• Public, private, secular • Variety of programs • Cost and access
Libraries and Public Information Access	• Library locations, hours, services, Internet access
Communication	• Public and private information and communication sources • Mail and courier services (public, private) • Telephone (landlines, mobile, access, emergency services, telephone chains) • Television, radio, newsprint, Internet • Newsletters, billboards, bulletin boards
Law Enforcement Services and Patterns (formal and informal)	• Police and special police services, animal enforcement, private security, neighborhood watch patrols, vigilante groups
Community Support Systems and Social Services (formal and informal)	• Social services (e.g., food and clothing banks, homeless shelters, adult day care, child care) • Nonprofit community service organizations • Neighborhood organizations • Pattern of emergency services responses (type, frequency, availability, response time)
Health Services	• Public, private for profit, nonprofit mix in community • Range of services (acute care, primary care, specialty care, home care, hospice, community clinics and home visiting, long-term care, occupational and rehabilitation services) • Access, cost, and quality of services

Health Services Access—Assessing the "7 As of Access"	• Is the individual, family, or population *aware* of their needs and services available in the community?
	• Can the individual, family, or population gain *access* to the services they need?
	• Are services *available* and convenient for the individual, family, or population in terms of time, location, and place for use?
	• How *affordable* is the service for the individual, family, or population?
	• Is the service *acceptable* to the individual, family, or population in terms of choice, satisfaction, and congruency with cultural values and beliefs?
	• How *appropriate* is the service for the individual, family, or population, or is there a fit?
	• Is there *adequacy* of service in terms of quantity or degree for the individual, family, or population?

Sources of Evidence:

Section 5. Policy and Interventions

Laws, Regulations, Ordinances	• Existing health, safety, social service laws, regulations, ordinances that impact health access and health delivery
Political Structures and Processes	• Elected and appointed officials (access and availability of officials and staff)
	• Political process cycle (elections, legislation, regulatory process and implementation, budgeting and allocation of funds, evaluation)
	• Lobbying groups and efforts
	• Coalitions and community organizing activities for social and political change
	• Community forums or public meetings
Current Health and Safety Issues	• Emerging, long-term
	• Identified community priority
	• Public consensus or disagreement on solution
	• Current actions or lack of action
	• Available funding or lack of funding

Sources of Evidence:

Part 2: Analysis of Population and Community Health Status

Section A. Health Statistics	
Birth and Death Rates	General and by age, gender, ethnicity, causes
Accidents and Injuries and Deaths related to Accidents and Injuries	General and by age, gender, ethnicity, location, type • Accidental • Intentional • Homicide and suicide
Communicable Disease Rates (top 10)	General and by age, gender, ethnicity, location
Immunization Rates	General and by age, gender, ethnicity, location
Non-communicable Disease Rates (top 10)	General and by age, gender, ethnicity, location • Medical diseases • Mental health • Acute illnesses • Chronic diseases • Disabilities
Health Risk Behaviors	General and by age, gender and ethnicity (i.e., smoking or chewing, drinking, drug use, obesity, drinking and driving, sexual behaviors and unprotected sex, use of seatbelts and helmets, interpersonal abuse, participation in antisocial or illegal behaviors)
Level of Independence	Adult population by age, gender, location, illness, and disability
Life Satisfaction	By age, gender, location, socioeconomic status, illness, and disability
Sources of Evidence:	

Section B. Determining Community Health Priorities	
Comparison of Populations	• Compare health risks and health status categories by key populations in community (age, gender, socioeconomic status, ethnicity, culture, location, health conditions) • Identify populations at risk and populations of interest

Identify Key Health Concerns	• Analyze by incidence, prevalence, patterns of increase or decrease, and severity
	• Analyze potential for harm to community as a whole
	• Compare with Healthy People 2020 goals and priorities or existing community goals and priorities
Identify Community Health Priorities and Establish Goals	• Establish community health priorities with community members
	• Align community health priorities with Healthy People 2020 goals and priorities or existing community goals and priorities

Source: Modified from Truglio-Londrigan & Lewenson, 2011.

> *Zack asked Shannon, "What did you do when you found out that you weren't seeing many young people with mental health problems?"*
>
> *Shannon responded, "We conducted some key informant interviews with the doctors, nurses, and social workers who were already working with this group. We also talked with the local police chief and the county attorney. We found that young adults with mental health problems often tend to fall through the cracks because, for the most part, they have not been diagnosed with a major psychiatric diagnosis like schizophrenia or bipolar or borderline personality disorder. Their problems are often perceived to be antisocial or criminal rather than medical, and many of them wind up in jail for drug use, disorderly conduct, assault, and other behaviors people find frightening. So the county decided to fund a demonstration project with a 25-bed halfway house for young adults with emotional and behavioral disorders who were living on the streets, in jail, or in and out of the hospital."*

At times PHNs and community agencies want to determine the health status of a specific population. This assessment can be conducted just like the community assessment, but with a more limited scope. For example, a school district might want to determine the health needs of its students, a homeless shelter might want to determine the health needs of the homeless it serves, or a senior housing agency might want to determine the health needs of its residents. The data from periodic health screening of individuals in a population, such as an elementary school, can be aggregated (combined) and the health of the student population assessed. See the following Evidence Example.

Evidence Example: Elementary School Health Assessment

Public health nursing students at a local college conducted a mass health screening of all students in a K–6 charter elementary school serving mainly African-American and Hispanic students. The health screening included height, weight, BMI, vision and hearing, dental, immunization compliance, and nutrition and activity level. Data were collected on individual students so that students with health needs could be referred to the appropriate health providers for further assessment and interventions. The major finding was that 80% of the students had unmet dental needs, with

20–30 % of the students having emergency dental needs. The health determinants that influenced the dental health status of these students included:

Personal-Behavioral

- Lack of family dentist
- Lack of awareness of resources
  - Dental insurance
  - Opportunities for free dental care
- Lack of transportation (no car available)
- 95% of families living in poverty
- Families at survival level with dental health a low priority
- Lack of toothbrushes and toothpaste
- Lack of knowledge about how to brush teeth
- English as a second language
- Parents not able to take children to dentist during normal Monday–Friday daytime hours
- Most parents are concerned about their children's health

Environmental–Physical

- The weather is cold with frequent rain and snow for 6 months of the year
- City buses are not accessible from many of the neighborhoods in which the children live
- Urban environment is dangerous for children out alone, so children would not be able to walk to dentist on their own

Environmental–Social

- Government financial resources for dental services for the poor is very limited
- A voluntary dental organization provides free dental service to children twice a year
- Local neighborhood clinic with ties to school provides dental care but only during Monday–Friday daytime hours
- High density of poverty
- Few dental clinics in older and poorer neighborhoods

These findings led to establishment of a dental health priority for the school.

Source: Schoon, 2010

ACTIVITY

Review the summary of the school health assessment in the previous Evidence Example.

- What health determinant protective factors were found?

- What health determinant risk factors were found?

- Which of these health determinants could be modified?

Zack commented, "So the young adults living in the halfway house can be considered a community or a vulnerable population. I guess we would need to modify the community assessment process somewhat, but I am not sure what we really need to find out."

Shannon responded, "The public health agency does need to know the residents' health status and what their unmet health needs are. We also need to know if the halfway house is able to provide the services needed and if any services are needed that can't be provided. We could use your help in collecting that information."

ACTIVITY

Zack is concerned about the community assessment that he and his fellow classmates will be conducting at the halfway home for young adults with emotional and behavioral disorders. How might he modify the community assessment process to fit the population and setting of the halfway house?

PHN Assessment at the Systems Level of Practice

Systems can be assessed to determine their ability to respond to public health priorities in the community. Systems that PHNs interact with on an ongoing basis include health care systems; public and governmental agencies; schools and school systems; community health and social service agencies; criminal justice system; local and state government, including elected and appointed officials; insurance companies; and faith-based organizations. PHNs assess systems to identify the extent to which systems can meet community health needs and, if they can't, to identify what resources are needed. In the case study about the halfway house, health care systems and providers were assessed to determine if they could provide the needed health care services for the young adults with mental health problems.

Identifying and Setting Health Priorities

PHNs employed in governmental public health agencies are accountable to the public for the health priorities they select, the populations they serve, and the services they provide. PHNs consciously make the connection between the health needs of the community as a whole and the health needs of individuals and families within the community. The priority health needs identified through the community assessment process help PHNs determine the most vulnerable and underserved populations in their communities in need of services and those with the greatest needs. The communities could be cities; school districts or schools; counties, states, or countries; or communities that represent a population with a specific health risk, such as those with mental illness, those lacking health insurance, or those with a specific ethnic identity.

PHNs also identify health priorities in the community by identifying health and illness patterns among their caseload and agency clients. PHNs look at multiple interacting health determinants including social determinants of health that allow them to identify population health patterns when working with individual clients and community partners (Meagher-Stewart, Edwards, Aston, & Young, 2009). Discovering and addressing underlying causes of illness, such as poverty and environmental hazards, was modeled by Lillian Wald. She was the founder of public health nursing who established the Henry Street Settlement House (Abrams, 2008). PHNs also conduct research to identify health concerns in vulnerable populations. A study of early childhood centers and education programs identified the following health needs of the centers and enrolled children: hygiene and handwashing; sanitation and disinfection; supervision; and safety of indoor and outdoor equipment (Alkon, To, Mackie, Wolff, & Bernzweig, 2010).

PHNs can determine community health priorities by reviewing the community assessment data to see which health problems have the greatest potential for harm and have effective interventions. A list of questions to consider when establishing health priorities follows.

1. What is the incidence and prevalence of major diseases, health risk behaviors, health concerns in the community (e.g., heart disease, teen pregnancy, drinking and driving, smoking, depression, influenza)?

2. What are the major causes of death and disability in the community (e.g., heart attacks, stroke, cancer, dementia, car accidents, and homicide)?

3. What populations in the community are most affected by these health problems?

4. What are the major health risks in the community (e.g., obesity, air pollution, homes with lead-based paint, seasonal flooding, homelessness, lack of health insurance)?

5. Which health needs are met by community resources?

6. Which health needs are not met?

7. Are there available, affordable, and effective interventions for these health needs?

8. Who is responsible for meeting these health needs?

PHNs are ever-vigilant community watchers who are often the first to notice when a new health concern emerges or a service gaps exists in the community. An example of a health concern identified by a PHN intake nurse, explored by agency staff, and taken to a group of community partners for a systems-level intervention is found in the following Evidence Example.

Evidence Example: Determining Population Needs in a Rural/Suburban County

The intake nurse at the public health agency was responsible for logging referrals and conversations of significant public health concern. The agency she worked at was small and without an on-site physician or walk-in clinic services. It was a 50-mile drive into a larger metropolitan community where low-cost clinics were available. Her log included the following:

10-01-2008	Adult Male	Uninsured	c/o prolonged diarrhea
10-02-2008	Adult Female	Uninsured	c/o URI
10-02-2008	Adult Female	Uninsured	Possible STD
10-03-2008	Adult Female	Insured	No well care. No physical exam for 10 years
10-03-2008	Adult Male	Uninsured	Diabetic. Needs glucose check.
10-04-2008	Adult Female	Uninsured	Pre-hypertensive. Needs BP check.
10-05-2008	Adult Male	Uninsured	Hypertension. Needs BP med refill.
10-05-2008	Adult Male	Uninsured	Unable to afford orthopedic shoes.
10-05-2008	Adult Female	Insured	No well care. No mammogram for 5 years.
10-05-2008	Adult Female	Uninsured	c/o abnormal vaginal bleeding
10-05-2008	Adult Male	Uninsured	Needs anti-depression med refilled.

Upon doing an analysis of incoming calls, the trend of increasing numbers of working adults lacking access to care was obvious. The intake nurse compiled a brief report summarizing 2 months of log entries and presented it to her public health director.

At the next community partner meeting with local medical clinics and hospitals, the director listened as the hospital CEO discussed the decision to place a social worker in the Emergency Department to assist families with completing financial aid applications. The director shared the summary provided by the intake nurse and inquired if the hospital had any data on unnecessary patient visits to the ER. As the group discussed this problem, they decided to form a smaller committee and to consult with other community partners, such as the local community action program director and the director of one of the largest faith-based clinics in the metro area.

This smaller committee led by the public health director met numerous times to discuss options for serving their community. One option that they investigated was the establishment of a nursing center, and upon presenting a proposal to the hospital CEO, they found the hospital was willing to fund the part-time center for one afternoon a week for 2 years. The nursing center was placed adjacent to the area employment and training center and was staffed by a PHN. Services focused on simple screening measures, referrals, and health promotion.

The committee met every 4 months to review data of clients visiting the nursing center. One outstanding need they identified was for services requiring the attention of a physician. The primary need was for obtaining refills of medications to prevent an exacerbation of existing medical conditions. As a result of these conversations, one medical clinic offered to see such patients free of charge if they were screened first by the nurse at the nursing center.

About a year later, another major health care provider had purchased a mobile health unit for doing mammography outreach in very rural parts of the state. The committee approached this provider about using the mobile unit for seeing patients in a community setting. It took extensive organizing by the public health department, but eventually the mobile unit and a physician were at several libraries and churches in the community each month. Physical exams and laboratory work could be done in mobile unit. These services were the direct result of systems-level collaboration and the determination to advocate for those lacking access to health care.

Source: Kleinfehn-Wald, 2010

Public Health Nursing Diagnoses

PHNs may use the classification system for nursing diagnosis developed by the North American Nursing Diagnosis Association (NANDA) when working with individuals, families, populations, and communities (Scroggins, 2008). A nursing diagnosis adapted for public health would include the components outlined in Table 3.4.

Table 3.4   Nursing Diagnoses Components for Public Health

Nursing Diagnosis Components	Examples
Diagnostic Concept	Coping, family process, homelessness, hope or hopelessness, health-seeking behaviors
Subject	Individual, family, population, community
Judgment (descriptor or modifier of concept)	Readiness for, impaired, compromised, altered, delayed, disturbed
Location	Site or place
Age	Biological stage (i.e., neonate, adolescent, older adult), individual or family developmental stage

Time	Acute, chronic, intermittent, continuous
Status	Actual or potential diagnostic condition, health promotion, risk or wellness diagnostic condition

- Health Promotion: motivation and desire to increase well-being and health

- Risk or vulnerability: exposure to factors that cause illness, injury, or condition

- Wellness: responses to level of wellness that imply readiness for enhancement or improvement

Modified from Scroggins, 2008

Nursing diagnoses are identified by their defining characteristics. These characteristics provide the evidence for the nursing diagnosis (Scroggins, 2008). The authors of the NANDA nursing diagnoses have discovered the diagnostic evidence through research or review of the literature.

- Actual, health promotion, and wellness diagnoses include defining characteristics or observable cues (signs, symptoms, behaviors).

- Health risk diagnoses do not include defining characteristics but do include risk factors (psychological, physiological, genetic, chemical, environmental (physical or social) that increase the vulnerability of the individual, family, population, or community to an unhealthful event.

Nursing diagnoses that are actual rather than potential also include related factors. These factors precede or contribute to the diagnosis and are often considered etiologies or causes.

When possible, a strengths-based diagnosis (wellness or health promotion diagnosis) should be developed. A strengths-based diagnosis leads to interventions that enhance potential for self-care and independence. Examples of strengths-based family diagnoses follow.

- Wellness Diagnosis: Readiness for enhanced family coping related to child with significant developmental delays, parental grieving, and anxiety as evidenced by parents enrolling child in early childhood education program, parents seeking counseling, and parents stating that they were adapting their expectations of child to child's current potential.

- Health Promotion Diagnosis: Potential for enhanced health-seeking behaviors related to inadequate family nutrition, loss of father's job, and lack of transportation as evidenced by parents signing up for county food assistance program, finding local food shelves on busline, willingness to use meat substitutes for protein and powdered milk.

ACTIVITY

Cherise wants to focus on Nicole's family's protective factors and strengths. She wants to enhance their ability to regain their independence. Cherise decides to write a strengths-based diagnosis. If you were working with Nicole's family what wellness or health promotion diagnosis would you develop?

Because public health nursing is interdisciplinary and occurs within the context of the community, we generally do not develop a nursing diagnosis at the conclusion of a community assessment process. The language we use must be clear and understandable to community members and to the interdisciplinary team. We often identify the public health concern or priority using population health terminology such as increase in SIDS deaths, increased teen pregnancy rate, and lack of community support and resources for the mentally ill. However, a nursing diagnosis could be used if it was understandable to all parties involved. An example of a wellness community diagnosis follows:

> Potential for enhanced community coping following natural disasters related to community-wide planning process, availability of community mental health resources, and state funding for recovery as evidenced by publication of state and county plans, list of mental health providers available for crisis intervention and counseling, and availability of funding for rebuilding damaged housing units.

Public Health Nursing Planning and Implementation Process

When the PHN is working with individuals or families in the community, determining priorities, clarifying the health need or nursing diagnosis, establishing goals, and developing an intervention plan are joint efforts between the PHN and the clients. Refer back to Table 3.1, *How the Nursing Process Occurs in Home Visits,* to review the process for planning and implementing interventions with families in the home or other community settings. The plan should be congruent with and integrated into the family's culture, lifestyle, daily routine, and be within the family's potential to achieve. The plan should enhance the family's potential for self-care and autonomy.

When the PHN is working with the community, the planning process, like the assessment process, involves an interdisciplinary team and key community members. After the team has established priorities and formulated clear statements of the health priorities to be addressed, it is time to determine goals.

Goals for health priorities are based on community values, beliefs, and the willingness of community members and elected and appointed officials to make changes; resources available; and a consensus of what is achievable in the given time frame. Specific outcomes are then established. Outcomes are statements that are realistic, understandable, measurable, behavioral, achievable, and time-limited. An example of a goal and an outcome for a community follows:

- Goal: Reduce obesity in our community.

- Outcome: Reduce obesity in adults in our community 10% by 2020.

The United States Department of Health and Human Services (DHHS) has released goals of Healthy People 2020 that are based in part on the level of achievement of Healthy People 2010 goals (Reinberg, 2010). See the following Evidence Example.

Evidence Example: Healthy People 2020 Goals

A recent news conference by the United States Department of Health and Human Services (US-DHHS) related that Healthy People 2020 goals would be more modest than the 2010 goals. Only 19% of Healthy People 2010 goals were met and progress was made on only 52% of them. Some, like obesity, have become worse since 2000 (25% in 2000 increased to 34% in 2010). Examples of some of the new goals for 2020 are:

- Reducing obesity 10%

- Reducing the number of smokers by 21%

- Reducing deaths from heart attack 20%

- Reducing cancer deaths 10%

Source: Reinberg, 2010

You might notice that the goals for 2020 include a measurable outcome that is time specific and stated as a percent reduction of a health problem. These measurable outcomes are called health status indicators. These outcomes are determined by reviewing existing population health outcomes, comparing specific population outcomes with outcomes from other populations, and reviewing evidence from the literature on acceptable outcomes. For example, scientific evidence suggests that obesity is a risk factor for many diseases, so reduction of obesity within a population would be a positive health outcome. At the same time, outcomes need to be realistic. Because U.S. obesity rates increased from 25% to 34% from 2000 to 2010, a 10% reduction in obesity over the next decade might be reasonable whereas a 25% reduction might be unreasonable.

PHNs often develop intermediate measures when the timeline for outcome achievement is lengthy or interventions needed are complex. See example of long-term outcome with an intermediate measure below.

Outcome – Student smoking rate will decrease by 30% by 2020.

Intermediate Measure – Smoking cessation program will be implemented by 2015.

ACTIVITY

Select a goal from the 2020 Healthy People Goals found at www.healthypeople.gov.

Review the literature related to the goal you have selected.

Does the evidence in the literature support the goal as reasonable and achievable?

Sometimes you might find it a good idea to select intermediate indicators of health outcomes. For example, it might be a good idea to gather data periodically during the decade between 2010 and 2020 to determine if the interventions selected to achieve the 2020 outcomes have actually been implemented and if they appear to be working. If the obesity rate has increased or stayed the same by 2015, a change in interventions might be in order.

Selecting and Implementing Best Practice Interventions

After the health status indicators, or measurable outcomes, have been determined, PHNs select the interventions. They select public health interventions based on evidence or "best practices." PHNs find evidence of effective interventions from journal articles, textbooks, and websites. PHNs also seek information and recommendations from colleagues who have been successful in working with specific populations to determine what factors have contributed to their success. Once "best practice" interventions have been identified, PHNs present their findings to other staff and administration to receive endorsement of the selected intervention approach.

PHNs worldwide use the seventeen interventions in the Public Health Intervention Wheel (MDH, 2001; Keller, Strohschein, Lia-Hoagberg, & Schaffer, 2004) as an intervention template. The 17 interventions of the Public Health Intervention Wheel are discussed in Chapter 2. These interventions are interdisciplinary in nature, which means that many health and helping professions use similar interventions. For example, health educators and social workers use health teaching and counseling as part of their discipline-specific practice as do public health nurses.

Each intervention selected has to fit the individual or family, population or community, situation, and health concern. Evidence of the effectiveness of a specific strategy should provide direction about what to do, how to do it, and how often. For example, the Advisory Committee on Immunization Practice (ACIP) recommends that all people aged 6 months and older receive the annual influenza vaccination (CDC, 2010b). However, not all children have ready access to the influenza vaccine. The following Evidence Example demonstrates that flu shots administered to children and adults in the home setting is an effective way for PHNs to increase the level of immunity in families living in poverty.

Evidence Example: In-Home Influenza Immunizations

The Minnesota Visiting Nurse Agency (MVNA) has been providing flu shots at public clinics and at contracted corporate sites for over 13 years but had not extended the program to in-home services. Family health nurses wanted to be able to give flu shots to family members of newborns and high-risk infants. New moms were getting flu shots before coming home with the baby, leaving the other family members (siblings and extended family) not protected and putting the infants at risk because they cannot receive the influenza vaccine until age 6 months. Many family members did not have health insurance. The family health nurses brought this unmet health need to the attention of their program managers. Working together, the family health managers, flu program managers, and MVNA administration developed a plan to purchase the needed coolers to transport the vaccine and to provide the nurses with the training necessary to give the shots and to complete the documentation for billing. MVNA was able for find donors who were willing to underwrite the cost of the flu shots for family members who were uninsured. Since starting this in-home immunization program, MVNA family health has given more than 400 flu shots to members of families with new infants in their homes.

Source: Lanigan, 2010

When working with families, PHNs select interventions that will enhance the family's capacity for problem solving and self-care. Health teaching, counseling, consultation, and case management are interventions commonly used to build on and enhance the family's strengths and encourage them to manage their health care needs. PHNs use mutual problem solving strategies with clients to foster self-efficacy. They use advocacy to facilitate the individual and family's ability to access health and social resources. They also use advocacy when populations are found to be at risk for a specific health hazard. The case study in the following Evidence Example illustrates how a small group of PHNs advocated effectively for an individual, a family, and an entire community.

Evidence Example: Advocating for All

A Story from "Getting Behind the Wheel"

I received a referral on a nine-month old little boy with a recent diagnosis of meningitis secondary to active tuberculosis. The child's parents were a young Hispanic couple who did not speak English. The child's mother was pregnant and stayed at home with her two small children. The family had no telephone, and neither parent had a driver's license. The entire family reacted positively to their Mantoux tests that I administered. At this point, I arranged an appointment at the local clinic for the entire family, complete with transportation and interpreters. The father was found to have active infectious tuberculosis. He was ordered not to return to his job at the meat packing plant and consequently lost his insurance. I assisted the family in applying for medical assistance and other services for which they were eligible.

At the same time I was advocating for this family, I was also involved with other PHNs in advocating for the health of the man's coworkers and overall community. The meat packing plant where the man worked employed over 1000 people who spoke 12 different languages. Initially the plant managers were more concerned about losing production than being exposed to tuberculosis. We worked with the managers to convince them that exposure to tuberculosis was a serious problem and that they could cooperate with public health and not lose production. Although the plant managers would not mandate testing, they did allow us to offer free Mantoux tests during work time on all three shifts to any employee who wanted to be tested. Over 700 employees were tested, with over 70 positives. Many of the employees with positive Mantoux tests lacked access to health care. We negotiated reduced clinic fees and secured community grant funds to pay for x-rays and prescribed treatment for infected persons who were uninsured and without resources.

Source: Minnesota Department of Health, 2006

Interventions are actions intended to improve the health of individuals, families, communities, and systems by altering a factor that affects a client's condition or health status. After the PHN has identified the client (i.e., individual, family, community, or system) and the health goal, then the level of intervention is selected. For example, if your goal is to increase the coping skills of a family, the level of intervention is the family. If your goal is to create community awareness of environmental hazards, then the level of intervention is the community. If your goal is to provide healthier food choices in a school cafeteria, then the level of intervention is the system (the school). See Chapter 1 for discussion of levels of nursing interventions.

Zack is working on the community assessment of the halfway house residents. He notices that many of the residents have unmet dental health needs. The residents all received toothbrushes, toothpaste, and dental floss when they were admitted to the halfway house. The staff reports that almost all of the residents brush and floss daily and are very concerned about having their teeth fixed. The staff members feel that improving the dental health and "smile potential" of the residents will improve their self-esteem. Zack thinks that providing accessible dental services for the residents will also help improve their sense of self-efficacy. He thinks dental services will make the residents feel more in charge of their lives. He wonders, "Do you think it would be a good idea to have the county mobile dental clinic visit the halfway house on a monthly basis?"

PHNs provide nursing care at all three levels of prevention, primary, secondary, and tertiary, although their primary focus is primary prevention. Review the discussion of prevention levels in Chapter 1.

ACTIVITY

When Zack considers having a mobile dental clinic visit the halfway house, what PHN intervention level is he practicing?

What level(s) of prevention would be accomplished through the mobile dental clinic?

How could Zack involve the residents in setting up and managing the dental clinic visits?

Public Health Nursing Evaluation

Before you implement interventions, you need to determine your evaluation measures. You want to measure outcomes whenever possible, rather than just the process of what you do. Evaluation is ongoing in public health nursing. After you implement your interventions, you need to regularly reassess the progress your clients are making toward goal achievement. Evaluation data can tell you if interventions are effective and if your clients have met, partially met, or not met expected outcomes. If outcomes have been met, you can choose to continue interventions or to cease interventions if achievements have resulted in optimal health outcomes for your clients. If outcomes have not been met or have only been partially met, you need to discover why this is so. The problem could be from inadequacies in any of the following: the assessment of the client's readiness or ability to change, the reasonableness and achievability of the stated outcomes, the measure used to evaluate the outcomes, or the appropriateness or effectiveness of the interventions used. Interventions not only need to be specific to the health determinants, but they also need to fit the characteristics of the clients (i.e., culture, ethnicity, developmental level, language literacy). Evaluation and reassessment take thought, time, and effort. After you have evaluated the reason outcomes have not been achieved, you need to revise your plan and interventions.

ACTIVITY

Write an outcome for dental health for the residents of the halfway house.

Zack has proposed the use of a mobile dental clinic. Think of the Public Health Intervention Wheel. List the interventions that would be involved in setting up and delivering dental services using the mobile clinic.

Determine how you would evaluate the effectiveness of the mobile dental clinic based on the outcome you developed.

At the beginning of this chapter, we discussed the importance of health information systems and electronic health records in data management and the evaluation of public health nursing interventions and client health outcomes. Automation provides an efficient and effective means for measuring individual client and family health outcomes and program outcomes. One HIS, the Omaha System, has been used effectively as a quality improvement strategy to promote excellence in client care; improve and ensure data quality; and increase data use of data analysis and reporting capacity (Monsen et al., 2006). The Omaha System has also been used to demonstrate how aggregation of data can be used within and across programs and agencies (Monsen et al., 2010). See the following Evidence Example for a discussion of this study.

Evidence Example: Comparing Maternal Child Health Problems and Outcomes across PHN Agencies

An exploratory descriptive study analyzed maternal child health data from four public health nursing agencies to determine the needs of maternal child health clients and to demonstrate outcomes of services provided. The four agencies developed and implemented a formal standardized classification data comparison process using structured Omaha System data. The Omaha System problems addressed most often by the four agencies were Growth and Development; Antepartum/Postpartum; Caretaking/Parenting; Family Planning; Income; Mental Health; Residence; Abuse; Substance Use; and Neglect. Significant improvement was demonstrated in 84% of the problems addressed. The greatest improvement was noted for Antepartum/Postpartum and Family Planning. The least improvement was noted in Neglect and Substance Use. Though there were some differences by agency, statistically significant improvement was consistent across all agencies (Monsen et al., 2010).

Though a few program evaluation studies use automated record systems, most program evaluations in public health nursing are still carried out by traditional research methods. Table 3.5 presents an example of a comprehensive program utilizing multiple public health nursing interventions to reduce repeat teen pregnancy. A global measure of pregnancy rate was the health outcome used to measure effectiveness.

Table 3.5   The Pregnancy-Free Club

Interventions	Outcome
Advocacy, case management, collaboration, community organizing, consultation, counseling, health teaching, policy development, screening, referral and follow-up	A public health agency, school, and local hospital collaborated in the development of a Pregnancy-Free Club to reduce repeat pregnancies among adolescent students. Following program initiation, the repeat adolescent pregnancy rate declined from 25% to 7.2% over a period of 9 years (Schaffer, Jost, Peterson, & Lair, 2008).

Putting It All Together

PHNs understand the interrelationships that exist between individuals and their physical and social environments. They understand the complexity of individual and family developmental needs. PHNs work within the community and the multiple systems that influence the health and wellness of individuals, families, and populations. They use a holistic public health nursing process to assess the complex factors that influence health and wellness. They weave a tapestry of interventions that provides a safety net for vulnerable individuals, families, and populations. The teen parenting program example (see the Evidence Example below) demonstrates the effectiveness of public health nursing practiced within the community.

Evidence Example: Public Health Teen Parent Program

In one metropolitan county, PHNs providing home visiting services to teens and their babies recognized that most teen parents were living in poverty with their primary source of income being federal assistance, including cash and food stamps. At the time, the rate of high school graduation or GED (General Education Development—five tests which are an alternative measure to determine high school graduation requirements) completion for teen parents was 34%. A study of teen parents and their dependence on federal and state funding showed that 50% of human service dollars spent in most counties in the state was expended on families with a birth to a teen.

Public health nursing, human services, and workforce services implemented a system of service delivery that promoted positive prenatal and postpartum outcomes, positive parental attachment and interaction, and utilized TANF (Temporary Assistance for Needy Families [pregnant women and families with one or more dependents]) System requirements to improve high school graduation or GED completion rates among teen parents. Public health staff analyzed agency data and found that the benefit of PHN services to teens was limited by teen parents' acceptance of nursing services while at the same time the literature reported the significant benefit of long-term, relationship-based services for teen parents.

Financial workers, child care authorizers, TANF workforce planners, and PHN staff initiated a collaborative effort to improve the health and well-being of teen parents and their children through systems change. Workforce planners approved budget allocations to improve services and move from a school-based delivery system to a PHN home-visiting model. Public health nursing became a mandatory service for teen parents receiving TANF funding. PHNs assumed responsibility for monitoring school attendance, working with teens to improve school attendance, and provided health assessment, teaching, and other interventions to improve the health status and well-being of the teen family.

Client satisfaction data and program evaluation data reflected significant systems change and significant teen parent outcome change. In 2009, 64.3% of teen parents enrolled in the program graduated or completed a GED compared to 34% in 2003. At exit from the program, the teen parents indicated that, based on their relationship with their PHN, they knew they could rely on their PHN for accurate information, health assessment, and teaching, advocacy, referral, and case management.

Source: Cross, 2010

Ethical Application

Community assessment involves collecting data on individuals. The data is aggregated which hopefully provides for confidentiality and anonymity. However, when group size is small or the members of the group are easily identified, ethical issues arise. It is important to protect the privacy rights of individuals.

> *Zack is collecting health data from the residents of the halfway house as part of his community assessment project. After analyzing the resident data, he will identify strengths of and health needs for the halfway house residents, work with them to identify their health priorities, and recommend interventions. The residents all have severe mental health disorders and are unable to live independently in the community. These residents are all considered vulnerable adults. Zack is concerned about ethical issues of informed consent, confidentiality, and autonomy.*

Use the ethical framework in Table 3.6 to determine how you would handle this situation if you were working with Zack.

Table 3.6   Ethical Application of the Nursing Process in Public Health Nursing

Ethical Perspective	Application
Rule Ethics (principles)	• Respect the rights of individuals related to privacy, autonomy, and self-determination.
	• Critique selected actions and interventions for possible unintended harmful consequences that might occur for diverse populations in a community.
	• Select interventions that promote justice through reducing health disparities.

Virtue Ethics (character)	• Maintain the dignity and confidentiality of individuals, families, populations, and communities when assessing their health needs.
	• Be honest in communicating purpose of selected interventions to individuals, families, populations, and communities.
	• Be an advocate for assessing public health needs of vulnerable populations.
Feminist Ethics (reducing oppression)	• Include voices of vulnerable populations in community assessment and in setting priorities for action.
	• Emphasize the contribution of the assets that communities and diverse populations bring to resolving public health concerns.

Table based on work by Volbrecht (2002) and Racher (2007)

Key Points

- Public health nurses use a strengths-based approach when working with individuals, families, and communities.
- The public health nursing process is an enhanced version of the basic nursing process.
- The public health nursing process is used to assess and intervene with individuals, families, communities, and systems.
- PHNs work in partnership with individuals, families, communities, and systems.
- PHNs use health data to determine the major health concerns in a community.
- PHNs use automated health systems to assist them in monitoring client health status, evaluating client progress, and determining effectiveness of interventions and programs.
- PHNs use 17 interventions to improve the health of the public.

Exercises

Learning Examples for Practicing the Public Health Nursing Process

Students learn best when clinical activities are meaningful and are directed at actually making a difference in peoples' lives. When students combine working with vulnerable populations and community organizations, conducting community assessments, and, intervening with individuals and families, they have the opportunity to develop public health nursing competencies at all three levels of PHN practice: individual/family, community, and systems. Review the following examples of student experiences and think about how the students used their public health nursing process skills at all three levels of practice.

PHN Clinical in Nicaragua (Ailinger, Molloy, & Sacasa, 2009)

- Students from the United States worked with vulnerable families in Nicaragua providing care to families, worked in clinics, provided health teaching to community groups, completed a community assessment, and held a health fair.

- Students learned about community health in a developing country, became more aware of social justice issues, and developed skills in cultural competency.

Population-Focused Analysis Project (PFAP) (Eide et al., 2006)

- Students working in small groups selected a vulnerable population to study.

- They researched the population using literature in print and on the web and by carrying out key informant interviews.

- Outcomes included 45-minute presentations to peers, poster session, and writing an advocacy letter to elected official, policy maker, or newspaper.

Combining Community Assessment and Change Projects to Make a Difference (Mansfield & Meyer, 2007).

- Students working in teams chose a community or population to assess and carried out a change project.

- Students completed a community assessment, selected a health problem to address, researched the literature for evidence of effective interventions, and developed and implemented a community-level intervention.

- Students learned that they could create meaningful positive change in community health and assume leadership roles in order to promote positive change.

Partnering with Faith Communities (Otterness, et al., 2007).

- Students working in teams carried out community assessment and provided interventions to populations within faith communities.

- The benefits to students included the ability to apply skills in real community situations; development of cultural awareness and competence related to faith communities; strengthening their critical thinking and communication skills; and learning how to work effectively in groups.

Development of a Clinic for Homeless Men (Wilde et al., 2004)

- Over a period of five semesters nursing faculty and groups of students developed a student nurses' clinic at a city mission for homeless men.

- During the first semester a community assessment was carried out. The clinic was developed in stages during the following four semesters with each group of students building on what previous student groups had accomplished.

Reflective Practice

Carrying out the nursing process with families in the home setting presents many challenges. PHNs need to be able to partner with the family, focus on their immediate needs and priorities, establish realistic goals, and implement interventions over time in a way that builds on family strengths and enhances their capacity for self-care. Review the following case study and think about what you would do if you were working with this family. Then answer the questions at the end of the case study.

"Getting Behind the Wheel"—Case Management Story

I received a referral on a 22-year-old and her 2-month-old baby. At my initial home visit the baby appeared overweight and overfed. The young mom had started him on rice cereal in a bottle at 2 weeks. Every time he cried she gave him a bottle, even though he often struggled and tried to pull away from the nipple. I talked to her about feeding the baby and my concern about his weight, but she responded with "once he starts moving around the weight will come off."

By 4 months of age the baby was 27 pounds. By now I was very concerned and called both the nurse and the doctor at the clinic, but no action was taken. Next, I arranged a joint home visit with a nutritionist from WIC. Both of us counseled the mom to feed the baby only when he was truly hungry.

Two weeks later I returned to do an NCAST feeding interaction and videotaped the mom feeding the baby. We watched the tape together and talked about hunger cues and how the baby did not appear hungry. The young mother listened but continued to feed the baby whenever he fussed or cried. It was as though she had no other way to comfort him other than to feed him. I was also becoming concerned about the baby's development as he exhibited several delays in fine motor and language when I tested him.

At this point I started visiting every 2 weeks and placed a family health aide in the home for 2 hours, 1 day a week. The aide's assignment was to role model appropriate parenting and feeding. I also arranged to get a high chair for feeding the child through a nutrition program grant. Currently, I continue to coordinate services from the clinic, nutritionist, and family health aide. At the present time the baby's weight has stabilized, and he has not gained any more weight.

Source: MDH, 2006

What family protective factors and risk factors can you identify that influence the baby's nutrition and growth and development?

_____

_____

How would you establish mutual priorities with the mother?

_____

_____

What would be an appropriate family nursing diagnosis?

_____

_____

What behavioral outcomes would you like to achieve?

_____

_____

What nursing interventions would you use to achieve these outcomes?

_____

_____

How would you determine the effectiveness of your interventions?

_____

_____

 ## Application of Evidence

1. What basic functions of the family (Clark, 2008) are you trying to strengthen?

2. What additional family assessment data would you like to collect for each of these functions?

3. What strategies would you use to have a good first meeting (Jansson, et al., 2001)?

4. What activities would you carry out in each phase of home visiting (McNaughton, 2005)?

 ## Think, Explore, Do

Activity 1: Obesity Prevention

Divide the class into small groups. Each group should select one of the following populations.

- Preschool children
- Elementary school children
- Middle school children
- Adolescents in high school
- College students
- Employees

- African-American women
- Latinos
- Middle-aged women
- Men

1. Review literature and Internet sources to identify known causes (health determinants) of obesity in the population you have selected.

2. Review literature to identify effective interventions for obesity prevention in population you have identified.

3. Select an intervention you would like to use with your client population.

4. Discuss how you would implement this intervention.

Activity 2: Electronic Health Records (EHRs) and Health Information Systems (HIS)

1. Find out if your clinical agency has an automated data management system for clients and services.

   a. If yes, talk with your clinical preceptor about the EHRs and HIS at the community agency. Observe your preceptor inputting data into the automated system. Ask about how the system is organized. Find out how your preceptor uses the system to monitor client progress and evaluate the effectiveness of interventions. Ask about the benefits and drawbacks of using the automated system. Find out if the agency is aggregating individual client data to evaluate program outcomes.

   b. If not, talk with your preceptor about the paper record system in use at the community agency. Review a client folder. How is the data organized? How does your preceptor use the paper record to monitor client progress and evaluate the effectiveness of interventions? Ask about agency plans to implement EHRs and HIS.

Activity 3: Shadowing PHN Preceptor

1. Talk with your preceptor about her job description and responsibilities.

2. Spend a day shadowing your preceptor. Identify the following.

   a. Your preceptor's client population

   b. The PHN interventions your preceptor uses

   c. The levels of interventions you observe

   d. The prevention levels you observe preceptor using

COMPETENCY #2:

Utilizes Basic Epidemiological Principles (the Incidence, Distribution, and Control of Disease in a Population) in Public Health Nursing Practice

By Carolyn M. Garcia

with Noreen Kleinfehn-Wald, Maureen A. Alms and Karen G. Lindberg

4

Elizabeth had worked as a public health nurse (PHN) doing home visits on the maternal child health team for approximately a year. One day as she was having lunch with her co-workers someone mentioned that an outbreak of pertussis had occurred in an adjacent county. In fact, there were 42 cases! Two days later, Elizabeth's supervisor asked if she could help the Disease Prevention & Control (DP & C) team investigate 10 probable cases of pertussis.

DP & C nurses operated the immunization clinic and worked with infectious disease issues like tuberculosis. Other than these activities, Elizabeth knew very little of what their day-to-day work was like. Her supervisor explained that a disease investigation was case management work. She would not be required to do any additional home visits, but would need to plan on a limited amount of time to place phone calls, review records, and work with community partners like school nurses. Elizabeth agreed to take the additional assignment and arranged to receive orientation from the lead nurse. During this briefing, the lead nurse explained the state data privacy laws, the state health department's infectious disease reporting requirements for pertussis, and the report form which needed to be completed for each suspect or confirmed case. This was a lot of new information!

ELIZABETH'S NOTEBOOK

> **Competency #2: Utilizes basic epidemiological (the incidence, distribution, and control of disease in a population) principles in public health nursing practice.**
>
> - Understands the relationship between community assessment and health department programs, especially the populations and programs with which the PHN works
>
> - Understands the relationships between risk/protective factors and health issues
>
> - Obtains and interprets information regarding risks and benefits to the community
>
> - Applies epidemiological triangle (host, agent, environment) when assessing and intervening with communities, systems, individuals and families

Useful Definitions

Agent: The primary cause of the health-related condition. Agents are most often classified into six main types: physical agents, chemical agents, nutritive agents, infectious agents, genetic agents, and psychological agents (Valanis, 1999).

Communicability: Likelihood that a pathogen or agent can be transmitted from a diseased or infected person to another person who is not immune and is susceptible (Merrill & Timmreck, 2006, p. 51).

Environment: The characteristics of the physical, biological, and social environment that contribute to health-related conditions. Environment might include pollution issues, microorganisms, social interactions, or cultural issues (Clark, 2003).

Epidemic: Occurrence in a community of cases of an illness, specific health-related behavior, or other health-related events clearly in excess of normal expectancy (Merrill and Timmreck, 2006, p. 5).

Epidemiology: The study of the distribution and determinants of health-related states or events in human populations and the application of this study to the prevention and control of health problems (Merrill & Timmreck, 2006, p. 2).

Epidemiological Triangle: Data are collected with respect to three elements: host, agent, and environment. The interrelationship of these elements results in a state of relative health or illness (Clark, 2003).

Host: The human being affected by the particular condition under investigation. Factors that the host brings to the triangle include intrinsic factors (age, gender, race, etc.); physical and psychological factors; and the presence or absence of immunity (Clark, 2003).

Incidence: The number of individuals who develop the disease over a defined period of time (Le, 2001) or the number of new cases of a particular condition identified over a period of time (Clark, 2003).

Life Course Epidemiology: The study of long-term effects on later health or disease risk of physical or social exposures during gestation, childhood, adolescence, young adulthood, and later adult life (Kuh, Ben-Shlomo, Lynch, Hallqvist, & Power, 2003, p.778).

Prevalence: The number of existing cases of a disease or health condition within a population at some designated time (Friis & Sellers, 1999, p. 97).

Protective Factor: Factors including characteristics of individuals and their lifestyle, the physical environment, the social environment, and characteristics of the agent that lessen risk for a disease or impairment.

Risk Factor: Risk is the probability that a given individual will develop a specific condition. An individual's risk of developing a particular condition is affected by a variety of physical, emotional, environmental, lifestyle, and other factors (Clark, 2003).

Using Data to Solve Health and Disease Mysteries

Nurses often want to know why something happens or does not happen. This inquisitive nature is useful when nurses are working to prevent something from happening, or to intervene before something gets worse. In some situations, if questions aren't asked, credible solutions might be overlooked, and health outcomes might not be optimal. In a worst-case scenario, lives might be lost or seriously harmed if status quo is maintained and curious questions aren't asked and acted upon. At the foundation of effective population-based public health nursing is the science of epidemiology. Epidemiology guides the questions that are asked by PHNs and the steps that are taken to find answers and solutions. Following is a list of questions nurses ask or should ask regularly.

- How did this occur?
- What could have prevented this outcome?
- When did the problem start (end, worsen, improve)?
- What has contributed to the change? Triggered a response?
- Why haven't there been improvements with x, y, z?
- Who do we need to involve who can contribute to the solution?
- Where are available resources to aid in addressing this?
- What interventions can we use to reduce the spread of this occurrence/disease?
- Will we be working at the individual/family, community, or systems levels?
- Are there any ethical issues I need to consider?
- How will I know if the interventions are effective?

At its core, epidemiology is the study of solving mysteries, of understanding where and to what extent diseases, events, and behaviors are influencing the health of populations. Epidemiology is more than simply understanding what is going on. It also involves acting on what is understood to prevent or control problems. Similarly, a PHN should be committed not only to understanding what is contributing to a problem and the extent of the problem, but also to identifying and implementing disease prevention and health promotion strategies. In fact, it is the use of core epidemiological pieces, namely mathematics and data analysis, that contributed to advancing the role and view of nursing in the 19th century (Earl, 2009). See the Evidence Example below to examine how Lillian Wald and Florence Nightingale used data gathering and analysis to understand and address key health problems. By doing so, they advanced the profession of nursing beyond what had, up until that time, been a fairly ill-considered occupation.

Evidence Example: Origins of Epidemiology and Nursing

Catherine Earl (2009) provides a fascinating and thorough historical article that describes the influence of epidemiology in the developing role of public health nursing. Beginning with the early 19th century, Earl presents a summary of history that reminds the reader of how far nursing and science have come in the past 200 years. Not that long ago, diseases were addressed solely within the individual, with little appreciation given for trends among the group or population. Advances in mathematic theories led this shift, notably when Pierre Charles Alexandre Louis, a leading 19th-century physician, declared that the practice of bloodletting (often with the help of leeches) was ineffective and used statistics to support his claims. It is intriguing that, according to Earl, the use of quantitative methods was not well supported at that time and was poorly understood. This is interesting, considering that today in the 21st century quantitative analyses are core to random-ized, controlled trials, which are considered gold standard methods for establishing evidence.

Lillian Wald used this advance in health and science to support her efforts working with families in New York. She advocated for nurses to live and work near and among those they were also serving. She used numbers to support her need for resources, including the number of nurses. Her successes are many, and they are in part based on her foresight and wisdom in recogniz-ing the need for data to accomplish goals and meet the health and social needs of society. Earl summarizes well the contribution PHNs, led by Lillian Wald, made in addressing tuberculosis because they collected and reported critical data. "Nurses' involvement in the care of TB patients in 1914 was considered a major advancement in the use of statistical methods, because nurses be-came involved in improving health through their role as data collectors" (p. 262).

Florence Nightingale, considered by many as the first biostatistician and the first epidemiolo-gist, also used data to support her efforts addressing health and sanitation. In her era, it was not common for women to receive education, yet her father encouraged her to learn varied subjects, including mathematics. As a result, Nightingale had skills that enabled her to identify causes of problems and to intervene not only to heal or cure but also to prevent. As Earl states, "With an epidemiological perspective and further discussions of mortality and morbidity rates and the importance of sanitary conditions as described by Florence Nightingale, the first preventorium, a program established to save children, was designed for the prevention, not the treatment, of TB [Tuberculosis]" (p. 263). Both Lillian Wald and Florence Nightingale contributed to a significant shift from solely focusing on treatment to giving attention toward prevention, which today is much of what is done by PHNs all over the world.

Although most PHNs are not epidemiologists, many activities that PHNs engage in parallel the work of epidemiologists. Often epidemiologists work at the systems level of a health care facility or state health de-partment and are responsible for the data collection, analysis, and program development related to a par-ticular health/medical issue. Conversely, PHNs are frequently found in the grassroot level of health care, working with local vulnerable populations and community partners, interpreting and promoting the rec-ommendations, protocols, and policies that have been developed by an authoritative body. See Table 4.1 for an example list of activities that an epidemiologist often engages in, and note the similarities to many public health nursing activities and interventions. The following Evidence Example further demonstrates the use of epidemiology specifically among rural public health nurses.

Table 4.1   Example Activities of Epidemiologists and Public Health Nurses

Epidemiologist Activities (adapted from Merrill & Timmreck, 2006, p. 3)	Public Health Nursing Activities and Interventions (from the Public Health Intervention Wheel)
Identifying risk factors for disease, injury, and death	Disease and Health Event Investigation
Describing the natural history of disease	Health Teaching

Identifying individuals and populations at greatest risk for disease	Outreach Screening Referral and Follow-up Advocacy Case Management
Identifying where the public health problem is greatest	Surveillance Disease and Health Event Investigation
Monitoring diseases and other health-related events over time	Surveillance
Evaluating the efficacy and effectiveness of prevention and treatment programs	Evaluation is a key part of the nursing process, but it is not a specific component of the intervention wheel.
Providing information useful in health planning and decision making for establishing health programs with appropriate boundaries	Consultation Collaboration Community Organizing Policy Development and Enforcement
Assisting in carrying out public health programs	Most interventions on the Public Health Intervention Wheel
Being a resource person	Consultation
Communicating health information	Outreach Health Teaching Social Marketing Consultation

Evidence Example: Epidemiology is Part of What PHNs Do.

A statewide cross-sectional study of PHNs was employed in rural and frontier solo (one-nurse) and multi-nurse public health nursing office settings across Idaho (Bigbee, Gehrke, & Otterness, 2009). One hundred twenty-four nurses responded to structured interview questions about experience, education, satisfaction, competency levels, and practice activities. Fifteen of the respondents were solo public health nurses. The services these nurses provided to their communities were extremely broad and included "epidemiology, family planning/STD clinics, immunization clinics, communicable disease surveillance, and school nursing" (p. 6). Interestingly, despite challenges associated with being in a solo work setting (e.g., isolation, communication), the solo nurses reported equally high levels of job satisfaction because of "benefits of autonomy, variety, and close community ties" (p. 7).

Historically, nurses participated in epidemiologic investigations to determine the cause of a recurring problem, such as cholera outbreaks. As part of that process very early on, nurses realized that often numerous risk factors contributed to the spread of disease. This realization led to creative interventions that had multiple components to aid those already sick or affected and to prevent others from becoming sick. Quarantine (i.e., forced isolation) laws are a good example of a specific effort to contain the spread of disease in the absence of other strategies. Interestingly, quarantine strategies are still used today because some infectious viruses take time to resolve and, during set time frames, can be easily spread from person to person. Examples of this in the 21st century include pertussis, chicken pox, and the flu. When a family member is diagnosed with pertussis and other family members have been exposed, they are strongly encouraged to stay "quarantined" away from the broader community until it is clear they have not become infected. Health care providers often recommend a specified duration of antibiotic treatment for the infected and exposed because this makes them no longer contagious; while on the antibiotics, individuals are asked to quarantine themselves in their home. Although quarantines are not always enforced as they were years ago, they can be effective when they are used and when individuals and families adhere to the restriction.

More broadly, Lillian Wald offers to us a great example of a PHN using a variety of intervention tools to address uncontrolled disease and unnecessary deaths in New York City tenements. Her efforts ranged from direct care of sick individuals in crowded apartments to community care of neighborhood children in need of a place to engage in physical activity to systems care through advocating for programs that would meet the needs of many (e.g., welfare, food accessibility, child labor laws). Today's PHN needs a repertoire of intervention strategies so that when health is improved, it can be maintained over time. This maintenance is hard to do. For example, if a child recovers from an illness that worsened as a result of malnourishment and lack of warmth, but the family home environment remains unchanged, the child's recovery might not be maintained. In this case, the nurse might provide a space heater as a temporary solution and connect the family to a food shelf. The nurse might begin to create long-term solutions by inquiring into the reasons for the lack of heat and might help adult family members explore financial management strategies, as well as possibilities for higher-paying employment or more affordable, reliable housing. Finally, the nurse might advocate for legislation that prohibits companies or landlords from turning off heat sources during cold winter months. Nurses encounter numerous possible mechanisms for influence when they face a problem that might appear to have a simple solution but often requires complex intervention approaches to keep that problem from recurring. Nurses deal with many complex challenges, and in the Evidence Example below there is an example of using an Ecological-Epidemiologic (Eco-Epi) model to understand and intervene in the complex factors influencing child failure to thrive.

Evidence Example: Caring for Children Using an Ecological-Epidemiologic (Eco-Epi) Model

In a study looking at children with nonorganic failure to thrive (NOFTT), Elizabeth Reifsnider (1995) describes the usefulness of an Eco-Epi model to PHNs caring for these children. She argues that the complexity of factors contributing to NOFTT occurring in a child requires a model that can lead nurses to identify and prioritize intervention strategies. In this model, the basic epidemiologic triangle (agent, host, environment) is represented by food, the child, and the home environment; this is examined in the context of influencing systems, including the child's broader community and interactions between influences such as parents, siblings, and others in the community. Reifsnider presents case study examples that demonstrate how PHNs can use this model during home visits to ensure that each influencing area is adequately addressed. For example, nurses address feeding practices to ensure that adequate food is available and offered on a regular basis. Nurses also assess the child, including factors such as personality, to help the family identify things that encourage the child to have an appetite. Also, the environment around the child might be distracting or not conducive to quiet, calm feeding sessions. Nurses can observe this situation and make recommendations to enhance the success of feeding sessions. The model is a useful guide that can encourage thorough assessment and intervention at home visits, which can be particularly helpful with complex, persisting challenges such as NOFTT in children.

Understands the Relationship between Community Assessment and Health Department Programs

Many public health agencies and community organizations use community assessments to prioritize the programs and services that are offered. A variety of strategies can be used to conduct a community assessment (e.g., needs assessment, knowledge-attitude-behavior [KAB] survey, windshield survey). The specific approach used is based on the key questions being asked. For example, if a public health department has recently received funding to implement an obesity prevention program, questions might focus on identifying the groups in the community at greatest risk for obesity (e.g., age, ethnicity, neighborhood). A KAB survey might be conducted to identify the most likely barriers to occur when the obesity prevention program is introduced. These data inform the steps that are taken to optimize successful implementation of the obesity prevention program. Often, PHNs are involved in every step of this process: (1) identifying the questions that need to be asked, (2) developing the data collection process, (3) collecting the data, (4) analyzing the data, and (5) using the data to inform future actions and program delivery.

PHNs work collaboratively in conducting assessments and using the resulting data for informing priorities and actions. Although it might be natural to focus on needs because the nurse is trying to address a problem, it is extremely valuable to take a strength- or asset-based approach toward the issue (Lind & Smith, 2008). An asset-based approach ensures that the assessment includes documentation of existing or potential strengths. In this way, the possible problem-solving strategies will ideally build on identified strengths and assets. If nurses focus only on problems, they might reach a solution that consists of outside resources rather than builds on what is available. Asset-based perspectives inherently encourage capacity-building as well as self-care among individuals and families, communities, and populations.

> *Elizabeth looked at the faxed pertussis report she had been given on 11-year-old Billy Johnson. Information included Billy's birth date, address, phone number, and laboratory results, which were positive for pertussis. Next, Elizabeth looked up Billy in the computerized state immunization registry. She saw that he had been vaccinated with five doses of DTaP vaccine, the last of which was administered at 5 years of age.*

ACTIVITY

Reflect on the following questions.

What has Elizabeth discovered so far?

What are the next steps?

Understands the Relationships between Risk/Protective Factors and Health Issues

No better classic example of understanding the relationship between a risk factor and a health issue exists than that of John Snow in London in the mid-1800s. For unknown reasons many people in London began to suffer and die as a result of cholera. People were fleeing the city because of fear, and without a known cause, the people had little confidence that the disease could be stopped or prevented. John Snow created a map that began to identify where the deaths from cholera were occurring across London. This now famous map (See Figure 4.1) yielded some clues for Snow because he managed to visualize the areas where the deaths were most heavily concentrated. He suspected a water source, and to prohibit people from accessing this source of "risk" he removed the water pump handle, as described below:

> **1854:** Physician John Snow convinces a London local council to remove the handle from a pump in Soho. A deadly cholera epidemic in the neighborhood comes to an end immediately, though perhaps serendipitously. Snow maps the outbreak to prove his point … and launches modern epidemiology (Alfred, 2009, p.1).

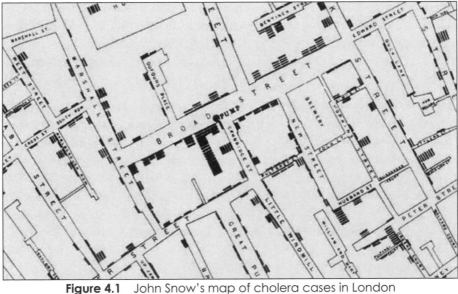

Figure 4.1   John Snow's map of cholera cases in London
Source: Alfred, 2009

Today in the 21st century, PHNs continue to solve mysteries in identifying and eliminating health risks. And though conditions have improved in many parts of the world, reducing the risks from unsanitary conditions, the improvements are not universal. Consider the following observation:

> The 2010 cholera epidemic in Haiti reminds us that cholera remains a deadly disease, not all that different from the time of John Snow. While Snow debated the appropriateness of the germ theory versus the miasmatic theory for the cause of the disease, current scientists are focusing on different, but related, hypotheses (UCLA, 2010, p. 1).

Indeed it is true that more than a century since Snow's solved mystery, we continue to seek clearer answers and solutions regarding the risks and diseases that are present in public health settings across the globe. In the United States, PHNs face complex challenges in meeting the needs of individuals, families, communities, and populations. Nurses need to identify risk and protective factors at multiple influencing levels. For example, a nurse might be working with a child recently diagnosed with asthma. The nurse needs to identify risk factors in the family environment that might be triggers for asthma episodes. Similarly, the nurse needs to assess for protective factors in the family, such as parental commitment to preventing episodes, which is an important asset the nurse can support with education and related tools. The nurse might want to go further and explore the neighborhood environment, including the school setting, for possible risks or protections influencing the child.

It can take time to carefully and thoroughly assess risk and protective factors using a strength-based approach. Usually, the time is well spent because the PHN will have a very clear picture of available assets as well as deficits to address when intervening on a particular health issue. Doing this proactively is a critical part of health promotion. Conducting assessments of risk and protective factors after a health issue has become apparent is important to minimize the effect of the health problem and to encourage positive intervention results. PHNs continually reassess for risk and protective factors because these factors can be temporal; one day a risk might exist (e.g., lack of health insurance coverage) and the following week the family might have new health insurance coverage. PHNs commit to efforts that routinely assess, intervene, evaluate, and reassess.

Elizabeth prepared to call Billy's parents. She placed the protocol nearby and had her report form ready. Elizabeth was lucky to find the mother answering the phone and introduced herself as a PHN who worked with infectious diseases. She explained how she had obtained a pertussis report on Billy and inquired if the mother had about 15 minutes to speak with her. Billy's mother stated that she operates a home child care, but most of the children had not yet arrived.

Elizabeth explained that the purpose of the call was to identify what could be done to prevent the spread of the disease. Elizabeth started with what she thought was the most logical question—When did this cough start? Billy's mother recalled that he started coughing on the 17th, and had a paroxysmal cough without a whooping sound. He occasionally coughed so hard that he vomited. About one week before his cough started, he had a low-grade fever and a runny nose.

Because his cough wasn't getting any better, his mother brought Billy to the clinic on the 26th. Billy did not have pneumonia, or any other complications of pertussis. He was given azithromycin antibiotic and was now on his third day of a 5-day course of treatment. Elizabeth jotted down a note that stated the period of infectivity started about the 10th of the month.

Next Elizabeth inquired how many other family members were in the home. Billy lived with his parent and had no siblings. Neither parent had been coughing. Elizabeth discussed with the mother the public health recommendation that other household members take a preventive course of antibiotics. The mother agreed to call the clinic for prescriptions.

Obtains and Interprets Information Regarding Risks and Benefits to the Community

PHNs need to have an understanding of how to find and use data. Data drive so much of what PHNs do. In fact, PHNs use data to determine health priorities by demonstrating the key problem areas or concerns. PHNs also use data to evaluate if interventions or programs are successful in reducing the risks or health problems in a local community. Unfortunately, data do not always come in ways that are easy to interpret or understand; data are often presented in formats such as tables, figures or graphs, or raw numbers. They might be posed as percentages or risk ratios. Although in-depth knowledge of data, formulas, and calculations is not necessary for entry-level PHNs, they will find some awareness of the data and data types useful.

Data Trend in a Graph

Often, data are presented over time using graphs to show what is happening in a community with respect to a particular health problem or population trends. For example, a PHN might be interested in exploring trends related to tuberculosis cases in the community over the past 6 years (see Figure 4.2). The data in a graph form provide a snapshot of how the cases are increasing, maintaining, or decreasing. In the tuberculosis example, it is apparent that active TB cases are relatively stable whereas latent TB cases are dramatically increasing. This information might lead the PHN to ask questions about population changes in the community and explore specific intervention strategies to reduce the number of latent TB cases over the next few years.

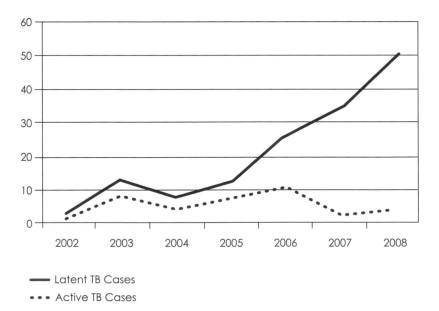

Figure 4.2   Example trend of active and latent tuberculosis cases in a community

Data Trend Per 100,000 in a Graph

Similarly, a nurse might examine the trend of Chlamydia cases over a period of 5 years. Rather than looking at the raw number of cases (as in the tuberculosis example), the PHN might prefer to examine the rate of cases. The case rate per 100,000 people helps the PHN to get a sense of severity in the population. The raw case number in the tuberculosis example does not give a picture of how serious the problem is because the graph does not indicate how many people are in the community. For example, if the community population count was 100, and the cases of latent TB were 50, the PHN would be much more concerned than if the cases were 50, but the community population was 100,000. Many PHNs use case rates to get a sense of the extent of the problem in a community. The case rate is always based on a ratio or number of cases per 100,000 persons. In the Chlamydia example, the rate of cases appears to be increasing, from around 90 per 100,000 in year 1 to nearly 140 per 100,000 in year 5 (see Figure 4.3). This increase is concerning by itself, but the PHN might want to compare the rate in one community with the rate in another community. Comparing rates in different communities or populations provides the nurse with perspective about the relative severity of the disease incidence or prevalence and helps in determining how to prioritize efforts to prevent the spread of Chlamydia.

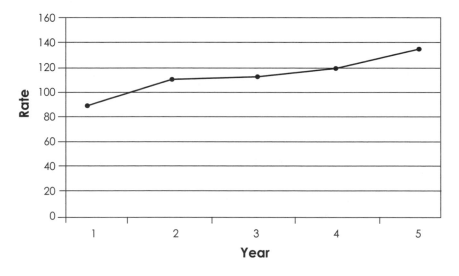

Figure 4.3 Chlamydia example of case rate per 100,000 over 5 years

In the following Evidence Example we observe the use of data in the form of rates to identify a problem and evaluate the impact of a system-wide intervention to reduce the rate of tuberculosis among inmates.

Evidence Example: Use of Epidemiological Tuberculosis Data to Inform a New York Corrections Intervention

In a study addressing tuberculosis, data were used to inform strategies to prevent increases of tuberculosis among inmates in New York State Corrections (Klopf, 1998). Data indicated that the incidence of tuberculosis increased over a 6-year period from 43 per 100,000 to 225 per 100,000. The data clearly indicated a serious problem that warranted intervention. Collaboratively, people from corrections, the local department of health, and the parole division developed a comprehensive TB control program that focused on the prevention and containment of disease. Importantly, they implemented a nurse-led case management program, using infection control nurses to carefully monitor and intervene on active and suspected TB cases. The program was truly comprehensive, including policies, development of a TB registry, surveillance, detection, and case management involving preventive and directly observed therapy among the inmates. The staff and inmates received education regarding testing, diagnoses, disease process, and treatment. It is believed that this comprehensive program contributed to the reduced incidence of TB. Six years later, the rate decreased from 225 per 100,000 to 61 per 100,000—a 73% decrease! The data informed the need for an intervention that relied heavily on nurses. The data also demonstrated, in part, the impact of the intervention program, with significant reduction in the new cases of TB among New York's inmates.

Data Comparison between State and National Sources

Comparing health and disease trends across communities can be challenging and can create turmoil if not done in a careful manner. No community wants to appear worse than another when it comes to a health problem or condition. On the other hand, if resources are scarce, a community might want to justify a greater need of resources. Careful comparison of data within and across communities is vital to ensure that public health priorities are appropriate and resource allocation is warranted. Comparison is useful because it can bring understanding of the severity or scope of a problem, especially if policymakers are unaware of the problem or not convinced it requires attention.

A good example of this is Lyme disease, which is contracted through exposure to ticks. From the Minnesota Department of Health, you can obtain the number of Lyme disease cases since 1986, ranging from annual cases of 67 to 1,299 (see Figure 4.4). However, without a comparison to another state, you would find it difficult to ascertain if the problem is serious or relatively consistent with national trends (which could also be serious, but at least then the state would realize the scope of the problem). So, the PHN investigating this issue might look beyond state-level data to what is occurring nationally. If the nurse reviewed national data provided by the Centers for Disease Control and Prevention (CDC), she would observe that in 2009 Minnesota had one of the highest density areas of Lyme disease cases, second only to states along the East Coast (See Figure 4.5). These data would support efforts by PHNs to bring attention to the problem, and to invest in preventive messages for Minnesotans regarding the spread of Lyme disease.

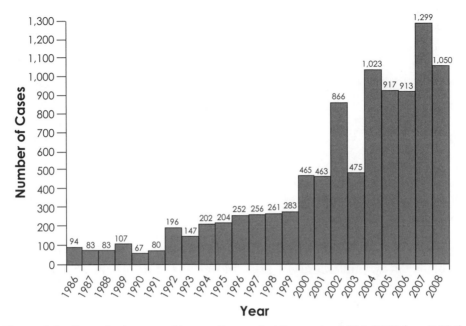

Figure 4.4   Reported cases of Lyme disease in Minnesota, 1986–2008 (n = 9,726)
Source: Minnesota Department of Health, 2010

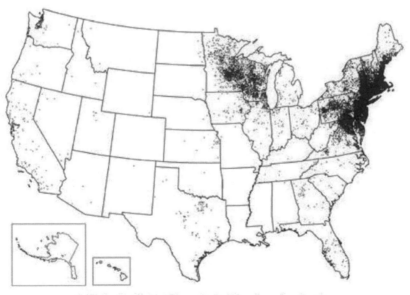

1 dot placed randomly within county of residence for each confirmed case

Figure 4.5   Reported cases of Lyme disease—United States, 2009
Source: Centers for Disease Control and Prevention (CDC), 2010

In this example, it is useful to point out that the data from the state and the CDC represent different years; the Minnesota data were reported through 2008, and the CDC data were from 2009. Often data are not easily and perfectly comparable between sources. An effective PHN tries to find the most comparable data possible and points out discrepancies that exist in incomparable data that might be presented by others. Using data that are not a perfect match is not wrong, but you need to point out differences so that people can make informed decisions based on the existing data. It might not be true that anyone can make data say exactly what they want it to say, but it certainly is possible to inadvertently or purposefully present data in ways that might not be entirely accurate. Therefore, PHNs need to spend time practicing how to present data in meaningful, representative ways, and equally vital, they need to have the ability to interpret and critique the data presented to them.

Data as Population Trends

Equally valuable are data that demonstrate population trends. These are most commonly presented in the form of a population pyramid, which at a glance provides a picture of population growth (see Figure 4.6). In this figure it is apparent that the Hispanic population is quite young, with a large proportion of the population under age 20. In contrast, the White population appears to be more evenly distributed among the age groups. PHNs can use this information collaboratively to prioritize prevention and promotion strategies with each of these populations. For example, PHNs might examine why there appears to be such a high reproductive rate among Hispanic women and explore data such as birth rates and birth outcomes to see if a need for interventions such as promoting prenatal care exists. Population data are important because they offer a glimpse into the big picture of how people are distributed, but the data by themselves might not be sufficient to guide intervention decisions or justify program budget priorities.

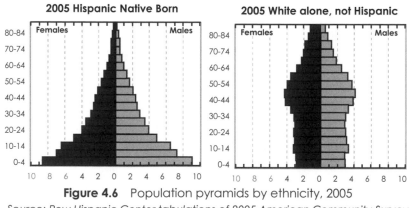

Figure 4.6 Population pyramids by ethnicity, 2005
Source: Pew Hispanic Center tabulations of 2005 American Community Survey

Data as Risk Ratios and Odds Ratios

Another very common tool used to examine the data regarding risks and health outcomes is a 2x2 table (see Table 4.2). This table aids in understanding how a disease is distributed in a population based on the presence or absence of a risk factor. From this table a nurse can calculate the rate of disease in each group; the risk ratio (RR), i.e., the rate of disease for those with the risk behavior divided by the rate of disease for those without the risk behavior; and the odds ratio, which is a regularly used number to describe the likelihood of contracting a disease for someone with the risk factor, compared to someone without. In the example shown in Table 4.2, the rate of disease for the "Yes" risk behavior group is 0.75 (75/100) and the rate of disease for the "No" risk behavior group is 0.02 (2/100). Already a relationship between the risk behavior and the disease seems obvious given the raw rates (0.75 versus 0.02). Taking this a step further, you can calculate the RR (0.75/0.02 = 37.5). By itself, the RR is not often used by PHNs, but it is an important calculation for those who might be interested in more in-depth statistical comparisons and analysis, such as chi-square analysis. PHNs might not routinely calculate these numbers, but they are often reading articles and consuming research data that include reported rates, risk ratios, odds ratios, chi-squares, and levels of significance (i.e., $p < .001$ or $p < .05$). It is beyond the scope of this manual to completely explain how to calculate each of these, but it is useful for nurses to have an awareness of what the numbers mean and how to appropriately interpret them.

Using Table 4.2, you can also calculate odds and an odds ratio (OR). This ratio is useful in identifying the odds of contracting the disease, given the presence or absence of the risk factor. For example, the odds of the disease in the presence of the risk factor is calculated by dividing the number of people with the disease and the risk by the number of people without the disease but with the risk (i.e., 75/25), or 3. Similarly, the odds of contracting the disease but not having the risk factor can be calculated (2/98), or 0.0204. The OR is calculated by dividing the odds with the risk factor by the odds without the risk factor (3/0.0204), or 147. In this example, someone with the risk factor is 147 times more likely to contract the disease than someone without the risk factor. A PHN with this information needs to make decisions on how to act based on many factors. For example, even though the OR is so high, the disease might not be life threatening or the risk factor might not be that common. The risk factor might easily be eliminated with an intervention, or the risk factor might not be easily identified, making it difficult to intervene. PHNs need to consider numerous factors when data are interpreted and then acted upon. PHNs have an important role in helping interpret data so that they are not misunderstood or inappropriately used to justify action or inaction, depending on the situation.

Table 4.2 Association between Risk Factor and Disease

Risk Factor	Disease		
	Yes	No	Total
Yes	75	25	100
No	2	98	100
Total	77	123	200

Innovative Data Collection

Data are typically collected through surveillance systems at the local, state, or national levels. Sometimes health care professionals provide the data, and other times, individuals are surveyed. Beyond these traditional mechanisms for data collection, new techniques are becoming available with technological advances. PHNs need to be aware of the variety of tools used to collect epidemiological data because they might participate in the data collection, interpretation, or dissemination. A geographic information system (GIS) is an example of a tool that is growing in popularity in the field of public health. Missouri is one state that is advancing use of GIS to track the health of communities across the state. GIS enables the state to compile data from numerous different places into a common website that the public can explore and search to identify priority problems, strengths, and a variety of related factors. As the Missouri website explains:

> GIS has been a vital tool in promoting quality of life and health at Department of Health and Senior Services [DHSS] since 1997. GIS specializes in combining data from multiple sources and displaying that data in a geographic context. Data such as demographic information, disease prevalence, and physical environmental factors can be analyzed with GIS to reveal relationships and trends that otherwise would be very difficult to find. GIS is also a valuable management tool for policymaking and resource management (MDHHS, 2010).

GIS data are also being used to carefully examine community-level assets and risks related to obesity prevention. For example, GIS data can aid in understanding how communities compare in terms of access to full-scale grocery stores, corner supermarkets, gas stations, or liquor stores. Additionally, GIS data can indicate the location of parks and transpose violent crime data, which might provide insights into why youth in certain neighborhoods are reporting higher levels of physical activity than youth in other neighborhoods. This is an example of how GIS tools can yield data useful to a neighborhood, community, state, or country in advancing public health priorities.

To further assess for close contacts, Elizabeth asked questions about Billy's school. Billy told his mother "a lot of kids" were coughing in his classroom. Elizabeth informed Billy's mother that state law allowed her to speak with the school nurse about a pertussis case in general, but she needed the mother's permission to use Billy's name with the nurse. Billy's mother was agreeable. Elizabeth stated that she would talk to the school nurse about sending a notification letter to the parents of the students in Billy's classroom. Elizabeth was careful to inform the mother that Billy would not be identified in the letter. Elizabeth explained that she would also be working with the school to identify children who sit adjacent to Billy, as they might also need preventive antibiotics.

Applies Epidemiological Triangle When Working with Individuals and Families, Communities and Systems

How a PHN comes to understand a problem, and possible causes and solutions, is somewhat dependent on the framework used by the nurse. An outdated model, popular for relatively straightforward disease transmission scenarios, is the epidemiological triangle. This triangle consists of identifying a host (e.g., person with flu), an agent (e.g., the flu virus), and an environment (e.g., crowded house in which the flu is transmitted). This model has been adapted to consider more complex scenarios that might be contributing to disease or illness (see Figure 4.7). It is an important adaptation because for most health problems addressed by PHNs, the contributing factors are complex and multifaceted. Illnesses result not merely from a simple transmission in the right time and place, but also because of factors not easily controlled or resolved (e.g., poverty, inadequate housing, food shortage).

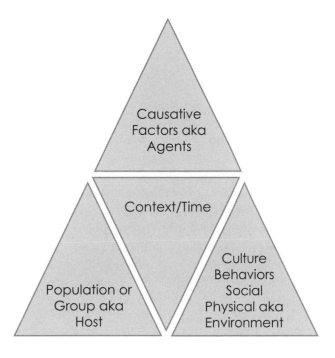

Figure 4.7   Epidemiological triangle in the 21ˢᵗ century
Source: Merrill & Timmreck, 2006, p. 15

For many in public health, the complex contributing factors to poor health or well-being have been informed by models such as the web of causation. The name itself implies greater complexity than the epidemiological triangle, yet this model is also not perfect. For example, imagine a spiderweb (where the name is drawn from) and how you might use the web design to identify all of the factors influencing the center of the web (e.g., the disease, such as cardiovascular disease or asthma or the social health problem, such as teen pregnancy). After you have drawn out the web you are faced with a dilemma, specifically, which related thread to address first. How do you decide whether to prioritize a biological related factor or a social-based factor? The web might help identify numerous potential causes, contributors, and influences, yet the model by itself does not yield readily apparent strategies or solutions. Over 10 years ago, Nancy Krieger (1997) identified these criticisms of the Web framework and proposed an eco-social framework for developing epidemiologic theories about public health problems and possible solutions. The central question answered using an ecosocial framework is, "[W]ho and what is responsible for population patterns of health, disease, and well-being, as manifested in present, past, and changing social inequalities in health?" (Krieger, 2001a, p. 694).

A shift in thinking about traditional epidemiology models has occurred with growing recognition of the importance of social epidemiology, the field that acknowledges and seeks to address the complex combination of biological and social factors influencing health and well-being. Social epidemiology was initially defined in the 1950s but has in more recent decades grown in popularity and use among public health professionals (Krieger, 2001b). PHNs need to be aware of the trends in public health as well as the theories that guide understanding of the risk-asset-problem-intervention relationships in public health.

For example, Krieger's ecosocial theory has shaped how many people are now addressing complex public health problems. She states that the ecosocial theory is a tool that:

> ... fosters analysis of current and changing population patterns of health, disease, and well-being in relation to *each* level of biological, ecological and social organization (e.g., cell, organ, organism/ individual, family, community, population, society, ecosystem) as manifested at *each* and every scale, whether relatively small and fast (e.g., enzyme catalysis) or relatively large and slow (e.g., infection and renewal of the pool of susceptible for a specified infectious disease) (p. 671).

Nursing practice should always be informed by theory. It is relatively easy in nursing practice to get caught up in the tasks one has to do and to forget, at times, to take a step back, reflect, and consider why something is being done a certain way or why things are occurring. Theories are always advancing, and an effective PHN strives not only to use theory, but also to keep up with theoretical ideas that guide and inform practice and the care of individuals, families, communities, and populations. Epidemiology is an ideal example of the value and importance of theory as a guide for understanding and intervening on extremely complex societal health problems and conditions. The following Evidence Example is one example of a complex health problem that is best considered using an ecosocial framework.

Evidence Example: Ecosocial Framework Applied to Childhood Lead Poisoning

In a study addressing childhood lead poisoning, a noninfectious disease that is directly the result of social environmental factors, not biological factors, Krieger's ecosocial framework was used (Aschengrau and Seage, 2008). It is more easily understood within an ecosocial framework than in a traditional epidemiological triangle or web of causation model. Indeed, the ecosocial framework aids in the recognition of numerous contributing factors to childhood lead poisoning, including direct, micro-level influences such as substandard housing (e.g., old home that landlord has not updated to remove lead-based paint sources) and workplace exposure (e.g., dad works with lead and wears clothing home that is contaminated with lead and exposes the children) and indirect, macro-level influences such as workplace policies and minimum wage laws that limit the families options with respect to the rent they can afford to pay. Numerous other factors can be considered in an ecosocial framework, yielding specific areas the PHN can immediately address and those that require more sustained advocacy and effort.

Another important theoretical framework in public health that PHNs should be aware of is referred to as life course epidemiology. Historically, as the focus of epidemiology shifted from infectious disease to chronic illness in the mid-20th century, new and expanded paradigms emerged to better recognize and understand the antecedents and causes of chronic diseases. The life course perspective views health not in stages (infancy, early childhood, adolescence, adulthood) separate from each other, but as a continuum. As Krieger (2001a), describes, "[L]ife course perspective refers to how health status at any given age, for a given birth cohort, reflects not only contemporary conditions but embodiment of prior living circumstances" (p. 695). A classic life course study was the research on the effects of the 1944–1945 Dutch famine that linked malnutrition with subsequent effects on human development and mental performance (Stein, Susser, Saenger, & Marolla, 1975).

Throughout the life course continuum, biological, behavioral, environmental, psychological, and social factors dynamically interact, contributing to one's health. As Matthias Richter (2010) summarizes, "This perspective was truly helpful to contribute to a better understanding of biological, behavioural and social influences—from gestation to death—for health as well as health inequalities" (p. 458). The impetus of life course epidemiology was chronic disease, and as such, the framework is grounded in a medical risk model, rather than an "ecosocial" model (Richter, 2010). Even so, PHNs gain benefits using a life course perspective when they are designing health promotion or disease prevention programs because they are encouraged to think about long-term implications and benefits. The increased thoughtfulness about impact over time can also enhance the sustainability of a program or the commitment of an agency to support a long-term intervention or screening program. The Evidence Example that follows relates the life course development model to maternal and child health.

Evidence Example: Building on Life Course Epidemiology: The Life Course Health Development Model

One model that builds on longitudinal connections is the Life Course Health Development model (Halfon & Hochstein, 2002). The model is an integrated framework that helps translate the life course perspective into interventions and policy recommendations designed to improve the long-term health of individuals and populations. The life course perspective has particular relevance to understanding health of Maternal and Child Health (MCH) populations. For example, in MCH, one of the problems with past research on birth outcome disparities comes from focusing on pregnancy-only factors, instead of looking at the entire life course of the mother (Lu, 2010).

These upstream determinants are factors largely shaped by families and communities, which have important implications for public health nursing practice.

In summary, public health nursing is grounded in the science of epidemiology. On numerous levels, epidemiological data help describe the scope of a problem, prioritize intervention strategies, and evaluate outcomes or trends over time. Data are presented and collected using many different formats; nurses need the skills to interpret and critique these data, regardless of how they are presented. PHNs also use epidemiological theories to inform actions and priorities for addressing public health problems. PHNs need to use and contribute to the development of theories that recognize the social complexities influencing public health problems in the 21st century.

The next area for Elizabeth to assess for close contacts was the home child care. Billy's mother stated that they have a split entry home and that the lower level is for the licensed day care. On a normal day, she has five children who stay until between 5:00 and 5:30 pm. In addition, a set of one-year-old twin girls stay until approximately 11:00 p.m. Billy's mother indicates that since Billy has been ill, he has stayed only on the upper level, away from the lower level child care children. However, the situation with the twins is different. Billy eats supper with them and plays with them until bedtime. The twins have been exposed, and according to the definition in the protocol would be considered face-to-face contacts.

Elizabeth asks if the parents of the twins have been told about Billy's pertussis. The mother states she has not told them because she is concerned about losing her child care clients and the potential lost income. Elizabeth explained that the public health recommendation would be that the twins receive preventive antibiotics because of their close contact with Billy. Billy's mother agrees to notify the twins' mother and tell her to call Elizabeth if she has any questions or if either of the twins develops a cough.

Ethical Considerations

As seen in the case study woven throughout this chapter, the day care provider was concerned about a loss of income and her reputation as a provider. Many times PHNs confront challenging situations in their practice. For example, reporting a nuisance house situation to the city building inspector might prompt the eviction of a renter or harassment from a landlord. Though the nurse is trying to protect children living in less than desirable circumstances, PHNs' actions might have unintended consequences for the entire family.

Similarly, interventions focused on reducing the exposure to lead paint in older homes might be embarrassing or financially difficult. Though the health department might offer a free home/environmental inspection for the detection of lead paint, this activity might force the family to temporarily leave their home. Many families perceive this as an invasion of privacy. Moving in with relatives for a day might be embarrassing for some, or for others, staying in a hotel might be beyond the family budget. Some health departments offer a free service to abate lead in a home if the family has not done so. Though this is helpful in covering up a lead source, the repainting services are often spotty and unsightly in appearance. The benefit of reducing lead exposure to children must be weighed against the other consequences for the family.

Table 4.3   Ethical Action in Using Epidemiological Principles in Public Health Nursing

Ethical Perspective	Application
Rule Ethics (principles)	• PHNs should use epidemiology to assess and develop interventions that promote beneficence.
	• PHNs can support the autonomy of those they are working with, even when uncomfortable changes are needed to minimize the spread of disease.
Virtue Ethics (character)	• PHNs need to demonstrate respect for individuals, families, and communities when suggesting promotion or prevention strategies; this can be challenging but necessary, especially when some might refuse to adhere to what is being recommended.
	• PHNs should be persistent in understanding the complexity of factors contributing to a problem so that potential solutions are comprehensive and yield lasting changes.

Feminist Ethics
(reducing oppression)

- PHNs can advocate for system-level changes that promote the well-being of those who often feel they have no voice (e.g., tenants who are unable to ask a landlord to maintain heat levels during the winter).

- PHNs should explore societal changes that can improve the underlying environment for people, such as increasing the minimum wage law so that families have additional resources to sustain and promote health.

Key Points

- Epidemiology is an important foundation to the work of PHNs.

- There is a growing shift from traditional epidemiological models toward more complex models that consider the social influences on health, such as a social epidemiological model.

- Epidemiological data, including prevalence and incidence data, help set national and local public health priorities.

- PHNs can and should use epidemiological data to advocate for health promotion priorities in their areas of influence.

Exercises

Learning Examples for Effective Use of Epidemiological Principles in Public Health Nursing Practice

The following learning example builds on the epidemiological concepts presented in the chapter and offers a real-life situation in which data were used by a public health nurse to address an important public health concern.

Somewhere County Learning Example: Using Population-Based Data

The following infectious disease data were obtained by the local PHN: 24 cases of Amebiasis, 169 cases of Chlamydia, 4 cases of Dengue fever, and 18 cases of Kawasaki disease. A quick review made it clear that Chlamydia is the most concerning infectious disease issue, based on the raw, or actual, number of cases. Using the United States Census Web site, the nurse obtained the estimated population for her jurisdiction (124,768). She was able to compute the rate of cases per 100,000 people as follows:

169/124,768 = 135 cases per 100,000

Next she gathered more data and determined the trend of cases over 5 years in the jurisdiction.

Year	Rate Per 100,000 Population
1	90
2	110
3	112
4	120
5	135

The incidence of Chlamydia was definitely increasing, but the nurse wanted a larger context or comparison, so she computed the rate per 100,000 for some neighboring jurisdictions.

Year 5	Rate per 100,000 Population
The nurse's area	135
Area to the south	123
Area to the west	143
Adjacent metro area	483

The nurse created this comparison table for each of the preceding 4 years. She discovered that overall the rate of Chlamydia was similar in her area to other adjacent areas, except the metro area where there was greater ethnic diversity, lower insurance rates, and more campus college settings (all of these being possible explanatory factors for the different rates).

The nurse then examined additional factors that were contributing to the snapshot of her jurisdiction. The following is her summary of the Chlamydia cases that occurred in Year 5 in her jurisdiction:

- 70% female

- 47% from Happyville, 21% from Somewherecity, and 21% from Wheresitville

- 61% Caucasian (including 1% Hispanic), and 8.3 % African-American

- Co-infection rate with Gonorrhea – 3.8%

- No co-infection with syphilis

- Heterosexual spread

- Top five diagnostic sites included sites outside of the jurisdiction. No cases reported from Wheresitville Clinic.

- Age distribution:
    - Age 15–19: 24.2%
    - Age 20–24: 37.7%
    - Age 25–29: 21.5%

Based on this summary of the nurse's analysis and comparison:

What next steps do you think the nurse should take in addressing the problem of Chlamydia in her community?

Who might she target for health education or screening activities?

Develop a plan of action she might implement with the goal of reducing the transmission of Chlamydia in her community.

 ## Reflective Practice

Investigating outbreak possibilities can be challenging, and it can present opportunities to practice great intercommunication skills. Elizabeth handled a situation that could have been extremely difficult in a professional, thoughtful manner. She asked the right questions and managed to express concern rather than judgment. By building a good relationship right away, Elizabeth received honesty from the child care provider and together they determined who had been exposed and an appropriate course of action. What do you imagine will be some follow-up steps that Elizabeth will take in this situation?

_____

_____

How can Elizabeth be a resource for the child care provider if the families grow angry when they are informed about the possible exposure?

_____

_____

Who might be additional partners to Elizabeth within the health department as she follows this case through until it is resolved?

_____

_____

How might Elizabeth address an ethical issue such as if some of the exposed refuse preventive treatment?

_____

_____

How will Elizabeth know this case investigation has been successful? What will be important for Elizabeth to document?

_____

_____

How will the numbers that Elizabeth has collected as part of this investigation be useful to others at her local health department? At the state level? At a national level?

_____

_____

Application of Evidence

1. What are some ways you can use the ecosocial framework to examine contributing and influencing factors on complex public health problems in the United States in the 21st century, such as obesity or adolescent pregnancy?

2. Examine the different types of data presented in this chapter (e.g., odds ratios, rates) and identify some of the pros and cons associated with the use of each of them.

3. As a public health nurse working in a community, identify three to five sources of state- or federal-level data you would want to use in demonstrating how your community issues compare to others.

Think, Explore, Do

1. Look through your local newspaper (or a national online news source) and identify all the articles that describe problems a PHN might be involved in addressing. How will the tools of epidemiology assist in identifying ways to intervene on the problems?

2. Develop an ecosocial model that portrays contributing factors to the problem of childhood obesity.

3. Visit a few websites about John Snow and learn about how he addressed the cholera outbreak in the 1800s. Develop a strategy that a modern day John Snow would use to address cholera outbreaks in the 21st century, such as the outbreak that occurred in Haiti in 2010.

4. Read _The Ghost Map: The Story of London's Most Terrifying Epidemic—and How it Changed Science, Cities, and the Modern World_ by Steven Johnson (2006; New York, NY: Riverhead Books) or _Flu: The Story Of The Great Influenza Pandemic of 1918 and the Search for the Virus that Caused It_ by Gina Kolata (2001; New York, NY: Touchstone) and reflect on whether or not PHNs should be concerned about these types of outbreaks occurring in the United States. What changes (positive or negative) contribute to your opinions (e.g., global travel in 21st century, communication capabilities via text, IM, etc.)?

COMPETENCY #3:
Utilizes Collaboration to Achieve Public Health Goals

5

By Marjorie A. Schaffer
with Joyce Bredeson and Rose Jost

Jake is a public health nursing student who has 10 years of experience in the acute care setting as an associate degree nurse. His expertise has been in the area of cardiac care working in the Coronary Care Unit at a local hospital. Jake has returned to school to complete a baccalaureate degree in nursing. The community surrounding the university that Jake attends has identified a need to address health care access for the homeless population. The university was approached by a local church to work with them to develop a clinic for the homeless by using resources in the community and students for the delivery of care for this underserved population. Jake's preceptor, Linda, a public health nurse (PHN), is representing the local public health department at planning meetings. Jake will have the opportunity to learn how professionals, community members, and organizations collaborate to contribute to the development of a community clinic that serves a vulnerable population. Jake has many questions. Who would he collaborate with to contribute to this goal? Who should be invited to be partners in the collaboration? How does such a diverse group work together? What is the responsibility of the public health nurse in collaborative work?

Before Jake attends the first planning meeting with Linda, he picks up his notebook to review the population-based public health nursing competency list and concentrates on Competency #3, which focuses on collaborative practice.

JAKE'S NOTEBOOK

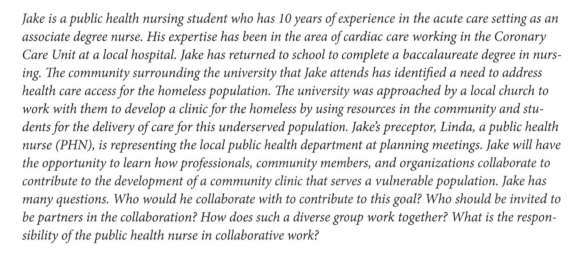

Competency #3: Utilizes Collaboration to Achieve Public Health Goals

- Demonstrates effective participation on interdisciplinary teams
- Develops relationships and builds partnership with communities, systems, individuals, and families
- Utilizes community assets to empower communities, systems, individuals, and families

Useful Definitions

Collaboration: Working together "to achieve a common goal through enhancing the capacity of one or more of the members to promote and protect health" (Keller, Strohschein, Lia-Hoagberg, & Schaffer, 2004, p. 456).

Interdisciplinary Collaboration: "Brings all members of the health team together," which is needed because "most health care processes involve more than one discipline" (Potter & Perry, 2009)

Partnership: "A close mutual cooperation between parties having shared interests, responsibilities, privileges, and power" (Seifer & Connors, 2007, p. 4).

Community Asset: "Anything that can be used to improve the quality of community life" including people, physical structures, businesses, and organizations (Community Tool Box, 2009)

Social Capital: Resources that promote a sense of belonging, including social networks, social support, reciprocity, and trust that lead to a socially cohesive society (McNeill, Kreuter, & Subramanian, 2006)

Accomplishing More By Working Together

Public health nurses work with many individuals and community organizations. Collaboration can be between two or more individuals or between organizations. PHNs collaborate with representatives of the population, other professionals, and organizations to contribute to health care planning and promote health (American Nurses Association, 2007; Chaudry, Polivka, & Kennedy, 2000). An important skill for PHNs is learning how to develop the collaborative community partnerships to bring about community and systems change for improving health (Fawcett, Francisco, Paine-Andrews, & Schultz, 2000; Franklin, Exline, & Stringer, 2002).

Building capacity for partnership and engaging community members is an important focus for PHNs. In a study of PHN practice, PHNs said their goal was to make a difference in the lives of their patients by focusing on "doing with" rather than on "doing for" (Aston, Meagher-Stewart, Edwards, & Young, 2009). They wanted to empower their patients to take responsibility and ownership for health decisions. The PHNs identified several strategies for empowering their patients: begin with the patient's perspective, tune into the readiness of the patient, assess holistically (refer to Public Health Nursing Competency #10 located in Chapter 12), and build rapport with their patients.

The study also suggested strategies to encourage community member participation in health programs and initiatives. The PHNs involved community members in decision-making groups, focused on community assets, and gave positive feedback and encouragement by affirming what was working well. The PHNs involved people who normally might not have the opportunity to participate in decision-making groups such as youth living in poverty and mothers who were isolated. At every group meeting the PHNs asked: "So who is missing and who needs to be here?" PHNs often initiate the process of joining people together around a problem they all care about. PHNs encourage group ownership and often look for community members to take the lead in problem solving. PHNs can assist with the group process, but ideally, community members should control the flow and process toward finding and implementing solutions. Collaboration works best when everyone has the opportunity to share thoughts and ideas. One nurse in the study used the word *catalyst* to describe an approach that brings in the voices and participation of community members. This means that someone needs to initiate the collaborative process, which then continues to develop with the input of the people who contribute their perspectives and skills to the collaboration.

The nurses in the study also talked about how important it was to connect community members and groups to existing social networks, which could be neighborhood groups, community organizations such as churches, or programs that provide food. The nurses talked about building these connections as "creating participatory infrastructure." This means the PHNs linked people and community organizations that were working on similar goals but had not yet worked together. PHNs created infrastructure by "building partnerships among clients, establishing self-help groups, advocating for clients by connecting them to other agencies, and linking together agencies to provide the best possible service for clients" (Aston et al., 2009, p. 30). One nurse talked about finding "the movers and shakers" in the community by reaching out to community groups such as men's or women's groups, church groups, and community health boards. These are strategies that encourage the collective voice of community members and foster citizen participation. PHNs can also bring their expertise in health promotion to existing collaborative groups that are already established in communities.

Collaboration Examples

Individual level: We know that PHNs collaborate with individuals, community groups, and systems. PHNs collaborate with individuals through mutual decision making about how to reach health goals. For example, a PHN might bring information to a family about where to find additional services for a child with special needs and work the family on their plan for finding access to those services.

Community level: PHNs work with many groups in the community and assist in establishing self-help groups. A PHN might find many elderly individuals in his or her caseload with adult children or spouses who are experiencing stress from the added caregiving responsibilities. After assessing the caregivers' needs for support, the PHN might connect with an existing community center for meeting space and bring together a community group with interested community members to discuss the need and strategies for establishing a caregiver support group. The nurse would work to have both community member voices and professional voices present such as a spiritual leader and a social worker

Systems level: PHNs can collaborate with systems that implement policy and program changes such as governmental organizations, schools, and hospitals. For example, the PHN might work with community leaders to institute a policy that addresses teen smoking.

All levels: In another example, a collaborative model was used to prevent childhood violence (Skybo & Polivka, 2006). Professionals in public health, primary care, and mental health specialties can work together to design interventions that reduce child exposure to violence. These interventions can be offered in a variety of organizations such as health departments, schools, community centers, clinics, and homes. Possible interventions include the following:

- Add screening questions that assess for exposure to violence in well-child and school health exams

- Screen for risk of exposure to violence in neighborhood

- Offer anticipatory guidance through health teaching in clinics and community settings—provide parenting information to decrease likelihood of physical discipline; offer group classes on parenting styles and discipline at community centers; provide information about preventing victimization by a bully, effects of violence in the media, and managing peer pressure

- Refer to a public health nurse when screening reveals a child is at risk for exposure to violence or to a program for mental health care for children who have been traumatized by violence

The preceding interventions contribute to the collaborative effort of reducing child exposure to violence and promote healthy relationships. Collaborative strategies have a greater influence on achieving the goal compared to the efforts of any one individual or organization.

The shared knowledge and expertise that comes from collaboration with other PHNs and interdisciplinary professionals and groups has the potential to create strategies and outcomes for improved population health status. Some examples of professional collaboration include sharing educational opportunities (emergency preparedness strategies), selecting a common screening tool to be used by all (assessment of child development), sharing knowledge about resources for referral (food programs), and linking to interdisciplinary referral options (social services).

Best Practices for Collaboration

Collaboration is important because with the input of several stakeholders (individuals and organizations), the pooling of expertise can lead to expanded ideas and strategies for improving public health. Collaboration might also lead to community organizing or coalition building that mobilizes a community to promote health (Findley et al., 2003). The creativity and synergy that can result from collaboration provide energy and a sense of purpose in reaching a common goal (Gamm, 1998). Together with community partners, PHNs strive to identify mutual goals for the collaboration and expected outcomes. The following list provides a summary of best practices for effective collaborative action.

- Effective leadership
- Commitment of the participants
- Shared values and a sense of purpose
- Linkages between groups and individuals
- Identification of strategies and resources to achieve the goals, a structure to support the collaborative work
- Internal systems to support the structure (for example, communication mechanisms, a place to meet, time available in assigned workload)

Demonstrates Effective Participation on Interdisciplinary Teams

The work of public health nurses is almost always interdisciplinary. Depending on their practice setting, they work with a variety of other professionals, groups, and organizations. For example, a public health nurse working in a school collaborates with teachers, families, students, school administration, physicians, other health and special education professionals, social workers, and groups that address health needs such as chronic illness and mental health services. The following are possible partners in public health nursing networks.

- Schools
- Child care programs and providers
- Physicians
- Nurse practitioners and clinical nurse specialists
- Dentists
- Native healers
- Clergy
- Psychologists
- Mental health centers
- Speech therapists
- Physical therapists
- Occupational therapists
- Audiologists
- Nutritionists
- Extension agents
- Early childhood development programs
- Businesses
- Social services
- Colleges and universities
- Special education
- Housing programs
- Battered women's shelters
- Service for children with special needs
- Financial assistance
- Food shelves
- Jobs and training services
- Transportation services
- Literacy programs
- English as a second language learner programs
- WIC
- Services for vision and hearing impaired
- Legal aid
- Ombudsmen
- Meals on Wheels
- Energy assistance
- Community service organizations (Rotary, Lions)
- City council
- Community residents
- Alternative therapy programs
- Head Start
- Community action programs
- Alcoholics Anonymous
- Chemical dependency programs
- Home-care agencies
- Law enforcement
- Congregate dining
- Homeless shelters
- Environmental health programs
- Vulnerable adult programs
- Child protection and welfare programs
- Planned Parenthood
- Volunteers
- Artists, Musicians

As a public health nurse, you are going to work with many people who have a different educational background, different experiences, and different philosophies of life from your own and from each other. As a result you are going to encounter many different perspectives about what issues are most important and what should be done to address specific health concerns. You need to become familiar with some common differences to avoid making assumptions about the viewpoints of community partners and members of the community. Sometimes tension and conflict occur as collaborators work through different perspectives and ideas about how to respond to the problem. However, in most cases the result of the Collaboration is more effective than what one individual or one professional group could accomplish. Conflict that can be worked through has the potential to lead to effective collaboration and positive change.

As you begin your practice, ask questions of persons with different educational preparation and roles about what they think about a situation. Also, do not be afraid to ask questions to learn about and from different perspectives or ideas. Differences can be as basic as using different terminology for similar work, practices, or interventions. What you call an assessment might have a different term in another profession. Take enough time to communicate and make sure all collaborators are on the same page. Time limitations and a sense of urgency in responding to a public health problem can sometimes create barriers to Collaboration. However, time spent in getting to know one another can prevent tension and conflict, which would likely take more time to resolve at a later point or result in a failure at collaboration.

When you collaborate with people representing different organizations, an understanding of group dynamics is useful for effective collaboration. A framework for understanding how a collaborative group develops the relationships and interaction patterns for working on a common public health goal is Tuckman's stages of normative group development (Figure 5.1): forming, storming, norming, and performing (Tuckman, 1965). In the *forming* phase, group members work to understand one another. They need to determine their boundaries and focus; group leaders emerge during the forming phase. Most groups will move through a *storming* phase in which conflict emerges; some resistance to following group direction forms and some "testing of the waters" and concern might occur about whether the focus and direction of the group is the right way to do things. Conflict management skills can be helpful in the storming phase to identify participant interests and positions, create new options through brainstorming, and negotiate a plan for moving forward (Bazarman, 2005). When the group reaches the *norming* stage, trust among membership develops. They identify themselves as a group and become cohesive in choosing the goal of the collaboration. Finally, in the *performing* stage, the group focuses on accomplishing specific tasks. The group has established rules for working together, formal or informal, but the rules are flexible rather than rigid. Group rules serve to help the group function and accomplish the public health goal. Whereas a dysfunctional group saps energy, a healthy functioning group creates energy that moves the group toward goal accomplishment.

Forming $\longrightarrow$ Storming $\longrightarrow$ Norming $\longrightarrow$ Performing

Figure 5.1 Normative group development

The first planning meeting Jake attended had 32 people present (including the pastor, assistant pas-

tor, a police liaison, two social workers, four nurses from various clinical backgrounds, two alternative healers, two chiropractors, two community members, two people from the churches board of directors, a director from a local clinic, a block nurse coordinator, three persons who are homeless, two faculty from the University Jake is attending, two staff from the surrounding homeless shelters, an insurance representative, a local physician, a musician, and two other nursing students along with Jake). It took most of the first meeting to introduce everyone and for each person to share what they felt the vision of the wellness clinic would be.

Jake was shocked to realize that for such a large group to come to a consensus about a vision about six meetings would be needed. He realized the group members needed time to talk so that they could determine their goals and how they were going to work together. During the initial meeting the police liaison, who was also a social worker and a member of the church, emerged as the natural leader of the project. His skills and experiences had prepared him for a leadership role. He also had experience working with the homeless population in the neighborhood. After the meeting Jake asked his preceptor, Linda, several questions. He wondered how a group of people who has such a variety of backgrounds and experiences could create one plan. What would the group do if everyone had different ideas about how to develop the clinic? What were the services the clinic needed to provide to meet the needs of the homeless population?

As the meetings progressed, some community members dropped out of the group, feeling frustrated, as they perceived their ideas were not being considered. As Jake continued to be a part of the planning team, he realized that conflict management skills and leadership skills were essential to work with such a large group. Jake marveled at the ability of the police liaison to calm the waters and keep refocusing back on the vision of the group to serve the homeless population through this community outreach project. Decision making involved negotiation and compromise among the group members.

New members came one meeting and were gone the next. This meant that at each meeting new members needed to be introduced and time was needed for explanations of vision and a review the group's planning phase. After about ten meetings, a core group of community members were identified through their commitment and attendance at meetings. Jake observed that the group came to a consensus about the vision and purpose of the project and that the members began to trust and understand their roles in the group.

Each group member was focused on the delivery of services to assist the homeless. Each member brought unique gifts and contributions to the table. Jake was excited to be a part of this collaborative endeavor. He was assigned a task to develop a flyer that would promote and advertise the wellness clinic that would be opening on Wednesday evenings.

 ACTIVITY

Identify the forming, storming, norming, and performing stages in the preceding scenario.

Develops Relationships and Builds Partnership with Communities, Systems, Individuals, and Families

Effective Collaboration and development of partnership requires equality among the partners (Kenny, 2002). Equality in collaborative relationships is promoted through listening, being respectful, appreciating differences, and developing trust. To encourage effective collaborative relationships with communities, professionals need to give up control, set aside the "rightness" of their view of health care, and trust the process of community participation (Clatworthy, 1999; Lindsey, Sheilds, & Stajduhar, 1999). Collaborative relationships work best if they are nonhierarchical in nature. Power to influence the collaboration is based on knowledge or expertise rather than on role or function (Henneman, Lee, & Cohen, 1995).

Community-Campus Partnerships for Health has developed key partnership principles that provide an excellent guide for establishing and maintaining partnerships with communities (Seifer & Connors, 2007). See the following list for the CCPH Principles of Partnership. In addition to being characterized by respect for all involved, partnerships for promoting the health of the public are undergirded by distributive justice (assuring equality and fairness) and beneficence (ensuring good outcomes) in their interactions (Kang, 1995). Foss, Bonaiuto, Johnson, and Moreland (2003) suggested that ineffective relationships result from power inequities. To reduce power inequities, you need to pay attention to how the partnership is structured, who controls resources, and time commitments.

1. Partnerships form to serve a specific purpose and may take on new goals over time.

2. Partners have agreed upon mission, values, goals, measurable outcomes, and accountability for the partnership.

3. The relationship between partners is characterized by mutual trust, respect, genuineness, and commitment.

4. The partnership builds upon identified strengths and assets, but also works to address needs and increase capacity of all partners.

5. The partnership balances power among partners and enables resources among partners to be shared.

6. Partners make clear and open communication an ongoing priority by striving to understand each other's needs and self-interests and developing a common language.

7. Principles and processes for the partnership are established with the input and agreement of all partners, especially for decision making and conflict resolution.

8. There is feedback among all stakeholders in the partnership, with the goal of continuously improving the partnership and its outcomes.

9. Partners share the benefits of the partnership's accomplishments.

10. Partnerships can dissolve and need to plan a process for closure.

Source: Seifer & Connors, 2007, p. 12

Jake realized that the tone of the meetings had changed to a collaborative relationship of listening to each other, respecting differences, and valuing each other's input in the process—all representative of an effective partnership. The members who were homeless were key partners and helpful in identifying needs and offering suggestions for delivery of services. Jake felt the strength of the bond of the collaborative partnership team in a shared vision. Jake observed that the team members were sharing resources and ideas with the group and striving for positive outcomes for the wellness clinic.

When Jake's preceptor, Linda, asked him what characteristics and skills that he thought were needed for partnerships to be effective in planning such a challenging project, he answered that being committed, tactful, and persistent was important. He commented that it was really hard when people dropped out of the planning group in the early stage. However, the people who stayed with the project were committed and persistent. Jake also told Linda he thought it was very important to have people in the group who had some influence in the community.

Utilizes Community Assets to Empower Communities, Systems, Individuals, and Families

PHNs identify assets that exist within a community. In addition, they strengthen community assets through collaborating with others to build social capital (community resources). To increase inclusion of community assets when planning interventions, PHNs can use specific strategies such as neighborhood mapping and community-based participatory research.

Focus on Community Assets

To be effective collaborators, PHNs must recognize and emphasize community assets in planning interventions to promote public health. Community groups and organizations, such as churches, social service agencies, and neighborhoods, can identify assets within the community that provide building blocks for public health initiatives. Partnerships with social organizations, such as a neighborhood community center, can build community capacity to achieve public health core functions: assessment, policy development, and assurance (Kang, 1995). See Table 5.1 for an example of how using community assets can contribute to efforts to reduce youth violence. An intervention that builds on a foundation of community assets is sometimes referred to as a strengths-based intervention, which means an intervention is selected and/or enhanced because it is already a resource or strength that exists within the community.

Table 5.1   Building Community Capacity for Responding to Youth Violence

Core Function	Community Asset	PHN Action
Capacity for Assessment	Parents, schools, police department can provide data about youth violence in the community	Recruit key community members to form an advisory group, which can help interpret assessment findings

Core Function	Community Asset	PHN Action
Capacity for Policy Development	Community advisory committee has knowledge of key resources and possible solutions for creating effective programs and policies to reduce youth violence	Collaborate with others on advisory committee to identify recommendations for an evidence-based policy and/or program to reduce youth violence; communicate advisory group recommendations to decision makers (might be governmental or non-profit organizations)
Capacity for Assurance	Lay helpers and persons from the community can effectively deliver health messages; organizations such as churches, schools, and neighborhood centers can provide resources for supporting a policy or developing a program	Provide tools and evidence-based strategy ideas for community members who select the strategy that best meets the needs and characteristics of both the community environment and the population targeted for the program or policy change

Source: Kang, 1995

Social Capital

By emphasizing community assets, PHNs are working with other professionals, community members, and organizations to strengthen the social capital that is available to community members. Why is social capital important? Research shows that social capital (resources that promote a sense of belonging) contributes to health by serving as a protective factor against chronic illness; social capital is also associated with better access to health care (Ahern & Hendryx, 2005; Hendryx, Ahern, Lourich, & McCurdy, 2002). People mobilize their existing resources to achieve their goals, including health goals. "Connected communities are more likely to support an environment that makes it easy for people to engage in health-promoting behaviors" (Looman & Lindeke, 2005, p. 91). Socially connecting organizations such as churches, schools, and neighborhood groups encourages the interactions of group members both within the organizations and within the larger community. When illness, injury, or crisis occurs for individuals and families that are socially connected, these social connections in the community help them to cope with the stressors of life challenges. In addition, the available social support can reduce the health disparities that result from ongoing strain associated with poverty, discrimination, and other health-damaging societal conditions such as environments with heavy industry and high crime rates (Aronson, Wallis, O'Campo, & Schafer, 2007; Berger & Neuhaus, 1977; Kang, 1995).

Tools for Strengthening Communities

Neighborhood mapping: A technological tool PHNs can use when collaborating with communities to identify assets and needs within a defined geographic community is neighborhood mapping, which uses geographic information system (GIS) software (Aronson et al., 2007; Burtman, 2010). As a tool, neighborhood mapping serves to identify and locate physical characteristics of the community. PHNs can use the knowledge gained from neighborhood mapping to *advocate* for increased services for populations at risk.

Evidence Example for Neighborhood Mapping: Infant Mortality Prevention

Neighborhood mapping was used to evaluate the effectiveness of an infant mortality prevention program called Healthy Start. Baltimore City community residents were paid to collect data, which was combined with census data for the Healthy Start target areas by using a GIS software program. Data from walkthroughs done by the community residents included the condition of each block and addresses of vacant or boarded up buildings, businesses, healthcare providers, schools, and parks and recreational centers. They also collected data on where people gathered together such as liquor stores or in parks. Healthy Start program data included program participation and pregnancy outcomes. Program staff gained information that could improve recruitment of community members and suggest where to focus resources.

Source: Aronson et al., 2007

Community-based participatory research: PHNs can make the best use of community resources by selecting evidence-based public health interventions. Community-based participatory research (CBPR) is a research strategy in which PHNs can partner with community members and organizations to investigate interventions that will be most effective with at-risk population groups. CBPR requires establishing a trusting relationship with community partners and engaging in collaboration between researchers and community members as equals (Israel, Eng, Schulz, & Parker, 2005; Savage et al., 2006; Schaffer, 2009). The expertise of community members enriches and adds authenticity to research findings. CBPR methods help to overcome some of the challenges of conducting research with at-risk populations and are more likely to result in meaningful data that lead to effective strategies for improving health status in the community. See the following list for Principles of the Community-Based Participatory Research Model. PHNs can use this model to build evidence for their practice in communities.

1. A community is a unit of identity that is reinforced through social interactions and characterized by shared values and norms and mutual influences.

2. Activities should build on community resources and relationships.

3. Programs should establish equal partnerships in all phases of research.

4. Programs should promote co-learning that facilitates reciprocal transfer of knowledge, skills, and capacity.

5. Activities should achieve balance between research and action.

6. Research programs should address locally relevant health problems and consider the multiple determinants of health and disease.

7. Program development should occur through a cyclical and iterative process that includes ongoing assessments of successes and obstacles.

8. Knowledge gained from community research should be actively disseminated to all partners in language that is understandable and respectful.

9. Community-based research involves a long-term commitment.

Source: Institute for Clinical and Translational Science, 2009

Evidence Example for Community-Based Participatory Research (CBPR): Maternal and Infant Health

CBPR was the approach used to conduct a study to learn ways to improve maternal and infant health in an African-American community. The nurse researchers, a parish nurse, an African-American nurse, and community stakeholders interested in infant health came together with community residents to collaboratively complete their research plan and develop recruitment strategies. Community partners provided essential information about the neighborhoods and enhanced the interpretation of the data in ways that would not have been known by the researchers if they had worked independently. For example, a participant complained about "black bars" in the neighborhood; the community partners provided the explanation that black bars were actually black wrought iron fences that were placed in between buildings to provide a barrier to criminal activity.

Source: Savage et al., 2006

Following are examples of research initiatives and partnerships that have used an asset-based approach for identifying interventions to improve health in a targeted population. These initiatives have used strategies at individual, community, and systems levels.

*   **Asset-Based Approach to Promoting Healthy Eating Behaviors.** Gayle Timmerman (2007) explored barriers experienced by women who are underserved and attempted to adopt healthy eating behaviors. Collaboration occurred by involving women who are underserved in focus groups to understand women's experience with ways to improve nutrition. Key aspects of the collaboration included establishing a personal connection with the women, emphasizing respect, facilitating reciprocity, and providing feedback (Crist & Escandon-Dominguez, 2003). Timmerman explained that using an asset-based approach (as opposed to the traditional needs-based approach) led to identifying community resources that could help sustain change in behavior. Additional important components were having a shared vision and purpose for recommended changes in health strategies and employing workers from the community. The African-American participants in the focus groups suggested that churches should be a central place for health promotion activities because churches were viewed as trustworthy and convenient for participants (*individual and community levels*). Possible partners for nutrition interventions include local grocery stores, restaurants, schools, farmer's markets, food shelves, and public transportation to increase access to nutritious affordable food (*community and systems levels)* (Timmerman, 2007).

- **Partnership to Decrease Childhood Obesity.** An initiative to address childhood obesity used asset mapping to identify individual and community strengths in the targeted population, a public school district in upstate New York (Baker et al., 2007). The goal was to reduce television viewing time. Partners in the initiative included child care staff, school and college staff and faculty, primary health care staff, local businesses, social and faith-based organizations, the local library, and students from all educational levels. Partners networked to involve others in the community; community groups offered 40 different after-school and weekend activities in 11 public locations for preschool children and their families in a sponsored "TV Turn-off week." Community groups collaborated on a variety of family activities: sports, lessons, music, dancing, and arts and crafts. Outcomes based on feedback from questionnaires and partner debriefing sessions indicated more parents enrolled their children in programs that encouraged physical activity (*individual level*), the library continued to offer storytelling (*community level*), and childcare providers changed their policies for viewing media (*systems level*).

- **Building Community Assets to Reduce Health Disparities.** A community-based participatory research intervention was used to address health disparities in African American and Latino populations in Portland, Oregon by identifying and building community assets (Michael, Farquhar, Wiggins, & Green, 2008). Community health workers, selected from partner communities, connected with community members and organizations to identify health initiative priorities. The projects were unique, designed to meet the interests of the group, and empowered participants through increasing their involvement and leadership. Among the projects were a public safety committee, a diabetes support and education group, a homework club, a dance class, a chronic pain support group, and a peace campaign (*individual and community levels*). Evaluation of the interventions included a social capital survey and in-depth interviews. Following the interventions, more participants indicated they had a greater number of people who could provide them with social support; they self-rated their physical health at a higher level; and they reported decreases in depression, loneliness, feeling that everything was an effort, and viewing others as unfriendly. Churches were instrumental in providing structure and space for group activities, a social capital resource. Data from the in-depth interviews suggested social capital resources contribute to improving health such as access to food, assistance with employment, addressing addictive behaviors, and participation in a neighborhood cleanup (*individual, community, and systems levels*).

Jake realized the importance of knowing community assets and working with other professionals. The pastor knew the neighborhood and community well and had space and people resources for serving the meal on Wednesday evenings to the homeless. The social worker had experience with chemical dependency patients and the skills needed to address the homeless who had drug abuse issues or concerns. Another nurse was a mental health specialist who knew about useful resources for referring people who were homeless. The police liaison knew many people who were homeless and was very well respected in the community. The insurance representative could help find resources to increase access to health care by identifying funding options and programs. The PHN knew about social service resources and possible sources of funding for health care. Even Jake, as a student nurse, brought his gifts of delivery of care by doing blood pressure screenings, health teaching, and foot care at the wellness clinic. The programs planned at the wellness clinic were services the collaborative community members could offer or find others to come in and provide those services.

Jake was present the first night the wellness clinic opened. As he sat down to share a meal with some of the individuals that attended the wellness clinic, he realized the value in the statement, "It takes a community to take care of its own." The strengths of each of the collaborative partners were needed for development of the wellness clinic.

Ethical Application

When public health nurses collaborate with other professionals, community members, and community organizations, ethical concerns often center on selecting interventions that promote social justice for vulnerable populations that have fewer resources for improving their health. However, as PHNs work to promote a healthier life for community members, they must also consider how community members are going to view and experience the interventions they develop. In addition, collaboration often involves courage to work with others who have different views and persistence to keep working together even when disagreement and tension about the right way to proceed exist. All voices need to be heard in decision making. In collaboration, an emphasis on community assets leads to inclusion, diversity, empowerment, and advocacy. See Table 5.2 for application of ethical perspectives to collaboration.

Table 5.2   Ethical Action in Collaboration

Ethical Perspective	Application
Rule Ethics (principles)	• The goal is beneficence or promoting good (improvement in health status) for the community and community members. • Encourage autonomy of community members by ensuring that their perspective contributes input in determining interventions to improve health.
Virtue Ethics (character)	• Be courageous in working with those with different views and perspectives. • Be persistent in working through disagreement and tension in collaboration with others.
Feminist Ethics (reducing oppression)	• Encourage inclusion of the voices of all stakeholders in the collaboration. • Respect everyone. • Strive for equality in provision of programs and services. • Emphasize community strengths. • Advocate for individuals and community groups who have less power.

When Jake first started the community health course, he felt that, though important, the delivery of services to persons who were homeless was someone else's concern, not his. He also wondered why individuals who were homeless were included in the planning group. In the early meetings he observed that the group members who represented the homeless population were very quiet, so many other members of the group were talking about what homeless people wanted. In the third meeting, the police liaison who had emerged as the group's leader asked the members who represented the homeless population to offer their opinions on some of the ideas that had been expressed. He explained that they were "experts" on what it meant to be homeless and they would have good ideas about what services and resources would help meet their health needs. The police liaison also did not back away from conflict but continued to emphasize the common goal of the group.

After being a part of the project, and actually spending time with individuals who were homeless, Jake now understood why it was important to include persons who have experienced homelessness in planning the clinic. The planning group empowered the group members who were homeless to participate as equal partners and take a leadership role in creating solutions.

As Jake provided foot care for a middle-aged man one evening, the man shared his story of how he worked for a big company, lost his job as the company downsized, coped by drinking, then lost his house and his family, and finally lost his sense of self-respect. As Jake reflected on this story, he noted that each of us could find ourselves in a similar situation. Through collaboration, Jake realized that a community can use its strengths and resources to make a difference.

Key Points

- Public health nurses collaborate with many partners: other nurses, health professionals, lay workers, community members, health care and community organizations, businesses, and government organizations.

- Effective partnerships share a common goal and require respect for and equality of partners.

- Partnership development requires trust between partners and a commitment to spend the time needed to develop that trust.

- Collaborative partnerships for promoting the health of the public should integrate community assets that develop intervention strategies, which contribute to social capital; design interventions that will be accepted by community members; and garner the buy-in and contributions of community organizations.

- Tools for using community assets and building social capital are neighborhood mapping and community-based participatory research.

Exercises

Learning Examples for Effective Collaboration Strategies

You can find abundant examples in the literature of learning opportunities for collaborating with others to improve population health. The following illustrates a few examples that involve collaborating with other nurses, professionals, community members, or organizations. As you read through these examples, think about your community and how you could collaborate with other health professionals, people, and organizations to improve the health of the population.

Health Fair (Aponte & Nickitas, 2007)

- Offered health fair in a medical center for meeting needs of underserved community.

- Nursing students worked with faculty to offer educational sessions on nutrition, hand washing, medication review, and glucometer use.

- Partners included the American Heart Association and American Diabetes Association for educational materials, local hospitals and nonprofit organizations, a fitness center, and community sponsors such as a supermarket.

Asset Mapping (Williams-Barnard, Sweatt, Harkness, & DiNapoli, 2004)

- Used to identify formal and informal health and social services and community gathering areas as potential learning sites for students.

- Nursing students and faculty identified children and families who could benefit from nursing interventions not available from traditional health services because of economic constraints.

- Nursing students collaborated with several organizations—provided a health promotion fair for one school each semester, expanded tobacco prevention activities to schools and communities, and partnered with community mental health nurses to assess mental status of homeless individuals.

Prevention of Childhood Obesity (Brosnan et al., 2005)

- In conjunction with staff at a school district, nursing students conducted a literature review, participated in a screening program, and presented health education topics in schools.

Services for Teen Mothers (Foss, Bonaiuto, Johnson, & Moreland, 2003).

- Collaborated with a county health department and public school system to restore health care resources to support teen mothers in school.

- Nursing students partnered with teachers, counselors, social worker, and nursing staff at an alternative school to provide teen moms with health education, health counseling, parenting education, and referral services to community agencies.

Collaboration in School District (Kreulen, Bednarz, Wehrwein, & Davis, 2008)

- Nursing students were assigned to a classroom, grade level, or specific school population

- They completed projects in oral health screening and education with a refugee population, nutrition and first aid education, teacher training on emergency preparedness, and childhood safety for preschool projects.

Reflective Practice

Developing a clinic for the homeless is a complex project that involves many stakeholders and community organizations. Before partners begin to collaborate, reflecting on the goals of the collaborative project is essential. When partners are gathered together, they need to reach consensus on a shared goal. Now that you have learned about collaboration and the knowledge and skills needed to collaborate effectively, consider the following questions.

What does Jake need to consider about effective partnerships before collaborating on developing a clinic for the homeless?

_____

_____

What information about the population and community organizations will be needed for planning? What is an effective way to gather the information?

_____

_____

What would be important to include on the agenda for the first planning meeting?

_____

_____

What additional questions will you need to ask to partner effectively to develop a clinic for the homeless population?

_____

_____

After you have worked through these questions, develop an outline of possible partners, relevant Public Health Intervention Wheel interventions that will be part of the planning process, and level of practice. Consider the following questions for guiding implementation of the plan. You can find additional "Think, Explore, Do" questions at the end of the chapter.

Application of Evidence

1. What responses would you expect from the planning group based on Tuckman's phases of group development?

2. Which of the CCPH principles of partnership do you think are most applicable to the scenario of developing a clinic for the homeless?

3. How does your plan build capacity for core functions of public health: assessment, policy development, and assurance?

4. In what ways could you build in the following strategies for utilizing community assets and building social capital: neighborhood mapping and community-based participatory research?

Think, Explore, Do

1. What previous experiences have you had with Collaboration or working in a partnership to promote health (student work groups or task forces)? What do you think went well and what did not go well? What factors contributed to the success of the partnership?

2. How have you been included or excluded as a collaborator in contributing to improving your own health?

3. What responses from others help you to feel respected and included?

4. What are the assets in the community that you live in that you think promote population health?

5. What organizations in the community or state could provide additional resources to promote the health for the homeless population in the scenario?

6. What actions do you think are essential for developing an effective partnership?

7. What can you do to promote equality when power differences exist among partners?

8. What can you do to promote buy-in to the partnership among community members and organizations?

COMPETENCY #4:
Works Within the Responsibility and Authority of the Governmental Public Health System

By Marjorie A. Schaffer
with Bonnie Brueshoff

Dan was recently employed as a public health nurse by a county health department. After 2 months on the job, he was asked to staff a clinic to respond to the vaccination needs for the H1N1 flu virus. The county health department had received a limited supply of vaccine. The state health department directed that the vaccine first be given to children age 9 and below. To reach a large number of children and maximize available staff, the public health director (acting as incident commander) made the decision to offer two mass clinics at health department sites.

Dan had never worked for the government. Through the orientation process he began to wonder if he would ever understand how the different levels of government worked together. He referred to his orientation materials for population-based public health nursing competency #4, which focuses on working with governmental systems. He commented to his supervisor, Carol, "This competency has so many parts. How will I ever understand what all these terms mean for the work I am doing?"

DAN'S NOTEBOOK

Competency #4: Works within the responsibility and authority of the governmental public health system.

- Describes the relationship among the federal, state, and local levels of the public health system

- Identifies the individual's and organization's responsibilities within the context of the essential services of public health and core functions

- Recognizes that public health has statutory authority such as public health nuisance, quarantine, and commitment

- Differentiates the public health model from the medical model

- Understands the independent public health nursing role as described in *Public Health Nursing: Scope and Standards of Practice*

- Describes the role of government in the delivery of community health services

- Is aware of components of the health care system

- Funding streams

- Programs of local health departments

- Community resources

- Understands legal issues such as data privacy and mandated reporting

Useful Definitions

Local Public Health Department: An "administrative or service unit of local or state government concerned with health, and carrying some responsibility for the health of a jurisdiction smaller than the state" (NACCHO, 2008a).

Statutory Authority: A "specific set of rules or a statute that gives an agency general authority to adopt rules to carry out its assigned duties" (Minnesota Rulemaking Manual, 2009).

Funding Stream: Source of revenue for public health programs and services.

Medical Model: Focuses on the individual; concerned with restoring health for individuals who seek care.

Public Health Model: Focuses on the health of populations; concerned with promoting, protecting, and maintaining the health of every citizen.

Taking Responsibility for Improving Population Health

You can find public health nurses (PHNs) working in all levels of government; in urban, suburban, and rural settings; and in a variety of community agencies and organizations. Federal, state, and local governments all provide essential resources for contributing to the health of the public. In this chapter you will learn about how levels of government work together to promote public health and how PHNs work with the government to deliver public health services.

How Are the Federal, State, and Local Levels of Public Health Connected?

At the *federal* level, the U.S. Department of Health and Human Services (USDHHS) oversees many other agencies that focus on the health and well-being of U.S. citizens. One of these agencies is the Centers for Disease Control and Prevention (CDC). The CDC keeps track of disease outbreaks and health statistics and protects the health and quality of life for U.S. populations. The CDC website is a good source for statistics and other information you need for public health interventions (www.cdc.gov). For example, a public health nurse could use the CDC website to find updated statistics on state and national obesity trends and evidence-based strategies for obesity prevention.

Other examples of agencies that come under the USDHHS umbrella are those that oversee Medicare and Medicaid Services; research and health care quality; substance abuse and mental health services; and the safety of food, cosmetics, medications, biological products, and medical devices. For example, a public health nurse could access information on food safety alerts. Past examples include the contamination of ground beef (salmonella, typhimurium) and salad bars (norovirus).

State health departments often work with both the federal and local levels of government. State health departments regulate facilities and organizations that impact health as well as health professionals, including nurses. State functions include financing and administration of programs (Stanhope & Lancaster, 2008) and also offer technical assistance to local health departments for program development and services (Minnesota Department of Health, 2009a). The organization and functions of state health care departments can differ greatly among the states. Regardless of the organizational structure, a strong partnership between the state and local health departments is essential. For example, the local public health departments in Minnesota use the Community Assessment and Action Planning process that was jointly developed by state and local health departments to assess and prioritize the health needs of their communities (Minnesota Department of Health, 2009b).

Local health departments offer specific programs and services. Some examples of local health department responsibilities and activities are as follows:

- Provide vaccinations to fill gaps for underserved populations

- Provide directly observed therapy for tuberculosis

- Investigate public health nuisances (for example, garbage accumulation, rodent infestation)

- Promote healthy communities by addressing injury prevention, child growth and development, nutrition, and by preventing unintended pregnancy

- Improve emergency response capability

- Help to implement Freedom to Breathe Act—smoke-free workplace requirements (Minnesota Department of Health, 2009a)

Local public health departments display considerable variability in the populations they serve and how they accomplish their work. A 2008 study identified the following characteristics of local health departments (NACCHO, 2008a):

- Population size of communities served varied from less than 1,000 to more than 9 million.

- Annual budgets ranged from less than $10,000 to more than $1 billion.

- Jurisdiction types varied from county, to combined city-county, to local boards of health.

The study (NACCHO, 2008a) also revealed that nursing staff made up 21% of the workforce, and 57% of the departments had an emergency preparedness coordinator. In addition, study findings show that emergency preparedness has become an important responsibility of public health. The skills and expertise of public health nurses are valued and needed to effectively deliver public health services, including emergency preparedness. See Table 6.1 for an example of how the three levels of government worked together during the flu pandemic.

Table 6.1   Example: Three Levels of Government Working Together

2009–2010 H1N1 Flu Pandemic: Dakota County's Response

Background
On April 27, 2009, the CDC declared a public health emergency.
On June 11, 2009, the World Health Organization (WHO) determined there was adequate scientific evidence to declare the H1N1 virus as the first global pandemic of the 21st century. The Dakota County Public Health Department collaborated with the Minnesota Department of Health and other health agencies to implement the pandemic flu response plans that had been previously developed.

Governmental Actions
Federal—CDC ordered H1N1 vaccine from manufacturers and identified priority groups for vaccine (initially pregnant women and children).
State—Minnesota Health Department gave direction to local health departments.
Local—Dakota County Public Health Department coordinated plans with community organizations and worked with health clinics and providers in county to redistribute vaccine doses.

Dakota County Response
Opened a Department Operations Center (DOC) to monitor the situation, coordinate response efforts, and provide updates to community stakeholders (schools, clinics, hospitals, long-term care facilities, police, fire, and emergency response).
When manufacturing problems delayed vaccine delivery, the local health department identified priority risk groups as caregivers of infants, pregnant women, health care workers, and first responders.
Provided vaccinations at scheduled immunization clinics, H1N1 appointment and walk-in clinics, and four mass vaccination clinics.
Established a telephone and appointment system with recorded messages in English and Spanish to respond to surge of phone calls.
Expanded groups eligible to receive vaccine as vaccine supplies increased.

Outcomes
Dakota County Public Health Department distributed 12,494 doses of vaccine by March 31, 2010.
Minnesota ranked 8th in the nation for percentage of residents who had received the H1N1 vaccine.
Minnesota ranked 1st in the nation for vaccination of people aged 25–64 who have medical conditions placing them at a higher risk for H1N1 flu-related complications.

Source: 2009–2010 H1N1 Flu Pandemic: Dakota County's Response.

How Do the Essential Public Health Services and Core Functions Guide the Public Health Department and My Work as a Public Health Nurse?

You first learned about the essential public health services and core functions in Chapter 1. The following section shows how public health nurses accomplish the work that is outlined in the essential services and core functions and contributes to the well-being of populations. In a survey of 57 PHNs working in local and state governments and representing 28 states, nurses identified the amount of time they spent providing each of the essential services. The percentage of time spent on each essential service ranged from 7% to 14% (Keller & Litt, 2008). See Figure 6.1.

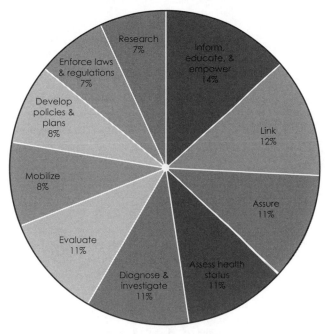

Figure 6.1   Percentage of PHNs' time dedicated to essential services (n=57)

Dan remembered seeing the Public Health Core Functions in his orientation manual—assessment, policy development, and assurance. He said to Carol, "Let's see if I understand how this works. For the H1N1 flu clinic, I can see assessment happening when we are identifying how many children in the targeted age group live in our county. For policy development, we are following the directives given by CDC and the state department of health for vaccine administration. I can see how we are working with and through others to make sure as many children as possible have access to the vaccine. Assurance happens when we make sure the vaccine is accessible to the population groups that need to be vaccinated and that the vaccine has been administered to them. Our health department redirected vaccine supplies to many area medical clinics so they could provide vaccinations."

Carol affirmed Dan's analysis of how the core functions were represented in the vaccine availability and distributed by the health department. Dan then said, "I am not sure about all those essential services. Do they all happen with our H1N1 response?"

Carol answered, "Let's analyze how each of the essential services happen when our health department responds to the H1N1 pandemic. Let's develop a handout to put into the orientation manual to help everyone understand how we are providing the essential services." See Table 6.2 for the handout developed by Dan and Carol.

Table 6.2   Essential Services in H1N1 Flu Clinic

Essential Service	Application Example
1. Monitor Health	Monitored county-specific data on school closures, hospitalization, and fatalities.
2. Diagnose and Investigate	Communicated with school nurses about H1N1 flu symptoms and reporting requirements.
3. Inform, Educate, and Empower	Worked with local media outlets to advertise H1N1 flu clinics and communicated educational information about protective measures such as hand hygiene and "cover your cough."
4. Mobilize Community Partnerships	Worked with Medical Reserve Corps volunteers to assist in mass clinics.
5. Develop Policies	Adopted policies from CDC and state department of health on priority setting of who should first receive the vaccine.
6. Enforce Laws	Activated Emergency Response Plan following the CDC declaration of a public health emergency.
7. Link to/Provide Care	Referred population to state flu telephone line to be assessed for influenza-like symptoms; local health department engaged local pharmacies to participate as dispensing sites for anti-viral medications.
8. Assure Competent Workforce	Provided training for staff prior to and day of mass clinics to ensure competence for roles and responsibilities.
9. Evaluate	Held "hotwash" after each clinic (people in command positions identified what worked well and what needed improvement); completed formal "after action report" (AAR).
10. System Management & Research	CDC provided information about system effectiveness in reaching population for administration of H1N1 flu vaccine.

How Do Public Health Nurses Use Statutory Authority?

Statutory authority refers to the rules or statutes (laws) through which government gives authority to agencies to carry out specific duties. In the public health arena, PHNs are responsible for following public health laws that have been enacted to protect and promote the health of communities (NACCHO, 2010). Public health laws might be federal, state, or local. Many public health laws are carried out at the local level. Examples of laws concerned with public health include public health nuisance; quarantine; mandated reporting of communicable disease; mandated reporting of suspected abuse and neglect of children, disabled, and elderly; and commitment.

PHNs can collaborate with environmental health staff to investigate *public health nuisances*, which are conditions that threaten the health of the public, including garbage accumulation, sewage, noise, junked cars, abandoned swimming pools, rodent infestation, and faulty electrical wiring or plumbing (Minnesota Department of Health State Community Health Services Advisory Committee, 1992). The top three complaints for public health nuisances investigated by local health departments in Minnesota in 2007 were garbage houses, mold, and improper sewage disposal (Minnesota Department of Health, 2009a). In some communities, vacant properties might also be a public health concern. Think about how each of these community concerns impacts the health of populations in the community.

Quarantine laws provide for isolating individuals and/or groups to prevent the spread of communicable disease. A quarantine is a "restriction, during a period of communicability, of activities or travel of an otherwise healthy person who likely has been exposed to a communicable disease to prevent disease transmission during the period of communicability in the event the person is infected" (Minnesota Statutes, 2005, Section 144.419). Historically, quarantining people with communicable disease was an important intervention when vaccines did not exist. Quarantine laws are in place as a measure to reduce the effects of bioterrorism or pandemic events such as the spread of avian influenza (Minnesota Department of Health, 2005a).

States have laws that mandate reporting of communicable diseases so that surveillance of the occurrence of the disease can be monitored. Minnesota law provides a ruling that lists each of the communicable diseases that must be reported (Minnesota Department of Health, 2005b). During the H1N1 epidemic during the fall of 2009, surveillance of incidence of H1N1 cases was important for determining the number of flu clinics that needed to be offered and provided data for determining whether schools needed to be closed.

PHNs might need to use the law on *civil commitment* when working with vulnerable individuals who are mentally ill. Commitment is the process of obtaining a court order "to treat persons with mental illnesses when they are unable or unwilling to seek treatment voluntarily and/or to protect the person with mental illness and others from harm due to the illness" (National Alliance on Mental Illness, 2006, p. 2). The purpose of the law is to protect mentally ill individuals from danger to themselves or others. PHNs collaborate with family members, other health professionals, community agencies, and the government in the civil commitment process.

What Is the Difference Between the Public Health Model and the Medical Model?

As you think about how government organizations guide and deliver public health services and the responsibilities of the government and public health nurses for improving the health status of individuals and populations, consider how public health nurses use a public health model in contrast to a medical model. One difference is that the public health model focuses on populations, whereas the medical model focuses on individuals. Another difference is the public health focus on prevention of disease as opposed to the medical model focus on treatment of disease. In the public health model, health care is viewed as a right, whereas the in the medical model, health care is a service. Public health nurses can use the public health model (see Table 6.3) to help frame their practice as prevention-oriented and population-based. You must consider how the public health model is different from a traditional medical model when planning interventions to improve health status among populations to ensure that interventions are consistent with the mission of public health.

Table 6.3 Differences Between the Public Health and Medical Models

Public Health Model	Medical Model
Mission is to promote, protect, and maintain the health of every citizen.	Mission is to restore health to those who seek care (i.e., treatment and cure).
Focuses on the primary health needs of communities and populations.	Focuses on the primary health needs of individuals.
Health is seen as a birthright of every citizen.	Health care is seen as a service to be sought.
Goal is client/family, population self-sufficiency.	Goal is providing quality service to meet immediate medical care needs.
Focus is on prevention.	Focus is on treatment.
Seeks to protect the public's health before problems arise.	Seeks to meet the needs of patients who present for care of an existing problem.
Reaches out to identify individuals, families, and populations with service needs (case-finding).	Addresses the needs of patients who present for care.
Focus is on populations, the community, and the family.	Focus is on the individual.
Provides services that others cannot or will not provide.	Generally provide services that are reimbursable.
Seeks social change to improve the health status of populations.	Seeks change to improve status of an individual.
Provides services primarily in community settings.	Provides services primarily in health care facilities.

Public Health Model	Medical Model
Provides services in the home that are holistic in nature; might provide services for medically necessary needs or refer those individuals with medically necessary needs to a home care agency.	Provides home care services for medically necessary needs related to disease and disability.

Some services might be provided in both public health and medical settings, but the approach to health care differs. For example, home health care and childhood screening are offered in both settings. In home visits to an elderly client, the PHN focuses on the holistic needs of the elder, the home environment, family support environment, and available community resources. The PHN considers how the community provides resources for supporting the population of community-dwelling elders. If an elder receives a home visit from a nurse from an agency that follows the medical model, the focus might be limited to the elder's physical care needs related to illness or disease. The home care agency is reimbursed only for disease-related necessary treatment because it is reimbursed by private insurance, Medicare, or Medicaid. The public health agency, visiting nurses association, or non-profit home care agency might provide additional health promotion and disease prevention services because their diverse funding provides coverage for services other than medically related care.

In another example, childhood screening is provided in public health programs to improve the well-being of the population of children in the community. From the perspective of the medical model, the child is screened on routine visits in a clinic to evaluate the child's health status.

Evidence Example: Public Health vs. Medical Model: Childhood Obesity Prevention

Marlene Schwartz and Kelly Brownell (2007) contrasted the public health and medical models in their analysis of childhood obesity prevention. The medical model frames childhood obesity as a physical problem for an individual child. The response to the problem is treatment of the individual, using clinical services. The treatment usually involves a cognitive-behavioral intervention that focuses on behavioral change and personal responsibility. From the public health perspective, childhood obesity is a disease that affects a population, resulting from individual vulnerability and environmental factors. The environment is viewed as a major driver of prevention. Interventions are targeted toward changing environmental factors, such as policymaking that creates guidelines for nutritious day care and school lunches and snacks to contribute to the reduction of childhood obesity.

For the preceding evidence example, consider how a public health nurse could provide interventions that are consistent with the public health model. At the community level a school nurse could consult with school administration and teachers on the implications of policies and guidelines for nutrition for school children. The action of consultation in this situation is focused on the health of the school population and promotes health through nutrition guidelines. The school nurse could use social marketing to communicate the benefits of healthy eating. Social marketing about healthy eating is intended to influence social change in food consumption to improve the health of the school population and the community. At the individual level the school nurse could provide health teaching to groups of school children on fun ways to eat healthy, which is consistent with the goal of protecting the public's health before problems develop. In the public health model, the focus of the school nurse is on providing interventions to populations at the individual, community, and systems levels. A public health approach often involves a greater number of interventions in a holistic and environmental approach to promoting well-being.

After the flurry of the response to the flu pandemic had subsided, Dan reflected on how his work differed from his previous position as a nurse for a pediatric clinic. Dan commented to his supervisor, Carol, "I never realized how the government is responsible for public health. I now think about people who need the flu vaccine not as individuals, but as populations. We prioritized which populations should receive the vaccine first—those who had the greatest need for protection from complications of influenza. We also made sure that the vaccine was available to everyone, whether or not they could pay for the vaccine. In the clinic we followed a medical model that approached clients as individuals."

Carol added, "Yes, the public health model is oriented to finding people that need health services, rather than always waiting for persons to identify the need. In addition, public health is oriented toward changing health and social systems to create environments that encourage improvement in health status. By reaching out to those populations most in need of the flu vaccination, we have actually created an environment that will help keep people healthy in the communities served by our agency."

How Do the Scope and Standards of Public Health Nursing Guide the Public Health Nurse in Independent Practice?

The American Nurses Association published an updated version of *Public Health Nursing: Scope and Standards of Practice* in 2007. This publication explains the professional role expectations for public health nurses. It has two sections—standards of practice and standards of professional performance. The standards of practice detail how the nursing process is applied in public health nursing (see Table 1.2 in Chapter 1). The standards of professional performance address professional role expectations: quality of practice, education, professional practice evaluation, collegiality and professional relationships, collaboration, ethics, research, resource utilization, leadership, and advocacy. Review Table 6.4, which analyzes how each of these role expectations took place in the implementation of an H1N1 flu clinic.

Table 6.4 Standards of Professional Performance—Application to H1N1 Flu Clinic in Dakota County, Minnesota

Standard	Example
Quality of Practice	Contracted with Minnesota Visiting Nurse Agency to provide vaccinations, which received the *Mark of Excellence Award*, Minnesota Department of Health flu shot provider award.

Standard	Example
Education	Provided education on roles, responsibilities, and incident command structure for staff working in the H1N1 mass clinics.
Professional Practice Evaluation	Completed After Action/Improvement Plan that follows guidelines from the Homeland Security Exercise and Evaluation Program.
Collegiality and Professional Relationships	Discussed the formula to use for distribution of limited supply of vaccine within the region during the early phase of the pandemic.
Collaboration	Worked with another county to share utilization of Medical Reserve Corps for staffing clinics.
Ethics	Decided and adhered to prioritization plan for which groups received the vaccine first.
Research	Accessed information from CDC for vaccine safety and adverse reactions.
Resource Utilization	Worked with local city police department for security and assistance with traffic during mass clinics.
Leadership	Activated Department Operations Center to coordinate the response and work with local organizations.
Advocacy	Provided outreach throughout the county to promote and encourage vaccination and communicate flu clinic schedules.

How Is the Government Involved in the Delivery of Community Health Services?

All levels of government deliver community health services under the framework of core functions: assessment, policy development, and assurance. Consider how core functions apply health promotion for school children at the systems level. The core function of *assessment* involves determining the important health problems and what needs to be done in response to the health problem. Assessment took place when a local health department surveyed school nurses and other health staff about the health conditions of students, health interventions provided by nurses and health staff, and referrals made to other agencies. Next, health department staff in collaboration with schools participated in policy development by making a decision about what needed to be done. The school nurse district coordinator presented the assessment data to the school board, and the public health nurse advocated for district policy to require parents of children with asthma to complete an Asthma Action Plan. Assurance means either doing the activity or enacting policy effectively or making sure someone else carries it out effectively. Assurance took place when school staff audited health records to determine that 100% of students with asthma had an updated Asthma Action Plan. The government was involved in promoting the health of school children through all three core functions.

What Should the Public Health Nurse Know about the Health Care System?

Public health nurses need to have specialized skills and knowledge to effectively meet the expectations for their role, including knowing how public health is funded, having the skills necessary to function in specific public health programs, and understanding the referral process for connecting people with community resources. Funding of public health impacts the ability of state and local health departments to provide adequate public health services. In your work as a PHN you might be called on to contribute to planning and writing grant applications for funds for specific public health programs. In larger health departments, you might become more specialized with skills and knowledge for a specific public health program, such as follow-up of clients with tuberculosis or family planning clinics. In rural health departments, your skill set and knowledge have to be broader because you might work in a variety of programs and settings. Also, you would be expected to have knowledge about the many resources that are available to individuals, families, and communities and the referral process needed to receive services from those resources.

Funding Streams

Funding for local public health is from a mix of local, state, and federal funds and fees and reimbursements. For example, for the state of Minnesota, 2009 local public health funding sources included the local tax levy (33%); other locally generated funds (35%); federal funds, including Medicare and Medicaid (20%); state general funds (7%); other state funds (5%); and client and non-client fees (Minnesota Department of Health, 2009a). Because of the multiple sources of funding for public health, budgets for services are complex and vary each fiscal year. Funding sources are often focused on responding to current crises such as the federal funding that was made available for the H1N1 pandemic response. Public health funding is dependent on a flourishing economy; a downturn in the economy means that public health resources might be more limited.

Another example of funding streams is the provision of home visits to high-risk families, which involves a mix of public and private funding. A family home visiting program provided by a visiting nurse agency focuses on pregnant and parenting families and children with illness. The population lives in a large metropolitan area. Public health nurses staff the program at 7.7 FTEs (See Table 1.2 in Chapter 1). Funding sources for the home visits from PHNs include third-party reimbursement from Medicaid and insurance companies (55%), funds from the city local government (33%), special project funds (1%), and funds from United Way, which is a community resource (11%). For this program much of the reimbursement from insurance comes through state public programs that contract with the insurance company to deliver health care services for a specified population. Special projects focus on a specific service that is provided, such as one-time assessment of pregnant women. PHNs provide a specified number of visits to meet program costs that are reimbursed by the funding sources (Lanigan, 2010).

Programs of Local Public Health Departments

Although variation among programs provided by local public health departments exists, some public health services are more frequently provided, such as immunizations and surveillance and epidemiology for communicable/infectious disease. In addition, population-focused home visiting programs can be offered that target specific vulnerable or high-risk populations such as parenting adolescents, aimed to improve the health status of the population of adolescent parents and their children. Figure 6.2 shows the services and activities offered by local health departments. In 2005 the National Association of County and Health Officials (NACCHO) conducted the National Profile of Local Health Departments study, using a stratified random sample by population size, to develop a comprehensive description of local health infrastructure and practice. They had responses from 2300 local public health departments, a response rate of 80% (NACCHO, 2008a).

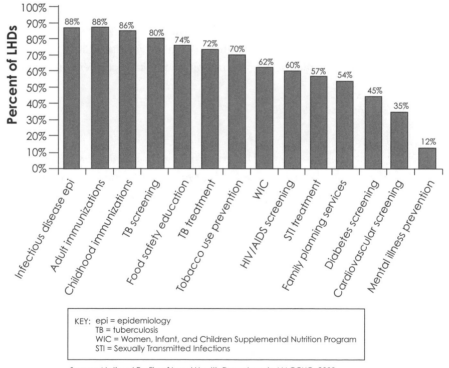

Source: National Profile of Local Health Departments, NACCHO, 2008

Figure 6.2 Evidence example: Activities of local health departments

Community Resources

Local health departments cannot carry out their mission without community partnerships and resources. PHNs build cooperative partnerships with community agencies, organizations, other professionals, and community groups to respond to community health concerns. Vital partners that assist in working on and achieving public health goals include many non-profit organizations. Non-profit organizations provide services that contribute to the well-being for persons, communities, or society and do not aim to make a profit. They might be funded by grants, donations, and sometimes receive funds from governmental organizations. For example, the Minnesota Visiting Nurse Agency was invaluable as a partner in providing the nurse staff capacity for mass clinics in response to the H1N1 pandemic. In many communities, the visiting nurse agency is a primary provider of community health services.

Evidence Example: American Lung Association Open Airways for Schools

For children with asthma, the American Lung Association is a non-profit organization that provides important information to schools, nurses, and parents about responding to asthma. The American Lung Association Web site offers classroom kits that include a curriculum guide, posters, activities, and handouts. The curriculum, available in English and Spanish, offers an interactive teaching approach that helps children and parents learn about self-management of asthma. A study of program effectiveness was conducted by Columbia University with a diverse group of 239 children from 12 elementary schools in New York City. Results showed that the school children who finished the program managed their asthma more effectively, had improved school performance, and had fewer episodes of asthma. Parents were also more involved in helping their children to manage asthma and the school environment increased their support for children with asthma.

Source: American Lung Association, 2010

Dan noted that nurses from the Medical Reserve Corps were volunteering to help staff some of the flu clinics. He asked one of the nurses, Grace, about how she became involved in the Medical Reserve Corps. Grace commented, "I have a regular job at the hospital in my community, but when I heard about the Medical Reserve Corps, I decided I wanted to help my community if a disaster occurred. I am a volunteer. I found out about this organization when some of my friends went to New Orleans to help with the health needs after Hurricane Katrina."

Dan later spoke with his supervisor, Carol, about the Medical Reserve Corps (Minnesota Department of Health, 2008; NACCHO, 2008b). Carol said, "Since Hurricane Katrina, many health care workers in our state have signed up to be in the program, and now there are over 7000 volunteers. This program strengthens the public health response, which we call public health infrastructure, when there is a disaster. Local coordinators oversee the program and provide training and support so that volunteers are ready to respond to the disaster. Our health commissioner can mobilize volunteers when they are needed."

Dan responded, "The Medical Reserve Corps is a great community resource. I am going to tell my friends from my last job at the hospital about this wonderful volunteer opportunity."

What Legal Issues Are Important for Public Health Nurses to Understand?

A fundamental responsibility of the government is to protect the health of the public. Each state has statutes that outline the broad and specific powers and duties granted to state and local government. Examples of authority include the following:

1. Planning and reporting

2. Regulating and enforcing health and sanitation laws, ordinances, and codes

3. Investigating disease control and enforcing laws

4. Ensuring that health services are accessible to all persons based on need (Minnesota Statutes 145A.03–145A.10, 2009)

Data Privacy

The Health Insurance Portability and Accountability Act of 1996 public law (HIPAA) is administered by the federal government. Public health nurses are accountable for ensuring the data privacy aspect of HIPAA. You are certainly familiar with this law from day one of your clinical experiences or working in a health care setting. State laws often specify that information important for assuring public health can be disclosed. For example, Minnesota's Data Sharing Law allows the sharing of immunization data with schools and child care providers without parental permission (Minnesota Department of Health, 2003b). In addition, health care providers can share information about communicable disease with the state health department without patient permission (Minnesota Department of Health, 2003a).

Mandated Reporting

All states have laws that protect abused children and require certain professionals, including nurses, to report suspected child abuse. Many states also have civil immunity for people who make reports and/or penalties if suspected child abuse is not reported (Pozgar, 2005). Although the first case of child abuse was addressed under a law that prevented cruelty to animals in the 1870s, it was not until the 1960s and 1970s that all states had mandatory reporting laws (Encyclopedia of Everyday Law, 2010).

Evidence Example: Child Protection

A qualitative study with ten Australian nurses from acute and community settings explored nurses' perceptions about how they protected children and the barriers they experienced (Land & Barclay, 2008). Nurses understood their accountability to report physical child abuse but were less certain about suspected abuse, emotional abuse, and neglect. They reported two major barriers to effectively carrying out their responsibility to protect children. They experienced communication barriers that decreased effective interdisciplinary collaboration and reported that professionals were unaware of one another's roles in child protection. They also described a fear factor. Nurses were concerned they would have to appear in court, and they were concerned about their personal safety, fearing retribution if they reported abuse. Authors of the study recommended that nurses needed education about their legal responsibilities for child protection and that organizational changes in structure and culture were needed to promote interdisciplinary collaboration and sharing of health information between professionals.

School-Entry Laws

PHNs who practice in school settings are involved in the enforcement of school-entry laws, which mandate evidence of vaccination for specific communicable diseases or a legal exemption signed by a parent. School entry laws have been in existence since the 1960s and have increased vaccination rates and decreased rates of childhood communicable disease (Horlich, Shaw, Gorji, & Fishbein, 2008). Some parents might object to compulsory vaccination for their children, believing that the government is taking away their authority.

Ethical Application

One of the ethical problems involved in implementing flu vaccine clinics is prioritizing which populations should receive the vaccine first. This sometimes creates an ethical problem when the benefits for the many (the population group) are deemed to be more important than the needs or interests of one person. Another ethical problem that PHNs might encounter regarding immunizations for children is that some parents are concerned that immunizations can cause their children harm, for example, the worry about the measles vaccination causing autism. An important role for PHNs is to be knowledgeable about evidence on the effects of immunizations to communicate to parents.

Another area that can create an ethical problem for PHNs is the enforcement of public health law, such as mandated reporting of child abuse. The preceding evidence example on child protection identifies concerns that can lead to ethical problems. The PHN might worry about losing the trust of parents following a suspected child abuse report. However, the well-being of the child is more important than losing the trusting relationship. The challenge creates more tension when the PHN is uncertain about whether child abuse is occurring. See Table 6.5 for the application of ethical perspectives to mandated reporting of child abuse.

Table 6.5   Ethical Action in Mandated Reporting of Child Abuse

Ethical Perspective	Application
Rule Ethics (principles)	• Promote justice by following the public health law, which specifies that nurses and other professionals must report suspected child abuse. • Prevent harm to the child by reporting the suspected child abuse.

Ethical Perspective	Application
Virtue Ethics (character)	• Consider how reporting child abuse will impact the relationship with parents of the child. • Be courageous in stepping forward to report the suspected child abuse. • Provide care for both the parents and the child.
Feminist Ethics (reducing oppression)	• Be aware of using authority in a manner that oppresses parents. • Encourage parents' voices and perspectives in decision making about what to do.

Key Points

- All levels of government (local, state, and federal) have responsibility for promoting public health and often work together.

- There are ten essential services and three core functions of public health that determine the goals of public health departments.

- Public health nurses who are employed by governmental agencies are responsible for upholding specific laws that protect the health of the public.

- The public health model focuses on populations and prevention in contrast to the medical model, which focuses on individuals and provides health care services that respond to illness and injury.

- Funding for public health comes from public and private sources and determines the programs and services that can be provided by local public health departments.

- Local public health departments work with non-profit organizations to improve the health status of populations.

Exercises

Learning Examples for Working with Governmental Systems

Following are four learning examples. The emergency preparedness example is described in the literature. In addition, learning activities are suggested for updating immunization records, nutrition policy for school children, and reducing youth access to tobacco. Useful websites from governmental organizations that provide additional information and strategies are listed to help you generate evidence-based approaches to the public health concern.

Emergency Preparedness (Carter, Kaiser, O'Hare, & Callister, 2006)

- Participate as a volunteer in a mock pandemic or biological terrorism event; reflect through writing or in a clinical conference discussion about the effectiveness of the governmental response to the event.

- In a clinical group, review the emergency response plan of a selected agency in the community. Evaluate the plan and summarize what the group has learned. Evaluate or develop a risk communication plan.

- Study a natural disaster (hurricane, tornado, or flood) and review the literature about the governmental response.

Updating Immunization Records

- Update immunization data on student health records at a charter school by accessing the immunization database on the state health department website.

- Review data privacy and requirements for immunizations for school children.

Implementing Nutrition Policy for School Children

- Review the following governmental guidelines and educational strategies for promoting healthy eating:

  - U. S. Department of Health and Human Services. (2009). Dietary guidelines for America. Retrieved December 28, 2010 from http://www.health.gov/dietaryguidelines/

  - Centers for Disease Control. (2008). Make a difference at your school: Key strategies to prevent obesity. Retrieved December 28, 2010 from http://www.cdc.gov/HealthyYouth/KeyStrategies/

  - United States Department of Agriculture, Food and Nutrition Service. (2010). Nutrition Education. Retrieved December 28, 2010 from http://www.fns.usda.gov/fns/nutrition.htm

  - Minnesota Action for Healthy Kids. (2006). Healthy foods for kids: Guidelines for nutrition at school. Retrieved December 28, 2010 from http://www.actionfor-healthykids.org/assets/clubs/mn1-nutritionatschool.pdf

  - Institute of Medicine of the National Academies (2007). Nutrition standards for food in schools: Leading the way toward healthy youth. Retrieved December 28, 2010 from http://www.iom.edu/~/media/Files/Report%20Files/2007/Nutrition-Standards-for-Foods-in-Schools-Leading-the-Way-toward-Healthier-Youth/FoodinSchools.pdf

- Discuss how each of the three levels of government would be involved in implementation of nutrition policy for school children.

- Identify interventions from the Public Health Intervention Wheel that you find represented by suggested strategies.

Reducing Youth Access to Tobacco

- Review the following resources and information about strategies for reducing youth access to tobacco.

- Minnesota Department of Health. (2002). *Minding the store: Curtailing the sale of tobacco to Minnesota teens.* Retrieved December 28, 2010 from http://www.health.state.mn.us/divs/hpcd/tpc/youth/mindingthestore.pdf

- Centers for Disease Control. (2010). Healthy youth: Tobacco use. Retrieved December 28, 2010 from http://www.cdc.gov/healthyyouth/tobacco/

- Identify PHN interventions for reducing youth access to tobacco.

- Identify governmental and community resources for reducing youth access to tobacco.

Reflective Practice

Governmental organizations develop and enforce regulations and laws to prevent disease and promote the health of populations. They also provide the resources needed to improve the health of the public. These resources include staff members with expert knowledge and funds to support public health programs and services. As a public health nurse working for a governmental organization, it is both a responsibility and honor to contribute to improved population health through one's expert knowledge and skills. Consider the public health response to the disaster of a flood occurring in a community and answer the reflective practice questions that follow. Review these resources prior to answering the following questions.

Minnesota Department of Health. (2010). Information and guidelines for healthcare facilities and providers in the event of spring flooding or other natural disasters. Retrieved December 28, 2010 from http://www.health.state.mn.us/divs/fpc/profinfo/ib10_2.html

Minnesota Department of Health. (2010). Floods: Protecting your health. Retrieved December 28, 2010 from http://www.health.state.mn.us/divs/eh/emergency/natural/floods/index.html

Minnesota Department of Health. (2010). Floods: Caring for yourself. Retrieved December 28, 2010 from http://www.health.state.mn.us/divs/eh/emergency/natural/floods/selfcare.html

Minnesota Department of Health. (2009). Food safety during a flood. Retrieved December 28, 2010 from http://www.health.state.mn.us/divs/eh/emergency/natural/floods/food.html

What are the responsibilities of the local, state, and federal levels of government in responding to major flooding in a community?

_____

_____

How could community resources be involved in responding to the consequences of the flood in the community (disease prevention and health promotion)?

_____

_____

How does a PHN use expert skills and knowledge to respond to this disaster? (See the following Public Health Nursing Story.)

_____

_____

Public Health Nursing Story—2007 Flood in Southeastern Minnesota

In August 2007 after extensive rainfall in southeastern Minnesota, the resulting flooding damaged or destroyed 1500 homes in Winona County. Two emergency shelters were opened, feeding stations were set up, and a massive cleanup was initiated. The 18 PHNs from Winona County's Community Health Services responded along with other government employees to prevent disease and promote the health of community residents. The nurses immediately became involved and acted. They:

- Credentialed volunteers by providing just-in-time training (Community Organizing)

- Collaborated with sanitarians and law enforcement to inspect and code damaged homes for habitation within the first 72 hours following the flood

- Gave information on clean-up methods and mold abatement (Health Teaching)

- Visited area shelters and connected with them daily (Consultation)

- Assisted medical providers in giving tetanus injections (Delegated Functions)

- Canvassed flooded homes to offer tetanus vaccinations, distribute cleaning information and supplies, and assess emotional health (Outreach, Screening)

Source: Minnesota Department of Health. (Winter 2008 – Spring 2009). Winona County story. Public Health Nursing Newsletter. Retrieved from http://www.health.state.mn.us/divs/cfh/ophp/resources/phnnews/phnnew0609.pdf

After you have discussed these questions, analyze how guidelines, standards, and public health law guide how the government and how you as a public health nurse will respond to the disaster.

Application of Evidence

1. Which essential services would be most relevant in responding to the natural disaster of flooding in a community?

2. Give a practice example that illustrates each of the three core functions for responding to a flood in a community.

3. Refer to Table 6.4 that identifies the ANA Standards of Professional Performance for Public Health Nursing. How are the following standards illustrated in the public health nursing story found above: education, collaboration, resource utilization, leadership, and advocacy?

4. For the same flooding scenario, what public health laws and legal issues do PHNs need to keep in mind when responding to a flood disaster?

 Think, Explore, Do

1. Choose a public health concern applicable to a population group. Analyze how the three levels of government are involved in responding to the public health concern.

2. Locate the annual report for the local health department (city or county) in which you have your clinical experience or where you live. (Annual reports are usually available on health department websites). Find the financial report and identify revenue and expenses for provided services. Analyze the sources of public and private funding streams for public health in the county or city.

3. Discuss the mandate for reporting suspected child abuse, which is a responsibility of the professional nurse. What public health interventions would the PHN use in working with a family in which child abuse might be occurring? How could community resources contribute to prevention of child abuse?

4. Make a list of public health programs and services provided by the local health department in which you work or have your clinical experience. Analyze how the programs and services are consistent with the public health model. (See Table 6.3 for how the public health model contrasts with the medical model).

COMPETENCY #5:
Practices Public Health Nursing Within the Auspices of the Nurse Practice Act

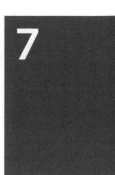

By Marjorie A. Schaffer
with Carol Flaten and Patricia M. Schoon

Jennifer, a public health nurse (PHN), has worked for the Weaver County Health Department for 10 years. Jennifer's first nursing position after completing her Bachelor of Science in Nursing (BSN) and passing nursing boards was on a medical-surgical unit in large metropolitan hospital. Since her public health experience in nursing school, she had been anxious to find a PHN position. In her search for a PHN position, Jennifer focused on three states in the midwestern part of the United States that interested her. Within several months she found a position at a small local health department in the town of Aurora, the county seat of Weaver County.

Aurora is surrounded by an agricultural community. Corn, soybeans, and sugar beets are the major crops. Cattle are also raised in this area. The town of Aurora has a population of 15,000. German immigrants settled Aurora in the 1850s. Today, Aurora is a multicultural community. The racial makeup is 91% Caucasian, 2% African-American, 2% Hispanic or Latino, 1% Native American, 1% Asian, 1% Pacific Islander, and 1 % other. The median income is $30,000.

Weaver County has a significant population of migrant workers from Mexico who provide a large portion of the workforce for many farms in the area and also provide the labor for a poultry processing company located on the northern edge of the county. This processing company opened 10 years ago. The town has needed to learn to adapt to a new cultural group.

Sarah, a public health nursing student, has been assigned to Jennifer to complete her public health nursing field experience. She is excited to start this experience. Sarah is completing her undergraduate BSN degree at a university about 45 miles from Weaver County. She is familiar with Weaver County through the media reports of the difficult racial issues in the county over the past years. Sarah grew up in an urban area, where a variety of cultures and races were represented. She is Korean and was adopted into an American family as an infant. Sarah is eager to learn not only about the role of the PHN, but also how the community environment affects the work of Weaver County Public Health Department and the work of public health nurses.

As Sarah has been reflecting on her public health nursing class, she remembers the three core functions of public health—assessment, policy development, and assurance. Along with this underlying framework, Sarah also knows the importance of the Cornerstones of Public Health Nursing. She is particularly interested in learning about how independent nursing practice is carried out and how public health nurses use the Public Health Intervention Wheel in Weaver County. Sarah will spend 5 weeks with Jennifer learning as much as possible about public health nursing.

SARAH'S NOTEBOOK

Competency #5: Practices within the auspices of the Nurse Practice Act

- Understands the scope of nursing practice (independent nursing functions and delegated medical functions)

- Establishes appropriate professional boundaries

- Maintains confidentiality

- Demonstrates ethical, legal, and professional accountability

- Delegates and supervises other personnel

- Understands the role of a public health nurse as described under public health nursing registration

Useful Definitions

Confidentiality: Non-disclosure of health information that is considered to be private information.

Delegation: "The process for a nurse to direct another person to perform nursing tasks and activities" (National Council of State Boards of Nursing and American Nurses Association, 2006).

Independent Practice: Professional decision making guided by professional standards of the profession; scope of practice that includes independent functions might also be defined legally.

Nurse Practice Act: State statute that describes the practice of nursing; describes scope of professional nursing practice.

Professional Boundaries: Limits that allow for safe connections and situations in professional interactions with clients; in the professional relationship, expert knowledge is assumed on the part of the professional and the relationship is directed at meeting the needs of the client, but not the needs of the professional (Gallop, 1998; Jacobson, 2002).

Public Health Nursing Registration: Requirements for practicing public health nursing, which are not universal across all states.

Supervision: "The active process of directing, guiding, and influencing the outcome of an individual's performance of a task" (National Council of State Boards of Nursing and American Nurses Association, 2006).

Understanding Public Health Nursing Roles Ethically, Legally, and Professionally

In this chapter you will have the opportunity to learn about the Nurse Practice Act and how state legislation guides independent practice in public health nursing. Every state has a Nurse Practice Act that lays out legal specifications for definitions, titles, licensing, and other legal parameters for the practice of nursing. Because much of public health nursing involves independent decision making on the part of nurses and in collaboration with others, PHNs need to be aware of how the Nurse Practice Act for the state guides the professional role and defines professional accountability.

When PHNs practice independently, they make decisions based on their own expert knowledge and skills, professional standards, and the best evidence that guides nursing practice. Independent practice in public health settings differs from the experience of nurses in hospitals and other structured settings, in which medical orders are required for many nursing tasks. On some occasions in public health settings a physician's order is needed for reimbursement from insurance, Medicare, or Medicaid for provided services. Also, a physician's order, although not legally required, might be necessary to make a referral for public health nursing services to obtain reimbursement. PHNs might refer to other members of the interdisciplinary team, such as lactation consultant or physical therapist, but again, a physician's order might be required for authorization of payment.

What Is the Scope of Public Health Nursing Practice?

Chapter 1 explained that the scope of practice refers to the boundaries of safe and ethical practice. The Public Health Intervention Wheel describes what PHNs do and further explains activities that fall within the scope of public health nursing practice. In public health nursing, nurses often collaborate with staff from different disciplines. Clarifying job descriptions and professional roles so that each discipline makes the best use of their specific expertise as they work together on reaching a common goal is important. Janet Schneiderman (2003, 2006) gave an example of nursing roles and accountability in scope of practice in an application of the Public Health Intervention Wheel to a California program in which PHNs provided case management to children in foster care. The PHNs collaborated with foster caregivers and social workers to help the children obtain needed health services. The PHNs assisted with interpretation of health care reports, development of health plans, referral for care, and evaluation of the placements in meeting health care needs. To be effective in working in the multidisciplinary model, the PHNs needed skills and knowledge that included flexibility, clear communication, the ability to prioritize, and an understanding of health and social services at the county and state levels. The analysis by Schneiderman revealed that PHNs provided all 17 interventions from the Public Health Intervention Wheel in their case management of foster care children. See the following specific examples for disease and health event investigation, health teaching, and case management:

- Disease and Health Event Investigation—The PHNs identified at-risk preschool foster children for lead poisoning (related to living in older housing).

- Health Teaching—The PHNs instructed foster families on ways to prevent lead exposure.

- Case Management—The PHNs connected foster families to health providers to ensure the continuation of child's seizure medication.

In Schneiderman's (2003) study of 12 nurses working in the child welfare system and the school district, school nurses most often used the interventions of screening, health teaching and surveillance, whereas the child welfare nurses more often used the interventions of consultation, referral and follow-up, surveillance, and case management. Interventions used vary according to the population served and the job responsibilities of the PHN. Schneiderman recommended that the collaborative work of PHNs within the child welfare system is enhanced by developing clear job descriptions, by having a structure that identifies the workflow for PHNs, and by providing education for other professionals on the competencies, skills, and knowledge of professional nurses.

In another study on the work of public health nurses, Linda Olson Keller and Emily Litt (2008) used an online survey to complete a task analysis of 60 PHNs who represented 28 states. Many of the tasks identified were consistent with the interventions from the Public Health Intervention Wheel and represent the scope of public health nursing practice. See Table 7.1 to find out which interventions were used most often by PHNs in the study.

Table 7.1   Task Analysis and Frequency of PHN Interventions (n=60)

Public Health Intervention
Health Teaching • Individuals and Families (100%) • Groups (82%) • Educational classes, meetings, workshops for providers (73%) • Health education classes (47%)
Referral and Follow-up (100%) Case Management (88%) Counseling (individuals and families) (88%) Disease and Health Event Investigation (78%) Screening (78%) Advocacy (70%) Community Organizing (60%) Policy Development 　　• Present information to decision makers (37%) 　　• Promote or lobby for public health legislations (20%) 　　• Testify for public health issues to policy makers (13%)

In the report of study findings, Keller and Litt highlighted PHN accomplishments and activities for some of the interventions. For disease and health event investigation, the two most common events investigated by PHNs were tuberculosis and vaccine-preventable disease. PHNs completed several activities within this intervention, including finding contacts, making sure clients complied with treatment, and making sure specimens were collected. Other common diseases and health events investigated by public health nurses included sexually transmitted diseases, food-borne diseases, lice, elevated blood lead, vector-borne disease, animal-borne disease, and HIV/AIDs (Keller & Litt, 2008).

For referral and follow-up, on average, the PHN participants made seven referrals and received five re-ferrals in a one-week time span. PHNs are experts in linking individuals, families, and groups with com-munity resources. PHNs consulted with a variety of groups and community members on a broad range of public health issues. They provided consultation to other health department staff, child care providers, clinic and hospital staff, school nurses and teachers, social workers, physicians and nurse practitioners, community leaders, and long-term care facilities (Keller & Litt, 2008).

For the intervention of advocacy, PHNs functioned as a liaison to agencies or professionals to advocate for vulnerable individuals and populations; made physician appointments and arranged transportation; connected families with services for meeting basic needs (food, housing, clothing, transportation); and arranged for interpreters. The PHN goal is to contribute to the development of self-reliance for vulner-able individuals. PHNs worked with others in the community to develop coalitions to respond to a health concern. Examples of coalitions identified in the study include the Healthy Family Coalition, Rural Health Coalition, Asian Immunization, and Childhood Obesity Coalition (Keller & Litt, 2008).

Evidence Example: The Independent Practice of Public Health Nurses

Researchers conducted a study with 23 focus groups in 6 Canadian geographic regions to identify organizational attributes that contributed to a successful experience in providing public health nursing interventions. Focus groups were held with 156 PHNs and were divided into staff PHNs and PHNs who were in management or policymaking. These groups were also divided by place of practice—urban or rural/remote. Analysis of focus group data revealed that organizational lead-ership needed to support PHN practice autonomy, which is consistent with independent practice. Staff PHNs wanted nursing management to trust the ability of the PHNs to work independently. Although they wanted clear guidelines and specified roles for their work, they also wanted flex-ibility in deciding with their clients the best approach to use because different ways of reaching the same goal exist. The focus group data revealed the importance of defining roles in terms of "what" needs to be accomplished rather than focusing on "how" an outcome should be accom-plished. The study also recommended that "champions" are needed at the organizational level to increase public awareness of the work of public health nurses.

Source: Meagher-Stewart et al., 2009

Sarah's first day of public health nursing clinical experience with Jennifer began right away on Mon-day morning (See Table 7.2 for Jennifer's schedule). Sarah met Jennifer at the Public Health Office at 7:30 a.m. She had met Jennifer briefly a week earlier, but this would be the first time that Sarah would have the opportunity to observe nursing through the eyes of a public health nurse. Sarah was on time and ready to enter the building at 7:28 a.m., but the door was locked! Sarah worried. This never happened at the hospital. She tried to open the door several times. It did not budge. She checked her calendar to be sure she had the correct day and time. She did. Within a minute, Jennifer drove up. They were off to their first visit.

Sarah rode with Jennifer. Jennifer had three home visits scheduled for the morning, followed by two home visits in the afternoon. At the end of the day Jennifer had a planning meeting for a health fair.

Jennifer briefly described the three morning home visits were to families that she knew from previous visits: 1) a 93-year-old woman with congestive heart failure who lived alone, 2) a toddler with an elevated lead level whose parents had emigrated from Mexico last year, and 3) a 17-year-old teen with a 3-month-old girl. After the morning visits, Jennifer planned to return to the office for a short time to make any follow-up phone calls and review plans for the afternoon home visits. The last hour of the day, they would meet with the new director of an alternative learning center in the school district who had identified a need among her students for a health fair that focused on healthy foods.

Table 7.2   Jennifer's schedule

Day/Time	Monday	Tuesday	Wednesday	Thursday	Friday
8am – 9am	Home visit: Hanson	Staff Meeting	Immunization Clinic	Women Infants and Children Clinic	Alternative Learning Center Health Fair
9am – 10am	Home visit: Vu	Diversity Coalition Meeting	Immunization Clinic	Women Infants and Children Clinic	Alternative Learning Center Health Fair
10am – 11am	Home visit: Loften	Diversity Coalition: Collect county data for grant application	Inventory and Order supplies for Immunization Clinic	Women Infants and Children Clinic	Alternative Learning Center Health Fair
11am – 12pm	Office: Follow up on calls, new referrals, plan for Health Fair	Office: Phone Triage	Meet with Program Manager to Determine Funding for Asthma Coalition	Women Infants and Children Clinic	Office: Phone Triage
12pm – 1pm	Lunch	Lunch	Lunch	Lunch	Lunch
1pm – 2pm	New Referral	Home visit: Ahmed	Prep for Foot Clinic at Community Center	Office: Follow up on phone calls and referrals. Pack up supplies for Health Fair	Write report for Alternative Learning Center Health Fair
2pm – 3pm	New Referral	Home visit: Johnson	Foot Clinic	Home visit: Wallis	Immunization Clinic

Day/Time	Monday	Tuesday	Wednesday	Thursday	Friday
3pm – 4pm	Meet with Director of Alternative Learning Center to Plan for Health Fair	Home visit: Freeman	Foot Clinic	Home visit: Froeland	Immunization Clinic

Expanded Description of Activities

Alternative Learning Center Health Fair: The alternative learning center is part of the public school system. It offers middle and high school curriculum for students who benefit from smaller class sizes and alternative methods of course content delivery. Many of the teachers at the school felt a need to provide "healthy lifestyle habits" information to the students. The school nurse contacted the public health office to collaborate with the PHNs to design a morning "Health Fair." The focus will be on including healthy snacks and exercise in your day, with demonstration stations on how to make a snack, followed by an opportunity for the students to make their own snack and eat it.

Asthma Coalition: One of the school nurses in Aurora noticed that more and more children with asthma were coming to her office over the past few years. She mentioned this concern to a local physician who also was aware of an increase in pediatric patients needing care related to asthma. The school nurse contacted the public health department to learn if they were aware of an increase in asthma, county-wide or statewide. The timing of that call was good. The public health nursing director had just learned of funds that were available for starting a coalition related to asthma in children. The state and county statistics were showing an increase in asthma cases over the past 5 years. Out of these conversations a coalition was formed. Currently one of the PHNs is the chairperson of this coalition, which meets monthly to identify ways to increase public and provider awareness of methods to manage asthma. This coalition is made up of school nurses, nurse practitioners, physicians, public health nurses, coaches, and parents of children with asthma.

Diversity Coalition: This is a group of community partners (educators, health care providers, local business owners) who are interested in supporting the various groups represented in Aurora. The overall goal of this group is to make Aurora a welcoming community for all. One of the elementary school teachers in town initiated this group as he was observing segmentation of racial groups not only in the elementary school that lead to tension, but also in the community at large.

Foot Care Clinic: Twice a month the PHNs hold a clinic to provide foot care for senior citizens at the community senior center. The PHNs worked with a podiatrist in the community and the public health medical director to develop a foot clinic protocol and referral system. Because an identified need existed in the community to provide basic skin and nail care and assessment for elderly citizens, this has been a very popular clinic. Two PHNs staff this clinic.

Immunization Clinic: Each week the public health office holds an immunization clinic where people can receive low-cost vaccinations for their children, or adults in their families. The clinic is held at the local health department, which is centrally located. No appointments are required. It is a walk-in clinic. Each public health nurse takes a turn staffing the clinic. One PHN oversees the clinic, ordering vaccines, following current protocols for administration, and informing the PHNs of updated information.

Phone Triage: All of the PHNs take turns on "phone triage." During this time the PHN works on documentation or projects at his/her desk and answers calls that come to the agency that require a PHN to assess and provide feedback. Calls can range from a parent needing to know which immunizations her child needs and a low-cost place to get those vaccinations to a landlord worried about bedbugs in a vacated apartment unit.

WIC Clinic: Women, Infants and Children is a federally funded food program administered by states and counties that provides screening, nutrition counseling, and health referrals for pregnant and breast-feeding women and their children birth to 5 years of age. In Aurora, public health nurses and nutritionists from the health and human services department staff this clinic twice a month at the public health nursing office. Jennifer's role is to provide height and weight checks of the children and review immunization status.

Sarah's assignment for the day was to observe Jennifer's communication and actions. Sarah planned to take notes about her observations and communication between the PHN and client. See Sarah's notes.

SARAH'S JOURNAL

Activity	Sarah's Observations
Visit 1: Lily Hanson, a 93-year-old woman with congestive heart failure. Lives alone.	Arrived at a fourplex apartment building. The yard and building are maintained well, with big shade trees, grass, and flower beds surrounding the building. Lily's apartment is on the first floor (no steps). Jennifer knocks on the door and opens it slightly; Lily calls to Jennifer to come in. Lily is sitting at the dining room table, neatly dressed, with her pill bottles lined up and using her portable oxygen. The apartment is well-kept, with many photos on the walls.
	A fan is running quietly in the corner of the living room. Jennifer completes a heart and lung assessment and asks Lily about her activity level. Lily reports that even in the hot, humid weather, if she stays indoors with the fans running she feels comfortable. Jennifer fills Lily's pillbox for the week. Jennifer also asks Lily about alternate plans if her apartment becomes too hot for her to tolerate. Lily reports that she had a window air conditioner, but it broke and she does not have enough additional money to buy a new one. Jennifer

suggests Lily call the County Senior Support Network (SSN). The SSN has funds for elders in need of basic housing supplies. In this heat wave Jennifer has learned that SSN will provide air conditioners.

Jennifer talked to Lily so naturally. Jennifer explained that she had known Lily for 3 years. The first year she came to visit, Lily was not friendly at all. She thought Jennifer was visiting to get information that would cause her to go to a long-term care facility. After that first year and many short conversations, Lily accepted that Jennifer was trying to help her maintain her independence so she could continue to live in her apartment. Jennifer hypothesized that her persistence and nonjudgmental attitude helped Lily realize she was there to support her.

Visit 2: Toddler with an elevated lead level whose parents emigrated from Mexico last year	Drove to an older part of town. There are many single-family homes. Much of the paint has worn off or is peeling. In most of the yards the grass is worn away, and there are many children's toys. Jennifer rang the doorbell, knocked, and called in the front window. But there was no response. There was no response to a phone call either. Jennifer explained that sometimes families might not be at home although an appointment had been made for the visit. Persons living in poverty experience more frequent crises and with few resources might live from day to day, with less emphasis on future planning.
Visit 3: First-time 17-year-old mom, Ann, who has a 3-month-old girl	Stopped at an old apartment building. Broken glass on the front steps. Entry security system working. Ann responded cheerfully to Jennifer. Ann lives on the third floor. No elevator. Smells musty. Ann has the door open for us. It is 90 degrees out at 10 a.m. Ann has the shades pulled to keep the sun out, but there are no air conditioners or fans in the efficiency apartment. Jennifer focused this visit on baby Kayla's development. She used the Ages and Stages Questionnaire that has questions specific to development expected for the age of the child. I noticed Jennifer also gave some suggestions to Kayla's mom about what she could expect to happen in Kayla's development over the next few months.
Office (and lunch)	Jennifer checks for messages and has a message from the Garcia family. They will not be home today. Completes some charting. Checks for new referrals. Makes calls to these families.

New Referral: Active case of tuberculosis (TB)	Met Mr. Adams at his house. Mr. Adams was diagnosed with TB (tuberculosis) about 4 months ago. He likely acquired TB working overseas in a disaster relief effort. He recently moved to Aurora to be near his aging parents. Jennifer will be providing Directly Observed Therapy (DOT) for Mr. Adams. In DOT, Jennifer will observe Mr. Adams to make sure he takes his medication correctly. When too many people are inconsistent in taking their TB medication, the TB bacteria can become resistant to medication.
	In comparison to Jennifer's interaction with Lily earlier today, this was a very formal meeting. Jennifer asked questions to get the intake information. She also inquired about Mr. Adams' preferences for the DOT therapy. After the discussion and a brief health history, Jennifer observed Mr. Adams taking the medication and left.
New Referral: Postpartum visit	We met Amy Chan. She is 2 weeks postpartum. Her baby boy is doing well. However, Amy is anxious and nervous about her son as her first child died of Sudden Infant Death Syndrome (SIDS) 3 years ago. Jennifer provided positive feedback regarding the care that Amy was doing for her son. Short messages and positive feedback seemed to help Amy. Jennifer suggested a support group for Amy.
Met with Director of alternative learning center	Jennifer met with the director, two of the teachers, and the school health aid. The director is very concerned about the nutritional status of the students. Many of the students drink sodas and eat chips for snacks at school and often skip lunch. Jennifer suggests planning a health fair that will focus on healthy snacks and provide samples.

Sarah spoke with Jennifer after the first day of her clinical experience. Sarah commented, "I don't know how I will ever become independent in my decision making about what to do."

Jennifer suggested, "Let's review the day and look ahead to the week. Then we can analyze what we did today and which independent public health nursing interventions were accomplished. Also I will have you look ahead at my schedule for the rest of the week. You can begin to think about what interventions you would consider to be independent practice and how you might collaborate with others. We can discuss the skills and knowledge a PHN needs for these interventions."

ACTIVITY

Review Jennifer's schedule for the week (Table 7.2). Answer the following questions:

What public health interventions from the Public Health Intervention Wheel did Jennifer use?

Analyze which interventions were independent and which were delegated functions.

What skills and knowledge enabled Jennifer to practice independently?

How did Jennifer collaborate with other individuals, groups, professionals, or organizations?

How Do I Establish Professional Boundaries in Public Health Nursing?

On Tuesday Jennifer has a visit scheduled with one of her favorite clients, Mindy, who is 16 and lives with her mother. Mindy has a 6-month-old baby girl. Mindy's former boyfriend, the baby's father, had been physically abusive to Mindy during her pregnancy. Mindy has developmental delays and struggles with school and fitting in. Mindy was referred to public health nursing after her first prenatal clinic visit when she was 6 months pregnant. Mindy and Jennifer have developed a good relationship. Mindy has worked hard to follow through with good parenting practices and has been receptive to Jennifer. Jennifer checked her Facebook account last night and Mindy had added her as a friend. Jennifer felt torn between the professional, therapeutic, and supportive roles she provided for Mindy.

Understanding professional boundaries is essential for all nurses. PHNs practice in environments that are sometimes more challenging for maintaining professional boundaries, such as in homes, schools, and other community settings that have different norms of behavior in contrast to the hospital setting. In the hospital setting, professional and client roles are more clearly defined. In community and home settings, relationships and the norms of interaction need to be differentiated from more casual social relationships. Sometimes students and PHNs find it difficult to keep from moving into a social friendship with the client as the relationship with the client progresses over time. PHNs must clarify their role and purpose for relationships with clients to maintain professional boundaries.

Gloria Jacobson (2002) identified potential areas for boundary violation that need clarification about the nursing role. Confusion about the nurse's role can occur in situations of gift-giving or offering money. Although PHNs do not wear uniforms, they need to choose professional-appearing attire that is comfortable. Individuals from some cultures might frown on clothing that they consider too revealing and might be reluctant to believe what the PHN is saying is important if the PHN is not professionally dressed. PHNs need to be alert for any situation or conversations that might result in self-disclosure. PHNs need to ask themselves if what they are doing is what a nurse would typically do. PHNs can use touch as a comfort measure but need to consider the meaning of any physical contact to the nurse and client. Touch and eye contact are not considered accepted practices in some cultures.

On some occasions physical assessment is required, and although it is a norm for adults and children to remove clothes for physical exams in the hospital and clinic settings, removing clothes is not a norm in a community setting. For infants and children who require physical examination, ask for parent permission, and ask the parent or the child, if old enough, to remove clothes for a needed physical examination.

Anne Clancy and Tommy Svensson (2007) found that one of the five themes in a qualitative study on the essence of ethical responsibility in public health nursing focused on boundaries. The PHNs in the study (n = 5) described the challenge of defining boundaries as they worked with clients. They described situations of being persuaded to do something and then feeling regret that they had not said "no." The authors of the study suggested that one's professional ethical responsibility does not mean doing what another demands. Closer relationships that develop over a long-term time period with clients can lead to a sense of duty, which can result in over-involvement and possibly developing a friendship, a potential professional boundary violation. Clancy and Svensson captured the challenge of balancing the management of boundaries and a sense of responsibility when working with individuals and families in public health settings:

> The clear-cut boundaries for involvement that nurses long for seem impossible to achieve. Each nurse has to make decisions that are not only based on quality standards, but also on their professional intuition and personal involvement. Boundaries in responsibility are not solid steel walls; they are more like a corridor of half-open doors, providing openings and opportunities, allowing for choices and adding to uncertainties (2007, p. 163).

Maintaining professional boundaries does not mean that one is detached. At the same time, the PHN does not fulfill the role of being a friend to a client. Kathleen Oberle and Sandra Tenove (2000) identified setting boundaries as one of the subthemes of the character of relationships in a qualitative study of the ethical problems experienced by 22 PHNs in Canada. PHNs who practiced in rural areas found it more difficult to separate personal and professional lives to keep client confidentiality. One PHN in the study discussed the challenge of wanting to be authentic with clients when they encountered them in personal situations.

Julie McGarry (2003) also identified maintenance of personal-professional boundaries as one of three key themes in a study of how district nurses (n = 10) in the United Kingdom defined their role. One reason given for maintaining a level of separation was a concern about the PHN giving too much emotionally and too much time, which could lead to negative consequences for both the nurse and the client. The client might become too attached, the nurse might become too vulnerable, and the boundaries might become blurred. The authors addressed the challenge of finding a balance between creating a participative, trusting relationship with the client while maintaining their own professional identity.

 ACTIVITY

When is it helpful to share something personal about yourself with a client? When is it not helpful?

What are some "red flags" that indicate you might not be maintaining professional boundaries with clients?

Is it a boundary violation to attend a patient's baby shower? A funeral for a client? Why or why not?

How do you think Jennifer should handle the Facebook request from Mindy?

How Do Public Health Nurses Establish and Maintain Confidentiality?

Confidentiality in public health nursing often goes hand in hand with professional boundaries. Maintaining professional boundaries requires that PHNs keep health information private. PHNs must consider who they talk to about clients and the confidentiality of the documentation process. The use of computers for documentation is subject to the same protection of privacy as written material. The Health Insurance Portability and Accountability Act (HIPAA), which specifies how health information is communicated, was discussed in Chapter 6. Respecting patient confidentiality is a professional and legal duty (Griffith, 2007). However, PHNs must also balance this duty against the need to disclose information to protect someone from harm, such as in situations of suicide ideation. When vulnerable adults or children are involved, the duty to protect outweighs the duty to keep health information in confidence. Competing interests can exist—disclosure can be justified for the public good, the protection of someone, or the prevention of or detection of crime (Griffith, 2007). See the discussion on mandated reporting requirements in Chapter 6 for more information.

Jennifer was well-known at one of the apartment buildings in Aurora where many elderly adults lived. Jennifer had made many visits to residents in this complex over the years. The residents, although not related, had become like family to each other and welcomed Jennifer. They had an informal system of checking on each other daily and helping each other with trips to the grocery store or pharmacy. Often as Jennifer exited a client's apartment after a visit, several residents would stop Jennifer to ask how her client was doing. The neighbors were genuinely concerned and wanted to be helpful in any way possible.

Question: *How should Jennifer respond to the residents' questions about the clients she had visited?*

Evidence Example: Maintaining Boundaries and Confidentiality in Working with Families with Intimate Partner Violence

Tracy Evanson (2006) investigated the role of PHNs who conducted home visiting with families who experience intimate partner violence. Thirteen PHNs who worked in urban and rural settings in a Midwestern state participated in two semi-structured interviews. The PHNs who worked in rural settings had more challenges in keeping confidentiality, helping women find resources, getting their own support, and keeping professional-personal boundaries. Although all PHNs viewed setting boundaries as an essential part of their work with families who were experiencing intimate partner violence, Evanson concluded that the boundaries between personal and professional lives for rural PHNs were less clear than those for the non-rural nurses. The rural PHNs had learned to be flexible with boundaries because they were highly visible in the community and often knew their clients personally through attending the same church, having children who were friends, or having mutual acquaintances. Personal ties were perceived as being a barrier to disclosure of the interpersonal violence. The need to maintain confidentiality limited opportunities for PHNs to discuss the stress of their work. Rural PHNs needed to be very vigilant about maintaining confidentiality and at times needed to withhold the truth. Evanson recommended that rural agencies need to provide support opportunities for nurses who work with families that have intimate partner violence to cope with the emotional labor of their work through staff meetings and case conferences.

What Do Ethical, Legal, and Professional Accountability Mean in Public Health Nursing?

Accountability in public health nursing practice is driven by ethical and professional standards and by legal guidelines. *Public Health Nursing: Scope and Standards of Practice* (ANA, 2007) specifies areas of accountability for PHNs (see Chapter 1). PHNs have more accountability to populations in comparison to nurses in other practice settings. The PHN is accountable for improving population health. Legal accountability has been previously discussed in Chapter 6. This chapter will focus to a greater extent on the ethical accountability of public health nurses.

PHNs consider individuals, families, and communities as their clients. PHNs might experience ethical problems when they have to consider the impact or benefits and burdens of their decisions on multiple clients, population groups, and communities (Racher, 2007). Culturally diverse societies and communities might have different moral standards from each other and also different from those of the public health nurse. These differences might lead to conflicts between the public health nurse and clients. Ethnic diversity in the community requires a complex ethical framework that includes the complementary approaches of rule ethics, virtue ethics, and feminist ethics (Racher, 2007; Volbrecht, 2002).

Rule ethics uses a framework of guiding principles for decision making (Racher, 2007). Examples of rules or principles include autonomy, beneficence (promoting good), non-maleficence (preventing harm), justice, loyalty, truth-telling, and respect (Aiken, 2004; Beauchamp & Childress, 1979; Purtilo, 2005; Scoville Walker, 2004). Rule ethics is based on a biomedical model of decision making.

In contrast, virtues ethics is based on good character (Racher, 2007). One's actions are evaluated in the context of one's community. Examples of nursing virtues include compassion, honesty, courage, justice, self-confidence, resilience, practical reasoning, and integrity (Volbrecht, 2002).

Feminist ethics focuses on building relationships and reducing oppression in society (Volbrecht, 2002). Key values in a feminist ethics approach are inclusion, diversity, participation, empowerment, social justice, advocacy, and interdependence (Racher, 2007). Table 7.3 provides additional explanation about these three ethical approaches.

Table 7.3 Ethical Framework for Public Health Nursing Practice

Rule Ethics
- Defines rules or principles that are based on perceptions of fairness.
- Ethical principles are standards of conduct that guide behavior and specify moral duties and obligations (Racher, 2007).
- Community rights might be given priority over individual rights in some situations.

- Resources are given based on need, and thus might be distributed unequally (distributive justice).

- Those who have been unfairly burdened or harmed are compensated (compensatory justice).

Virtue Ethics
- Identifies characteristics of the individual (moral agent) and that person's intentions and behaviors.

- Dictates individual responsibility to develop good character and good community (Volbrecht, 2002).

- Provides foundation for codes of professional ethics, which specify professional values and virtues.

Feminist Ethics
- A core ideal is achieving social justice; applies social justice and distributive justice to social structures and context.

- Focuses on characteristics of relationships; strengthens relationships and connectedness; eliminates oppression and realigns power imbalances.

- Committed to restructuring relationships, social practices, and institutions so that people can live freer and fuller lives (Volbrecht, 2002).

Public health ethics is driven by social justice. The aim is to create a flourishing community for all rather than satisfying individual self interests. A bioethics perspective focuses more on autonomy and individual rights (Easely & Allen, 2007). Ethical challenges in public health nursing can result from the conflict between protecting the community and respecting individual autonomy. For example, individuals might be required to take medication for treatment of tuberculosis (even when they would choose otherwise) to protect the health of others. Protecting individual rights to privacy might conflict with the need to share information for benefiting the health of the public, such as in the case of reporting communicable disease to the health department so disease incidence can be monitored (Racher, 2007).

In the study by Anne Clancy and Tommy Svensson (2007) PHNs expressed that they thought they had a greater sense of responsibility than hospital nurses because the PHNs primarily worked on their own. They expressed that they felt alone with their worries and their uncertainties about what to do. Ethical decision making does not occur in a vacuum. Resolutions will be better with input from other experts in the field. PHNs need to seek out collegial and organizational support for their decision making to ensure ethical, legal, and professional accountability.

Evidence Example: Ethical Problems in Public Health Nursing

A qualitative study of 22 PHNs in Canada (11 in rural and 11 in urban settings) revealed 5 categories of ethical problems experienced in their work: 1) relationships with health care professionals, 2) systems issues such as distribution of resources and consequences of policies, 3) character of relationships with clients, 4) respect for persons, and 5) putting self at risk, which involved value conflicts or potential physical danger (Oberle & Tenove, 2000). Most of the ethical problems identified by the PHNs focused on relationships. The authors of the study explained the ethical challenge:

"Decision making in public health might be equated with a juggling act in which the nurse tries to keep many balls in the air simultaneously, always in the interests of doing 'good' for the client. Difficulties arise in defining 'good' and determining whose good should be promoted. Moreover, good must also be defined in the long term, not just the immediate present" (p. 436).

Kathleen Oberle and Sandra Tenove recommended that PHNs should have opportunities for dialogue with administrative leaders, dialogue should be multidisciplinary, and public health nursing leaders need to provide support and mentorship for ethical decision making.

What Should I Know about Delegation and Supervision in Public Health Nursing?

Much of public health nursing is independent practice, but on some occasions PHNs perform nursing care activities delegated to them, such as giving immunizations or providing care activities ordered by the physician for community-dwelling elders. On other occasions, PHNs might provide supervision for health aides, LPNs, or community health workers. When PHNs delegate an activity or task to someone, 1) the task is for a specific patient, 2) the circumstances are specific, 3) the task is delegated to a specific person, 4) clear direction and communication is given, and 5) the activity is monitored and evaluated (National Council of State Boards of Nursing and American Nurses Association, 2006). Some tasks should not be delegated because they fall in the realm of professional nursing, for example, counseling; health teaching; and activities that require nursing knowledge, skill, and judgment based on evidence or data (American Nurses Association, 1992). Tasks that can be delegated are more often repetitive and supportive in caregiving (Williams & Cooksey, 2004).

ACTIVITY
Read the case study and analyze how a PHN could ensure the Five Rights of Delegation when delegating to the family health aide. Then complete the right-hand column in the following table.

Delegation Case Study

I received a referral on a 22-year-old and her 2-month-old baby. At my initial home visit the baby appeared overweight and overfed. The young mom had started him on rice cereal in a bottle at 2 weeks. Every time he cried she gave him a bottle, even though he often struggled and tried to pull away from the nipple. I talked to her about feeding the baby and my concern about his weight, but she responded with, "Once he starts moving around, the weight will come off."

By 4 months of age the baby was 27 pounds. By now I was very concerned and called both the nurse and the doctor at the clinic, but no action was taken. Next I arranged a joint home visit with a nutritionist from WIC (Women, Infants and Children Supplemental Food Program). We counseled the mom to feed the baby only when he was truly hungry.

Two weeks later I returned to do an NCAST* feeding interaction and videotaped the mom feeding the baby. We watched the tape together and talked about hunger cues and how the baby did not appear hungry. The young mother listened but continued to feed the baby whenever he fussed or cried. It was as though she had no other way to comfort him other than to feed him. I was also becoming concerned about the baby's development as he exhibited several delays in fine motor and language when I tested him.

At this point I started visiting every 2 weeks and placed a family health aide in the home for 2 hours 1 day a week. The aide's assignment was to role model appropriate parenting and feeding. I also arranged to get a high chair for feeding the child through a nutrition program grant. Currently, I continue to coordinate services from the clinic, nutritionist, and family health aide. At the present time the baby's weight has stabilized and he has not gained any more weight.

*NCAST (Nursing Child Assessment Satellite Training) is an objective and systematic assessment of interactions between parent and child (30 hours of continuing education). It can alert the nurse to areas of concern and the need for teaching. It has been used as legal documentation in court cases of child abuse

Source: Minnesota Department of Health, Office of Public Health Practice. (2006). Wheel of public health interventions: A collection of "Getting Behind the Wheel" stories 2000–2006.

The Five Rights of Delegation	Example from Case Study
The right task is delegated for a specific client.	
The right circumstances are specifically identified (consider setting and client safety).	
The task is delegated to a specific person with knowledge, training, and experience for safe performance of the task.	
There is clear and direct communication that explains task objectives, directions, and expectations in a safe and efficient manner.	
The activity is monitored and evaluated, including giving feedback and answering questions.	

Do I Need to Become Registered to Become a Public Health Nurse?

Public Health Nursing: Scope and Standards of Practice states, "the baccalaureate degree in nursing is the educational credential for entry into public health nursing practice" (ANA, 2007, p. 10). You can look at your state's Nurse Practice Act to determine if a baccalaureate degree is required for the practice of public health nursing in your state. Some states require certification or registration for the title of public health nurse.

Sarah is very excited about public health nursing and asked Jennifer how she could obtain PHN certification. Jennifer recommended that Sarah read the Nurse Practice Act in whichever state she practices nursing after she graduates with her baccalaureate degree in nursing. Sarah can also contact the Board of Nursing in that state to learn more about nursing practice specific to that state.

Examples of Legal Requirements in Nurse Practice Acts

- California, Hawaii, Iowa, Minnesota, New York, North Carolina, South Carolina, and Wisconsin require a baccalaureate degree for PHN practice.

- In California, Minnesota, New York, and South Carolina, licensure acts or rules have language that defines the scope of public health nursing practice and reserve the use of the title "public health nurse" for those professional nurses who meet specific criteria.

- In California, public health nurse certification requires training in child abuse and neglect, and a PHN certificate is needed to use the title of "public health nurse" (California Board of Registered Nursing, 2006).

Ethical Application

When working with individuals and families, PHNs often must balance acting in the professional role with building a trusting relationship. In the attempt to find this balance in working with at-risk families, a PHN might encounter tension between different ethical perspectives. If a PHN emphasizes the expert role, the client might feel inadequate or judged.

The client might need a "friend" and want to view the PHN as a friend. However, framing the relationship as friendship implies expectations of sharing and obligation that might fall outside of the professional role. Professional caring does not carry the responsibility of friendship but carries the responsibility of ethical action based on promoting good for the client, contributing to a flourishing community, and strategizing to reduce oppression for clients and families who receive public health services.

See Table 7.4 for an application of ethical perspectives to maintaining professional boundaries. Think about the related scenarios in this chapter: 1) the adolescent mother asked Jennifer to be her friend on Facebook and 2) residents in the apartment building where Jennifer visited several elderly clients asked her how her clients were doing.

Table 7.4 Ethical Action in Maintaining Professional Boundaries

Ethical Perspective	Application
Rule Ethics (principles)	• Use expert public health nursing knowledge to promote good and prevent harm to clients and families. • Keep health information confidential to protect the client.

Ethical Perspective	Application
Virtue Ethics (character)	• Be compassionate in recognizing the hardships and health challenges encountered by clients and families. • Use caring interactions to communicate confidence in the client's ability to make positive health decisions. • Focus on building trusting relationships as a basis for mutual goal setting.
Feminist Ethics (reducing oppression)	• Connect families to resources that reduce some of the inequities they experience because of poverty. • Establish a relationship with the client that communicates valuing others as equal individuals.

ACTIVITY

For either of the two scenarios discussed earlier in the chapter (the Facebook incident or apartment residents asking about the well-being of clients), analyze the resolution to the ethical problem by answering the following questions:

What values related to the situation do you see as important to you as a professional and as a person?

Who do you think you should be as public health nurse (important virtues)?

Based on your values, and who you should be, what would you do in this situation?

Which ethical perspectives (rule ethics, virtue ethics, and feminist ethics) support your chosen action?

Key Points

- Nurse Practice Acts in each state and the Scope and Standards of Public Health Nursing both provide expectations for the professional accountability of public health nurses.

- The Public Health Intervention Wheel defines the independent interventions that public health nurses implement in their practice.

- Professional boundaries can be more challenging to maintain in public health nursing, given the community setting and long-term relationships with clients.

- Protection of patient confidentiality can be more challenging for public health nurses to assure in rural communities where many residents know the public health nurse.

- The Health Insurance Portability and Accountability Act of 1996 (HIPAA) provides legal standards for handling protected health information.

- The National Council of State Boards of Nursing and American Nurses Association developed a joint statement that explains delegation and supervision responsibilities for all nurses, which also includes public health nurses.

- Reflecting about and discussing ethical challenges in public health nursing can help the PHN practice ethically.

Exercises

Learning Examples

The following learning examples can be used to expand your knowledge about public health nursing responsibilities covered in the Nurse Practice Act in your state. In addition, the examples will help you to think about maintaining professional boundaries and acting ethically in public health nursing practice.

Nurse Practice Act

- Locate a copy of the Nurse Practice Act from your state (Internet search).

- In a small group or pairs, explore implications of the Nurse Practice Act for public health nursing practice.

   1. How does the language in the Nurse Practice Act describe the scope of nursing practice?

   2. Do any requirements apply specifically to public health nurses? If so, what are the requirements?

   3. What does the Nurse Practice Act say about delegation and supervision responsibilities of the professional nurse?

   4. Are any specific educational requirements identified?

   5. What does the Nurse Practice Act say about the ethical and legal accountability of nurses?

Professional Boundaries and Ethical Accountability

- Analyze the following scenario from the rule ethics, virtue ethics, and feminist ethics perspectives.

- Do you agree with the actions taken by the students? Why or why not?

Scenario:

Two students went to make a visit to a single mother and her three preschool children. The mother was in the final trimester of pregnancy and had severe swelling of ankles and feet. She was unable to walk. She had not been able to use a cab or a bus to get to the grocery store and had no food in the apartment. The mother reported the children had not eaten for 2 days and were very hungry. The students knew that they were not supposed to give food to their clients; however, they were very concerned about the children. They went out to their car and got their bag lunches, made sure the food was appropriate for children, and, with the mother's permission, gave lunches to the children. They also called the police and the social service agency to obtain help for the family, but first they fed the children.

Reflective Practice

Nurses who practice in health care organizations such as hospitals are constantly reminded about rules and regulations that guide their nursing practice. They are surrounded by other nursing staff and supervisors who they can quickly ask about what to do in any situation that might seem confusing. In many situations, PHNs do not have the security of having other nurses and nursing administrators immediately available to them. School nurses are often the only nursing professional in the school building. PHNs who make home visits might feel isolated and unsure of what response comprises ethical and legal action. PHNs must be knowledgeable about the scope of professional practice and guidelines for ethical and legal practice. They need to provide rationale that is based on ethical, legal, and professional guidelines to support their choice of nursing actions.

Read the case study and write down your answers to the following questions. Then discuss with classmates.

You are a public health nurse with about 40 high-risk families in your caseload. One of your clients is a 17-year-old woman, Tiffany, who has an 11-month old baby boy whom she delivered at 34 weeks gestation with a birth weight of 4 pounds and 1 ounce. Tiffany lives in a trailer court off and on with an unemployed boyfriend who has struck her twice in the last month. She will not report the assaults because he is on probation for selling drugs and he would immediately go to prison. She states, "He has promised it will never happen again."

Your initial referral to the family was for the premature birth of Jeremy, the little boy, who had respiratory complications and spent 3 weeks in the hospital before he came home. Tiffany is estranged from her mother, reporting, "She kicked me out when she found out I was pregnant." She appears to have minimal parenting skills but is receptive to your visits and is working on developing parenting skills. She has declined your referral to Early Childhood and Family Education (ECFE) activities.

Jeremy was within normal developmental limits for the first 6 months of his life, but is now starting to exhibit some delays. You suspect that his frequent illness is contributing to the developmental delays. He suffers from chronic upper respiratory illnesses and otitis media. Tiffany smokes a half pack of cigarettes per day and has not been receptive to discussing smoking cessation.

Tiffany just told you she had a pregnancy test last week and is pregnant again. The smoking is putting both Jeremy and the unborn child at risk.

Source: Adapted from case study developed by Minnesota Department of Health

How does the scope of public health nursing practice (see Chapter 1) guide the responsibilities of the public health nurse in this case study?

_____

_____

What do you think are the most relevant interventions for the PHN to implement from the Public Health Intervention Wheel?

_____

What is the PHN's ethical and legal accountability for the boyfriend's domestic violence?

_____

_____

What concerns do you have about maintaining confidentiality and professional boundaries in this case study?

_____

_____

How would you ensure ethical practice on your part in working with this family?

_____

_____

Application of Evidence

Jennifer, the PHN from Weaver County Health Department, has received a referral from the county Child Protection Services. The referral was originally made by a registered nurse who worked at the local hospital and suspected possible child abuse in a 2-year-old named Marcie who had a minor injury that required a visit to the emergency room. The child protection worker did not find any evidence of child abuse or neglect but asked to have a public health nurse follow-up on promoting positive parenting practices with the child's parents.

1. What independent nursing interventions could Jennifer use in working with the child's parents? How are these interventions consistent with the Nurse Practice Act in your state?

2. What should Jennifer remember about maintaining professional boundaries as she meets with Marcie's parents?

3. During the visit, Jennifer discovers that Marcie attends the same community day care as one of Jennifer's children, although the 2 children are not in the same group. What will Jennifer need to do to maintain confidentiality in the small community setting?

4. How do rule ethics, virtue ethics, and feminist ethics guide Jennifer's interactions with Marcie's family as she balances developing a trusting relationship with the family, keeping information confidential, providing parenting guidance, and monitoring for possible child abuse or neglect?

Think, Explore, Do

1. Think of an ethical concern that you have encountered in your public health nursing clinical. How can you use rule ethics, virtue ethics, and feminist ethics to help you know how to act ethically in this situation? What ethical perspective offers the most guidance?

2. Think about a situation in which you were concerned about maintaining professional boundaries. What are some strategies you could use to avoid a potential violation of boundaries?

3. How do you think Facebook should be used in communication with your peers, teachers, and clients?

4. How will you balance expectations for independent practice with collaboration to ensure that you are ethically, legally, and professionally accountable in your practice?

5. How can you create a support system for yourself to ensure your actions are consistent with the Nurse Practice Act?

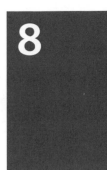

COMPETENCY #6:
Effectively Communicates with Communities, Systems, Individuals, Families, and Colleagues

8

By Marjorie A. Schaffer
with Rose Jost and Linda J. W. Anderson

Angie is a public health nursing student in a suburban public health department. Her public health nurse preceptor, Janet, asked her to create a poster for the WIC clinic (Women, Infants and Children supplemental food program) on dental health for children. Angie had no experience with creating a poster for display in a professional setting. She also could not remember learning anything about dental health in her nursing program. What does Angie need to know to create the poster, and what steps does she need to take to create a poster that effectively communicates the importance of dental health to the population served by the WIC clinic? In addition, Janet asked Angie to assist her with creating a PowerPoint presentation to update staff on new strategies to promote oral health, such as tooth varnishing.

Angie remembered that there was a population-based public health nursing competency that focused on communication in public health nursing. She pulled out her handout on Competency #6 to re-view the communication skills that would help her create a successful poster on dental health. Angie also realized she would need to update her computer skills on the most recent change in software needed to create a PowerPoint presentation.

ANGIE'S NOTEBOOK

Competency #6: Effectively communicates with communities, systems, individuals, families, and colleagues.

- Interacts respectfully, sensitively, and effectively with everyone

- Presents accurate demographic, statistical, programmatic, and scientific information

- Selects appropriate communication methods, such as audiovisual, technological, and multimedia tools

- Organizes written materials that are clear, concise, accurate, and complete

- Utilizes sound teaching/learning principles that consider specific characteristics of the community, system, individual, or family

- Communicates electronically using basic word processing, Internet, e-mail, Netiquette, attachments, and web-based systems

Useful Definitions

Health Literacy: The degree to which individuals have the capacity to obtain, process, and understand basic health information and services needed to make health decisions (Institute of Medicine, 2004).

Learning Styles: Processes by which you learn; these vary among learners.

Motivational Interviewing: A counseling technique that focuses on behavior change through emphasizing a side-by-side companionable approach that supports client's own values and reasons for change in contrast to a traditional approach of expert provider and passive recipient (Miller, 2004).

Social Marketing: "Utilizes commercial marketing principles and technologies, for programs developed to influence the knowledge, attitudes, values, beliefs, behaviors, and practices of the population of interest" (Keller, Strohschein, Lia-Hoagberg, & Schaffer, 2004, p. 456).

Reaching Populations with Health Messages

Learning communication strategies for working with individuals and families is an essential component of your nursing education. Also, you often learn about communicating with colleagues as you focus on leadership strategies, teamwork, and delegation in a leadership course. However, strategies for communicating with communities and systems involve additional skills. These skills include learning how to clearly organize and present data and health information, using technology in communication, and applying teaching-learning principles that integrate knowledge about the learner (individual or community group).

Interacting Respectfully, Sensitively, and Effectively with Everyone

PHNs use a repertoire of basic communication skills in all their work. Effective interpersonal communication, involving the use of self, is especially essential for the counseling and health teaching interventions. The purpose of the communication is to benefit the clients through increasing the clients' participation in decision making about ways to improve their health. Keep in mind that the client might be an individual or a family. The following list contains tips for effective communication with individuals and families.

- Use active listening.
- Model "I" messages (I think…, I feel…).
- Paraphrase and summarize message to confirm client's meaning.
- Pay attention to silence and nonverbal communication.
- Consider client's comfort with degree of physical space between persons.

- Ask open-ended questions.

- Consider context of communication environment—privacy and confidentiality.

- Use touch if it enhances the communication and is acceptable to client.

    Sources: Green, 2006; Public Health Nursing Section, 2001

Public health nurses (PHNs) can use motivational interviewing to encourage positive health behaviors (Shinitzky & Kub, 2001). Motivational interviewing is a specific kind of counseling strategy in which the professional assists clients to become aware of their values and the reasons they might have for changing their behavior. The purpose of motivational interviewing is to encourage clients to change from behaviors that hurt their health to behaviors that improve their health. Five steps are involved in behavior change:

1. Pre-contemplation to recognize the problem

2. Contemplation about making a change

3. Preparation or making a commitment to change

4. The action or the change itself

5. Maintaining the lifestyle change

    (DiClemente & Proschaska, 1998)

PHNs can determine the relevant step of behavior change the client is experiencing and then use motivational interviewing to encourage clients to change their health behaviors. Some clients might move through these steps quickly whereas others might remain at one step for a period of time. The PHN follows the cues of the client in motivational interviewing. Strategies include the following:

- Express empathy, which shows acceptance of the person.

- Develop discrepancies by asking questions about current behaviors and consequences of those behaviors that may be contributing to poor health.

- Avoid arguing about the client's beliefs, choices, or actions because disagreement will not lead to positive behavior change

- Roll with resistance to change by continuing to listen to the client and reflect on what you are hearing to facilitate working toward mutual determined solutions.

- Support self-efficacy, which means the client is responsible for choosing and initiating the behavior change (Shinitzky & Kub, 2001, p. 181).

The emphasis is on empowering clients to make decisions that benefit their health. Empowerment results in a sense of competence, a willingness to take action, and the opportunity to make decisions (Toofany, 2006). The example in Table 8.1 illustrates the use of motivational interviewing with a pregnant adolescent who smokes.

Table 8.1   Motivational Interviewing

Motivational Interviewing Strategy	Client Statement	PHN Statement
Express empathy	I started smoking when I was 15.	It can be difficult to stop smoking because the body is dependent on the nicotine in tobacco.
Develop discrepancies	I know I should stop smoking.	What have you learned about why it is important to quit smoking during pregnancy or around your baby?
Avoid arguing	I don't really think it is so bad. My best friend smoked during her pregnancy and her baby is fine.	I'm glad to hear your friend's baby is ok. Let's take a look at how smoking might affect your baby's health.
Roll with resistance	I just don't know if I can quit. I have so much going on in my life—smoking helps me feel more relaxed.	I would like to hear more about ways that help you to relax.
Support self-efficacy	I wish I could quit smoking.	It is your choice. What do you think you can do to have a healthy baby?

Effective, client-focused communication is essential for public health nursing practice. In a study based on interviews with 13 Norwegian PHNs (Tveiten & Severinsson, 2006), the nurses communicated and thought about their communication with families through 1) building a trusting relationship, 2) looking beyond the current situation, 3) creating partnership and equality, and 4) considering challenges in promoting the individual or family's best interests.

Building a trusting relationship. How do PHNs build a trusting relationship in client situations where they face a great difference in lifestyle and worldviews? The nurses in the study said they built trust with families by confirming and supporting them; sharing thoughts, experiences, and knowledge; and respectfully approaching the client (Tveiten & Severinsson, 2006). Listening to the needs of the family was a primary focus. One PHN talked about what she did as a dialogue as opposed to a monologue. The nurse used dialogue to create an opportunity to talk about health promotion while respecting the needs and family norms. Building trust means being honest about one's expert knowledge as well as lack of knowledge.

Joyce Zerwekh (1991) also identified building trust as a key competency that public health nurses displayed in working successfully with maternal/child home visit clients. The following strategies to build trust are grounded in basic therapeutic relationship techniques.

- Getting through the door—You are on their territory

- Backing off—Don't pressure

- Listening—Find out what their concerns are

- Discovering and affirming strengths—Look for the positive

- Not judging—Don't be shocked

- Persistence—Keep making contact

  Source: Zerwekh, 1991

Looking beyond the current situation. This means thinking about the "big picture." What is the best way to approach the family to achieve the goal? It often takes time to develop a relationship that makes it possible to work collaboratively toward that goal. Some clients might reach the selected goal in one or two months. Other clients might require many visits on a long-term basis (more than a year) for making progress toward the selected goal. Also, the goal might need to be revised over time to make it more realistic or possible for the client to achieve. By learning more about the client's outlook on life, the PHN can be more realistic about what change is possible and ensure a mutual goal-setting process (Carey, 1989). Listening and encouraging reflection about what the client needs helps the PHN to look beyond the current interaction. As part of the dialogue, ask, "Have we talked about what is important to you?"

Creating partnership and equality. The PHN uses communication strategies to strengthen the ability of the client to make decisions that improve health. The PHN listens, affirms, and supports positive coping strategies through dialogue. Also the PHN conveys the belief that the client will make good decisions.

Considering challenges in promoting the individual or family's best interests. In many situations, the PHN might have different personal values, such as the meaning of health and the importance of being on time, than what the client believes is important. As a public health nurse, you need to be aware of any assumptions or biases you might have about a client's lifestyle choices or cultural background. The purpose of the interaction is empowering the client rather than interacting with an attitude that you know what is best. Although we do not want to be controlling in our interactions, we must think about and resolve any tensions, such as disagreement about parenting practices or when a client does not follow up on a referral for health care, so that we can continue to work with the client. When is the PHN an expert and when is the client the expert? Keep in mind that, although as a PHN or nursing student you have expert knowledge about community resources and strategies for promoting better health, the client has expert knowledge about their life situation and motivation for changing health behaviors. You need to have expert knowledge but not be "a know it all" (Tveiten & Severinsson, 2006). When does the PHN encourage the client to act independently versus depending on the nurse? By reflecting on these tensions we might experience in our interactions with individuals and families, we can become more skilled in using communication to collaborate with clients on reaching their goals.

Presenting Demographic, Statistical, Programmatic, and Scientific Information

PHNs must be able to transition from communicating effectively in interactions with individuals and families to communicating information about data for making decisions about public health interventions that improve the health of population groups and communities. PHNs are called on to translate complex concepts and information into terms that are accurate and easily understood by the general public. Health data and scientifically based information must be reduced and reformatted to enhance understanding. Simplification of both verbal and written communication of information is required. When crafting messages, you need to engage the public to help identify the public concerns. To involve the public, PHNs can recruit community members for an expert advisory group to give input on how to respond to public health data about their community (Holmes, 2008).

The evidence example that follows, written by a public health nursing student, explains the process of translating data for public understanding and decision making. A student group completed an analysis of safe walking paths and made a recommendation for action to community decision makers. The student project was published in the local city newspaper and the city obtained a grant for improving walking paths.

Evidence Example: Presenting Data on Improving Walking Path Safety

We proceeded to plan how we would assess the walkability of the city, implement our plan, and eventually evaluate the results of our study. The purpose [was to identify] areas that could use improvement to increase the percentage of people who chose to walk, ultimately resulting in lower obesity rates and obesity-related health problems. We began to prepare for this project by doing background research on the problem of obesity, which health problems came from being overweight, and the role of walking in reducing these problems. After that, we planned how we would implement our study by looking at city maps and selecting the routes that we wished to walk. We also got a standardized survey to fill out as we went, which measured things such as the presence of sidewalks, behavior of drivers, and the aesthetic appeal of the route for an overall score on a scale of 1 to 30. Over a period of several weeks, we proceeded to walk each of these paths and mark down the positive and negative attributes of each as we saw them. After completing each route at least once, we began to evaluate our data. We compiled out results and came up with an average score for each of the five areas on the survey. Using these results, we were able to pinpoint a couple of areas that we thought could use the most work. More specifically, there was an overall need for more crosswalks and aesthetic appeal on several of the routes. The data were presented to a group of city officials along with our conclusions so they could have some data to help guide them in the use of their grant money. Evidence was needed to guide the use of grant money to improve the streets, hopefully increasing the physical health of the community members.

Source: Senior Public Health Nursing Student

Using Audiovisual, Technology, and Multimedia Tools

In today's technological world, we are bombarded with messages. What strategies are best for communicating health messages that people actually will hear and understand? Health communication involves the creation of messages that inform, motivate, and influence change for positive health behavior (Chaffee, 2000). These messages are created for organizations, such as schools, the workplace, and churches, and for the general public. The messages are intended to promote health and prevent disease with the goal of improving health status and quality of life for individuals living in communities. Six stages guide structured health communication messages:

1. Planning and strategy selection

2. Selection of communication channels, such as radio, television, newspapers, or pamphlets

3. Development of materials and pretesting how well they work

4. Implementation

5. Assessment of effectiveness

6. Feedback to refine the program (McGrath, 1995)

Skills needed to communicate health promotion messages to communities include presentation, group facilitation, and social marketing skills (Zahner & Gredig, 2005). PHNs are called on to present health data to local leaders, policymakers, and community partners and to interpret the meaning of the data in relation to the community's health status (Jakeway, Cantrell, Cason, & Talley, 2006). PHNs use group leadership and facilitation skills to bring to the table voices of all stakeholders to make decisions about community-level public health interventions.

Cultural variables influence whether the information is viewed as important—variables including unique health beliefs, values, norms, expectations, and language barriers (Kreps & Sparks, 2008). To increase the likelihood of successful communication, be sure to involve representatives from the cultural group in the design of the communication strategy and pretest it to ensure readability, understanding, and appeal. Feedback mechanisms such as consumer surveys, focus groups, hotlines, and comment cards can help to validate whether the strategy was effective or not and provide ideas for improvement (Kreps & Sparks, 2008).

Public health uses strategies from the commercial marketing field to design health programs that "influence the knowledge, attitudes, values, beliefs, behaviors, and practices of the population of interest" (Public Health Nursing Section, 2001, p. 285). In public health, this work is known as social marketing (see definition in this chapter's Notebook page) because messages are constructed to change social norms of unhealthy behaviors to create social environments that support healthy behaviors. For example, social marketing messages to prevent fetal alcohol syndrome (a possible consequence of ingesting alcohol while pregnant) might include radio and television ads, billboards, and posted messages at bars about the harmful effects of alcohol for the fetus (Public Health Nursing Section).

Social marketing messages should be delivered in the right context and channels to motivate recipients of the communication to pay attention to the health information (Evans & McCormack, 2008). PHNs often work with others in planning, implementing, and evaluating a social marketing intervention. In the planning stage, consider the social environment, target audience, priority health concerns, and effective evidence-based strategies for delivering messages. Develop a plan that includes attention to the "4 Ps"— product, price, place, and promotion. Flexibility in working with community partners and commitment to fulfilling responsibilities contribute to a successful implementation stage. In the evaluation stage, ask whether the intended behavioral change was accomplished (Public Health Nursing Section, 2001). Following are tips for effective social marketing.

- Involve opinion leaders (for example, community leaders, elders, and respected individuals whose opinion is valued by others)

- Promote active-learner involvement

- Provide for repetition and reinforcement

- Avoid message clutter and information overload

- Consider socioeconomic factors, cultural beliefs, values, geographic location, and local norms in speech and dress

- Use stories and anecdotes in the presentation of risk data

- Use several approaches (written, oral, or electronic)

- Engage the target population in the development process

- Anticipate and manage use of controversy and conflict

- Avoid messages that reinforce stereotypes or contradict verbal messages

Sources: Evans & McCormack, 2008; Public Health Nursing Section, 2001; Westdahl & Page-Goertz, 2006

Targeted health messages are developed for specific population groups. Tailored health communications are client-centered and involve customizing messages based on individuals' lifestyle, location of residence, and consumer habits. Possible social marketing communication channels include television, radio, Internet, posters, periodicals, and pamphlets and other written material. In addition to using mass media, you need to locate opinion leaders (persons who have social influence and have adopted the desired behavior or attitude). Opinion leaders act as catalysts for behavior change. Because humans are social beings, connection to social relationships influences adoption of healthy behavior (Levy-Storms, 2005). For example, to promote mammography screening for older women PHNs could focus on beauty salons where older women are likely to discuss health-related concerns or initiate a "Tell a Friend" campaign in which women name 10 friends to call about getting a mammogram (Calle, Miracle-McMahill, Moss, & Heath,1994). For mammography screening, the opinion leaders are older women who have knowledge about the effectiveness and importance of getting a mammogram for early identification of breast cancer.

Evidence Example for Social Marketing: Breast-feeding on a Navajo Reservation

Researchers evaluated individual, community, and systems interventions to improve breast-feeding decision rates among a Navajo population (Wright, Naylor, Wester, Bauer, & Sutcliffe, 1997). The Navajo Infant Feeding Project implemented the following interventions: 1) provided written and videotaped information on breast-feeding for prenatal and postpartum teaching (individual and family level), 2) created a positive view of breast-feeding through community empowerment techniques such as radio spots, infant T-shirts, billboards, and slide shows (community level), 3) educated health care providers to increase their knowledge and skills for the promotion of breast-feeding (systems level), and 4) provided visits on the maternity unit from a native bilingual "foster grandmother" to talk about her own breast-feeding experience and its contribution to children's health (opinion leader). Measurement of outcomes showed an improvement in breast-feeding rates. Both the initiation and duration of breast-feeding increased. Fewer infants were given formula in the hospital, and the mean age at which formula was introduced increased from 12 days to 48 days.

After reviewing evidence in her textbook on effective health education and social marketing, Angie decided she should make a list of the next steps needed to create a dental health poster for the WIC clinic. Angie knows that the population attending the WIC clinic has a high percentage of Latino families. In addition, WIC clinics are offered in several different locations in the county. What does Angie need to think about before she begins to work on the poster?

ACTIVITY

Based on what you have learned about social marketing, answer the following questions:

What are the questions that Angie needs to ask, and what information sources does she need to explore?

What does she need to do to create an effective poster?

Apply the six stages for guiding structured health communication messages to strategies you will use to create the poster.

What tips for social marketing did you find most useful for planning the poster?

Organizing Written Educational Materials

When crafting messages, PHNs consider the health literacy of the intended target group. Health literacy is the capacity that individuals have to find and understand information about health and health services that can be used to make health-related decisions. The inability to understand health information might mean individuals do not engage in effective self-care practices and increase the risk for hospitalization (Clark, 2008; Weiss, 2007). For groups with lower literacy, effective strategies for communicating health information include the following: 1) use plain language (nonmedical), 2) use visuals, 3) talk more slowly, 4), limit information (two or three key points that are repeated), 5) use a "teach-back" process when possible, and 6) encourage questions (Black, 2008; Weiss, 2007). In a teach-back process, clients are asked to restate the information in their words or demonstrate a specific skill to others, such as a peer group. To engage the reader in written information, give examples that reflect the age, gender, and culture of the targeted population group (DeBuono, 2002). You will find more information about health literacy in Appendix B.

In some settings, PHNs might work with a media or graphic design specialist to communicate clear, captivating, and motivating health messages. Effective messages result from clear and simple writing, using a layout that enhances readability, and adding pictures that enhance the message. Following is a list of tips to improve written messages.

- Use an active voice rather than passive. For example, use "Eat five servings of fruits and vegetables" rather than "Five servings of fruits and vegetables should be eaten."

- Use subheadings.

- Use short sentences of 8 to 10 words that are varied by a few longer sentences of 12 to 15 words. Use short paragraphs.

- Summarize main points to improve understanding.

- Use no more than 5 items in a list.

- Use underlining or bold to emphasize key points rather than italics or caps.

- Use large, easily readable font.

- Avoid large blocks of information and use white space to provide a more inviting space to the reader.

- Paper and ink should contrast for readability.

- Because pictures are remembered, show the behavior you want people to do.

  Source: Substance Abuse & Mental Health Service Administration Network, 1994. http://www.actforyouth. net/documents/YDM%20pdf6.4C%20handout.pdf

Using Teaching-Learning Principles

Public health nurses provide health education to promote better health for their clients. The goal is to motivate clients to learn about ways to promote their own health and then act on that knowledge. See the following list on health education tips that integrate important teaching-learning principles. Teaching-learning principles help you assess how the learner learns. Then you can plan the content and method of teaching that best fits the client situation.

- Target health education messages to the specific audience, rather than trying to cover all information.

- Learner readiness impacts what is learned—health status, health values, developmental characteristics, prior learning experiences.

- Motivation affects learning—use life goals, self-concept, responsibility, quality of life, and other factors that can "hook" and are meaningful to the learner.

- Active learning is best. Have the learner demonstrate or repeat learning.

- Use learning objectives to guide your teaching plan. Objectives should be written, clear, and measureable.

- Send a clear message that is easily understood. Avoid overwhelming the learner with excess materials. Avoid professional jargon. Use short sentences and simple, one- and two-syllable words.

- Use visuals to enhance printed materials and verbal messages.

- Create a comfortable learning environment that is free from distractions and interruptions (ask client to turn off the TV).

- When possible, integrate a variety of learning styles to deliver content.

- Base content on best evidence—review literature for most recent evidence-based information. Give credit to information sources.

- Link information to prior knowledge.

- Allow time for interaction to apply information.

- For written materials, use large type fonts, white space, and bulleted information to prevent readers from being overwhelmed by content.

- Reinforce written materials with verbal messages.

- Use multiple methods to assess understanding of content, such as questioning and demonstration.

  Sources: Clark, 2008; Kolb, 1984, 2005; Onega & Devers, 2008; Whitman, 1998

Consider the learning style that is predominant for the individual or group that you are teaching. Preferences for how, where, and when to learn differ from individual to individual and group to group. Because we all tend to teach from our own learning style, you must evaluate the style of the individual client or group members. When you adapt your teaching to the learner's preferred or natural learning style, the effectiveness of communication for health education is increased.

David Kolb (1984, 2005) identified four different learning styles: diverging, assimilating, converging, and accommodating. In the diverging style, individuals like to reflect about concrete experiences. They enjoy brainstorming, generating ideas, and working in groups. Assimilating learners are more interested in abstract ideas; they prefer lectures, reading, and having time to think logically. Converging learners like to apply what they have learned for its practical use and find solutions to problems. They are more focused on technology than on interactions with people. Finally, accommodating learners like to learn from "hands-on" experience. They rely more on people for information and like to take action. You can provide a variety of strategies to appeal to the variety of learning styles that individuals might have.

> *Angie is ready to design the poster. Angie decides to create a layout for her poster. She plans to ask a roommate who is a communication major to evaluate her planned layout. She also realizes that she needs to ask her public health nursing preceptor to evaluate her plan. She is not sure about the reading level of the population group who will be viewing the WIC poster. She knows that her preceptor is very familiar with this population.*

ACTIVITY

Design a layout for the poster on dental health for the WIC clinic. Consider the following:

How could Angie learn more about the population served by the WIC clinic?

What teaching-learning principles should Angie keep in mind as she designs the poster?

What tips for effective written communication will you use for the poster?

Communicating Electronically

Electronic communication includes word processing skills; Internet savvy; facility with e-mail, including knowing how to attach documents to e-mail messages; and the navigation of web-based systems. Protecting confidentiality and communicating respectfully are essential when you are sending e-mail messages. Because much of the professional communication in the public health setting involves e-mail, you need to practice ethical and respectful e-mail communication. Appendix B includes two resources for respectful e-mail communication. In addition, you can use the Internet to deliver public health information (Bennett & Glasgow, 2008). The Internet offers an option for broad dissemination to populations in need of health information who have online access. However, information on the Internet can also be overwhelming, sometimes contradictory, and in the worst case, inaccurate. A challenge for researchers is to determine the potential of Internet interventions to influence positive behavior change and improved health outcomes.

Evidence Example: Delivering Public Health Interventions through the Internet

Gary Bennett and Russell Glasgow (2009) reviewed the evidence on effectiveness of public health Internet-based interventions, including interventions that focused on smoking cessation, increasing physical activity, weight loss, and drug-abuse prevention. Health information delivered via the Internet has resulted in positive changes in knowledge, social support, health behaviors, and self-efficacy. High rates of attrition are reported, as high as 40% to 50%. Use of the website tends to drop off during the early weeks of the intervention. Improvement in use of the website occurred with reminders through postcards, e-mail, and phone calls. The authors of this study suggested that human counselor support could increase use of the website, but would add to the cost of the intervention. They also suggested that tailored messages and social networking might increase the amount of learning, but noted a lack of research on the contribution of social networking strategies to improved health outcomes. Most Internet interventions that have been evaluated are individually focused.

When Angie completed the poster, she remembered that Janet, her preceptor, had asked her to help prepare a PowerPoint presentation on oral health for public health staff. Angie decided to do some preplanning before her next meeting with Janet. Because of her work on the poster, Angie had accumulated a large amount of information on oral health from journal articles and government websites. However, she was perplexed about how to organize the content, how much information to include, and what information would be most useful and interesting to staff. Then she remembered the same principles she had used to guide her work on the poster were also applicable to creating effective messages in the PowerPoint presentation.

 ## ACTIVITY

Think about the PowerPoint presentations you have viewed. What did you like about the way content was organized and presented? What enhanced your learning? What aspects would you like to be different to increase your interest and learning?

Explain how the six stages for creating structured health communication messages apply to developing the PowerPoint presentation on oral health for staff.

Which tips for improving written messages do you think are most relevant for creating the PowerPoint presentation?

Which teaching-learning principles are important to remember in your planning for the presentation?

Ethical Application

When people communicate with one another, messages might be confusing, misunderstood, or responded to with a high degree of emotion, such as fear or anger. The public health nurse is accountable to provide professional communication that considers the consequences of the communication for individuals, family, communities, systems, and colleagues. See Table 8.7 on the application of ethical perspectives to communication.

Table 8.7 Ethical Action in Communication

Ethical Perspective	Application
Rule Ethics (principles)	• Maintain the confidentiality of private health care information. • Ensure the accuracy of health information, because wrong information could result in harm and/or legal liability. • Consider the impact of communication on others in the client's environment—evaluate whether communication could contribute to client harm (such as in situations of abuse). • When using an interpreter, explain that you expect a verbatim translation to avoid inaccurate or misleading messages.
Virtue Ethics (character)	• When collecting information from individuals and families and developing large data sets, collect only the information needed for decision making. This respects the time of clients and staff. • Be respectful of the clients and build on positives if change is needed. • In situations of limited time or limited client capability to learn, prioritize the most important health education needed to avoid overwhelming the clients. • Consider that clients might interpret health education as a criticism of their behavior.
Feminist Ethics (reducing oppression)	• Create an environment for the communication that is comfortable, welcoming, and affirming. • Consider client vulnerability in communication of sensitive information.

When Angie's preceptor saw the poster plan, Janet responded, "I really like the clear and simple messages. I can see that you have not overwhelmed your audience with too much information. I can see that you have emphasized the risk for 'baby bottle tooth decay.' I think that is very good but what you have written sounds negative, almost critical of parents. I wonder if you could approach this more positively and emphasize what the parent can do to prevent baby bottle tooth decay. I think the picture is good to include because that helps parents to know what should be prevented." Janet provided Angie with some additional resources:

- *Baby Bottle Tooth Decay—American Dental Association http://www.ada.org/3034.aspx*

- *Cavities/Tooth Decay—Mayo Clinic http://www.mayoclinic.com/health/baby-bottle-tooth-decay/AN01969*

ACTIVITY

How can you communicate the information on baby bottle tooth decay on the poster in a way that does not blame parents but helps them to know what they can do to promote dental health for their child?

What is an example of health communication that could promote harm?

After Janet and Angie discussed the revisions needed on the poster, Janet suggested that it would be helpful for WIC clinic participants to have a take-away pamphlet on dental health with some of the same information presented on the poster. Angie responded, "I'm not sure I have enough time to create a pamphlet. I don't know much about how to use the computer to create a polished pamphlet." Janet suggested that Angie work with the health department communications specialist who had expertise with software for creating pamphlets. Angie consulted with Joan, the Communications Specialist at the health department, about how to organize key oral health information in a simple and attractive pamphlet. They collaborated on the development of the pamphlet. Joan used Angie's ideas and created a draft of the pamphlet for Janet and Angie to review. Angie was excited when she saw the result. She commented, "Now, families who come to the WIC clinic can take information home with them about oral health and resources for dental health services."

Key Points

- PHNs need to develop effective communication skills at all levels of practice—with individuals, families, communities, and systems.

- Motivational interviewing is an effective strategy for promoting positive health behavior change.

- Building trust enhances healthy behavior change.

- Health education strategies are based on the characteristics, the motivation, and the learning styles of the client or group.

- Health communication messages are crafted based on the literacy level, cultural inclusiveness, and involvement of consumers in the development of messages.

- PHNs use social marketing to communicate health messages to targeted population groups.

- PHNs use interdisciplinary communication to collaborate with other public health experts in creating effective health communication messages.

Exercises

Learning Examples for Effective Communication Strategies

The literature has many examples of activities that provide opportunities to learn about effective practices for communicating health information. In addition, interdisciplinary learning activities are helpful in preparing you for the reality of working with different disciplines. You must learn how to come to a consensus on common goals and strategies to improve population health. Following is a list of learning examples for effective communication strategies.

- *Presented targeted health information at senior food commodity distribution centers* that included heart healthy recipes and samples made from the recipes (Sowan, Moffatt, & Canales, 2004).

- *Developed a Medicaid Dental Access Fact Booklet* with current information on how to access dental care (Sowan et al., 2004).

- *Interviewed key informants about concerns in the neighborhood* for a research study and discovered residents were fearful about gang violence (Ervin & Cowell, 2004).

- *Implemented a prevention project to reduce deaths from motor vehicle accidents* in a rural Appalachian county (nursing, medical, and public health students). Students interviewed key informants, worked with a community coalition on a media campaign, conducted a driver safety fair, and wrote articles for the local newspaper. The community had a reduction in automobile-related fatalities, and the state initiated an investigation on improving the roadway (Goodrow, Scherzer, & Florence, 2004).

- *Partnered with a community to implement health fairs at selected agencies*—a pregnant and parenting teen residential program, a community center that served an immigrant and refugee population, an alternative school, and a residential care home for elders nursing (social work, physical therapy, and medical students). In addition to presenting and providing targeted health information at the health fairs, the students learned group communication skills through e-mails and face-to-face meetings as they worked in interdisciplinary teams. Each of the interdisciplinary teams presented their health fair project at an evaluation dinner (Maltby, 2006).

- *Developed folic acid educational and supplementation initiative in Kentucky*—students implemented a program to provide evidence-based information to college women about the effects of folic acid in the reduction of neural tube defects and to encourage folic acid supplementation before pregnancy (Anderson, Richmond, & Stanhope, 2004).

Reflective Practice

Effective communication is foundational to the implementation of all 17 interventions of the Public Health Interventions. The necessary communication skills do vary according to whether the intervention is at the individual/family, community, or systems levels. Expectations for PHNs' skill base have grown with the development of communication technology. Local health departments often have staff members who are skilled in data management and analysis and have Social Marketing skills; however, PHNs needs basic word processing skills, the ability to work with spreadsheets and input data, and the ability to collaborate with information technology staff in development of health information materials. PHNs can bring expertise in understanding the needs of the population, teaching-learning principles, and knowledge about health and illness to Collaboration on creating health information messages for individuals, groups, and communities.

Use key concepts and ideas presented in this chapter to design a school campaign to decrease tobacco use among teens. You can use the following Teaching Plan template in Figure 8.1 for learner readiness assessment, identification of expected outcomes, key content, resources, and evaluation plan.

Student _____ Teaching Plan _____ Date _____

Educational Topic _____

Description of Learner(s) _____

Learner Readiness Assessment and Plan

PEEK	Learner Strengths and Barriers	Teaching-Learning Approaches & Strategies
P Physical	Cognitive Abilities Communication Abilities (verbal, non-verbal, written) Language Registry (formal versus informal) Developmental Level	
E Emotional	Current Stress, Coping, Resilience Motivation for Learning Readiness for Learning—Stages • Pre-contemplation • Contemplation • Preparation • Action • Maintenance	
E Experiential	Culture and Languages Spoken Past Experiences with Health Care/Specific Health Topic	
K Knowledge	Language Literacy Health Care Literacy Present Knowledge of Topic/Past Health Education	

Source: Shinitzky & Kub (2001)

(continues)

Goal and Learner Priorities for Teaching Module					
Time/ Pacing	Behavioral Outcomes At the completion of this presentation the learner will be able to:	Brief Content Outline	Teaching— Learning Resources	Evaluation & Documentation Methods—Measures
	Outcome #1			
	Outcome #2			

Figure 8.1   Teaching plan

Source: St. Catherine University, 2008. Developed by Lois Devereaux, Karen Ryan, and Patricia M. Schoon.

How will teaching-learning principles guide your campaign design (learner-readiness, motivation, active learning)?

_____

_____

How will consideration of health literacy influence your plan?

_____

_____

How will you use knowledge about learning styles in planning the campaign?

_____

_____

Who will you collaborate with to design the campaign?

_____

_____

How will you use social marketing principles to design the campaign?

_____

_____

What is the key health message that you want to convey to the teen school population?

_____

_____

What are some strategies that you can use to involve the teens in planning the campaign?

_____

_____

Application of Evidence

Janet's public health department has collaborated with the local hospital and county social services to establish a suicide prevention hotline. Janet is representing the health department in the Suicide Prevention Coalition that worked to establish the hotline. The coalition is now working on a strategy for communicating the availability of the hotline to the community. The coalition members decide that they need to use multiple methods to communicate this new community resource. How can the coalition members use the evidence on effective communication strategies to reach the community?

1. How should the school nurse at the local high school communicate the availability of the suicide hotline to students, teachers, and parents?

2. What data about suicide might motivate individuals and organizations in the community to be concerned about suicide as a health problem? How should the data be communicated?

3. What tips for effective social marketing should be used in communicating the availability of the suicide hotline?

4. How can the coalition use electronic communication to reach a larger community audience?

 ## Think, Explore, Do

Using the poster example discussed in this chapter, work through the following questions for dental health or a poster on another topic.

1. Who will look at the poster? Will it be only for adults, or will children be included?

2. What is the literacy level and languages of the viewers?

3. What are some sources of reliable information about the topic?

4. Where will the poster be displayed?

5. How far away will viewers be from the poster? How close can people get to it?

6. Is there room to have handouts nearby or on the poster for viewers to take?

7. How can it be designed to grab attention and pull people in to look at it?

8. How long is it expected that the poster will be used or displayed?

9. What are the key health issues to focus on in the poster? What key issue will you focus on, and what is the rationale for your choice?

10. What are the two learning objectives you want your target audience to achieve?

11. How can the poster be designed so that information is secure and firmly attached?

12. How could the presentation be interactive for the viewer?

13. What other health education activities could be used along with the poster to enhance learning?

14. How can the clinic environment be organized to focus attention on the poster?

COMPETENCY #7:
Establishes and Maintains Caring Relationships with Communities, Systems, Individuals, and Families

By Carolyn M. Garcia
with Christine C. Andres, Maureen A. Alms, and Cheryl H. Lanigan

Susan, a public health nurse (PHN) for a couple of years, has been developing her skills as a family home visiting nurse. She works with young families her supervisor has identified as high-risk. She has been slowly increasing her caseload. The population that Susan serves is composed of single, young mothers who need support with their parenting and identifying normal development for their children.

One of Susan's first families was a young mother named Julie with four children. Julie had her first child at 16 years of age and then proceeded to have two additional children before moving to the community Susan served as a PHN. Julie was not involved in a committed relationship and had no job. She became part of Susan's caseload when a Women, Infants and Children's (WIC) nurse referred her for a PHN baby visit after the birth of her fourth child.

At the baby visit, Susan established the foundation for a strong nurse-family relationship. Julie was open about many issues with Susan, including the fact that the two older children were not living with her, but with each of their fathers. She told Susan that she was unable to be a "good mother" to them. She was very excited about the birth of her new son. Susan explored Julie's strengths and needs. It was apparent that Julie could benefit from some parenting information and anticipatory guidance for the 2-year-old and newborn that she planned to parent. Julie was very excited about the program that Susan described, which entailed monthly visits until her newborn turned three or until she felt she was no longer benefiting from the program.

SUSAN'S NOTEBOOK

Competency #7: Establishes and maintains caring relationships with communities, systems, individuals, and families.

- Demonstrates trust, respect, empathy
- Follows through with commitments
- Maintains appropriate boundaries
- Demonstrates tact and diplomacy
- Seeks assistance when needed in managing relationships

> **Useful Definitions**
>
> Caring: "Means listening to 'more than what is said'" (Schulte, 2000, p. 7).
>
> "Facilitates the possibility for a client to feel hope for healing and comfort and/or develop resilience" (Warelow, Edward, & Vinek, 2008, p.146).
>
> "Creates a range of possibilities and can be the catalyst of change for the care recipient" (Warelow et al., 2008, p. 147).
>
> Professional Relationships: "Key elements include: the need to listen well, establish trust, offer respect and advocacy, avoid power-over interactions and care of self in order to offer care for others" (Jackson, 2010, p. 181).

Touching Lives Without Stepping on Toes

It is probably not an exaggeration to state that most individuals who choose to become nurses have an inherent desire to care for other human beings. In some ways, caring is synonymous with nursing. As a profession, nursing is a process of assessment, planning, intervention, and evaluation delivered in a context of caring with goals of prevention, healing, recovery, or peaceful transition. As a discipline, nursing is contributing knowledge and advancing science about the complex interplay of health-environment-person-nursing (Fawcett, 2000). Much of this knowledge generation would not be possible in the absence of caring relationships.

Public health nurses have unique opportunities to develop caring relationships with individuals, families, and groups (e.g., communities and systems). Lillian Wald emphasized caring when she said, "Nursing is love in action, and there is no finer manifestation of it than the care of the poor and disabled in their own homes" (Ridgeway, 2010, p.1). Although it can certainly be argued that a caring relationship can and should be established by any nurse in any environment, many public health nurses develop and maintain caring relationships with their clients over weeks, months, and years. This opportunity for lengthy caring relationships is not as pervasive in acute clinical settings but certainly can be observed in nursing care for the elderly (i.e., nursing homes) and terminally ill (i.e., hospice care; Othuis, Dekkers, Leget, & Vogelaar, 2006). Certainly, a meaningful caring relationship can be long or short, and challenges can be experienced in both situations. For new nurses, the desire to care, help, intervene, and be of benefit to a family can be a great asset, but can also present challenges because knowledge of how to establish appropriate boundaries might be still developing (for more on professional boundaries, see Chapter 7). Indeed, many nurses have learned about boundaries by experiencing what happens when boundaries are not established or appropriately maintained. Emotions, in moments of sickness, illness, or disease, are intense for families. Serving those families with an effective caring relationship can enable the nurse to optimally benefit and support families. This chapter explores Competency #7 from the Henry Street Consortium entry-level public health nursing competencies and offers strategies for establishing and maintaining meaningful, appropriate caring relationships in public health nursing. This chapter presents challenging situations along with preventive strategies so that, hopefully, some of these common pitfalls are avoided as you launch your nursing career.

To appreciate the nature of a "caring relationship" you need to first briefly look at a description of caring. A thorough analysis of caring in the nursing literature has demonstrated five conceptualizations, or expressions, of caring in nursing (Morse, Bottorff, Neander, & Solberg, 1991):

1. Caring as a human trait/state

2. Caring as a moral imperative

3. Caring as an affect

4. Caring as an interpersonal interaction

5. Caring as a therapeutic intervention

In essence, caring is an attribute that, for many, is inherent to who they are as a nurse and human being. Caring is also a behavior or emotion that is morally mandated or expected from nurses (Morse, Solberg, Neander, Bottorff, & Johnson, 1990). In addition, caring is an action between two or more people, and it is a way to intervene or act to improve the well-being of an individual or community. It is the last two points, interaction and intervention, that in essence reflect a "caring relationship" in nursing because these involve the nurse and another person or group of people.

ACTIVITY

How much do you agree with the above statements regarding caring and nursing? Do you feel it is possible to be an effective nurse and not care? Why or why not?

Do you feel it is possible to care too much? If so, how do you determine how much caring is appropriate?

Following Susan's initial visit, the next year passed with Susan visiting Julie and the children monthly. The relationship flourished as Susan provided Julie with parenting support and information to understand safety and the developmental milestones of her children. Susan worked with Julie to access community resources. At times, Julie would reveal pieces of her past that included mental health issues stemming from a childhood of molestation and abuse. Susan always listened without judgment. Susan realized how much she had come to care about this family and how Julie trusted her with caring for them.

Demonstrates Trust, Respect, and Empathy

Relationships—In every aspect of life, relationships exist: family relationships, casual acquaintance relationships, colleague relationships, distant relationships, and close relationships to name a few. In public health nursing, relationships can be built over minutes and often last for years. The variety of settings in which PHNs work is reflected in the diversity of their relationships. For example, a local public health department PHN administering flu shots might have only 10 minutes with a client whereas a PHN conducting weekly home visits with a pregnant mom on bed rest might be in that relationship for years. A PHN employed in a jail setting might develop an intermittent relationship with incarcerated individuals who are released and rearrested multiple times over years. Every relationship a PHN develops, regardless of how long or deep the relationship runs, can be a caring relationship.

A caring relationship can only exist when trust is present. An effective PHN builds trust in verbal and nonverbal ways that reflect awareness of the situation and the needs of the individual, family, or community. Practically, PHNs encourage trust when their actions are consistent, dependable, nonjudgmental, and sensitive to the needs or preferences of the other person. (See Chapter 11 for more information on nonjudgmental nursing.) Professional relationship building is described in the context of a program to prevent teen pregnancy. "The daily presence of the PHN is an important program component for the kind of information nurses provide … as well as relationship building with a professional who can be trusted and is not judgmental about the adolescent's problems and concerns" (Schaffer, Jost, Pederson, & Lair, 2008, p. 308, 310). Often, trust is developed with time and consistency. Diane McNaughton (2005) observed that for at-risk pregnant women, multiple nursing visits "were needed for clients to develop trust in nurses, discuss their problems, and utilize the services offered by nurses" (p. 435). (See the first Evidence Example below.) Some PHNs find themselves in situations where they are seeking to create relationships with individuals, families, or communities that might not want the relationship. This might occur when the PHN is working with families involved in child protection situations, necessitating thoughtful intention on the part of the PHN to develop a caring relationship. Establishing trust is critical, yet can be challenging because many families are vulnerable and powerless (Jack, DiCenso, & Lohfeld, 2005). (See the second Evidence Example below.)

Evidence Example: Phases of Relationship Building

McNaughton (2005) identified phases of building relationship between at-risk pregnant women and public health nurses, including (1) Orientation Phase—(nurse assessment, women answering questions, feeling anxious), (2) Working Phase—Identification (nurse providing information, women identifying problems, asking questions), (3) Working Phase—Exploitation (nurse providing mutual support, women describe using resources provided by nurse), and (4) Resolution Phase—Occurs when problems are solved or relationship ends.

Evidence Example: Theory of Maternal Engagement with PHNs

A grounded theory study was conducted in Canada to describe the process of mothers engaging with PHNs as part of a home-visiting program (Jack, DiCenso, & Lohfeld, 2005). Twenty mothers participated, and data were collected using interviews and record review. Key findings demonstrate the unique feelings of those receiving home visits from PHNs. Specifically, the mothers "felt vulnerable and powerless when they allowed the service providers in their home" (p. 182). The mothers described three phases to the process: overcoming fear, building trust, and seeking mutuality. Strategies to overcome fear included "'hiding nothing,' 'trying to measure up,' and 'protecting self'" (p. 185). For example, mothers cleaned their houses and made sure their babies were looking nice before the nurse visited their homes. When fears could not be overcome, the mothers were more likely to cancel appointments, drop out of the program, or withhold information from the nurse.

Trust levels ranged from no trust to tentative trust to strong trust, and the level the mother was at was largely dependent on her own characteristics and her perceptions of the PHN. The mothers wanted nurses they could relate to, thereby developing a sense of mutuality. The success of the relationship was also directly influenced by the nurse characteristics, the client characteristics, and the home-visiting context, including the frequency and duration of visits.

ACTIVITY

What might you do to encourage a client to feel secure and comfortable during an initial visit?

How will you acknowledge the sense of vulnerability and work with the client to move beyond the vulnerability to a trusting relationship?

Often, nurses are trusted more readily by families than other professionals (e.g., law enforcement or social work), although depth of mutual trust takes patience and time and might not be achievable in every situation (Jack, DiCenso, & Lohfeld, 2005).

After this first year, Susan started to notice a change within Julie. She started to "care" less about herself and would reveal to the nurse that she was not happy. Julie reported finding it difficult to get out of bed. Susan noticed the environment of the home changing, and Julie was beginning to miss appointments. Susan decided to have a "heart-to-heart," or deep conversation, with Julie because she felt their relationship was built on trust and honesty. As Susan revealed her observations, stressing the desire to help Julie feel better, Julie stated she felt her depression medication was not working anymore. Susan supported Julie and focused on Julie's strengths, one of which was seeking medical care when appropriate. Susan screened Julie for the safety of herself and the children. The plan made was for Julie to visit her primary care physician as soon as possible.

Evidence Example: Mothers' and PHNs' Perspectives on Empowerment

In a study with three mothers and three PHNs to explore the different perspectives of mothers and PHNs regarding empowerment during a home visit, in-depth interviews were conducted (Aston, Meagher-Stewart, Sheppard-Lemoine, Vukic, & Chircop, 2006). Interviews with mothers were conducted in their homes separate from the PHNs and lasted approximately 1.5 hours. Interview transcripts were analyzed using an inductive approach (i.e., themes were not preselected, but were identified as the transcripts were read and reread), yielding five overarching themes: (a) mothers' perceptions of PHNs, (b) normalization as problematic: the good/bad dichotomy, (c) professional/expert: the balance of power, (d) working the relationship, and (e) reflections on empowerment (p. 63). Mothers reported that the PHNs helped them to feel comfortable, supported, and not stupid when they asked the PHNs questions. They also indicated that they liked that the PHNs were accessible and competent. The PHNs talked about "massaging the relationship" by being aware of mother beliefs, social norms, and verbal and nonverbal communication and by using self-awareness and knowledge of best practices to deliver optimal care. For the PHNs, "starting "where the client was' and building on their strengths was important to supporting empowering relationships" (p. 66).

A framework has been developed for relational ethics (i.e., the ethics of relationships) that gives attention to what the PHN needs to do to establish or encourage development of a trusting relationship (Marcellus, 2005). The framework includes four themes: mutual respect, engaged interaction, embodiment, and creating environment. The first theme, mutual respect, is an interesting combination of respect and empathy; it encompasses respect for oneself and for the other, yet it also includes receiving respect from others (Austin, Bergum, & Dossitor, 2003). And, similar to empathy (described later in this chapter), mutual respect occurs when the PHN seeks to understand, though not necessarily agrees with, the actions or circumstances of the individual, family, or community.

The second theme, engaged interaction, means being responsive and sensitive in a manner that can counteract, to an extent, the powerlessness that some clients or communities might feel in relationship with a public health professional. This level of interaction can occur only when PHNs are willing and able to truly listen to those they are serving. Lee SmithBattle describes this as "listening with caring" (2003, p. 369); similarly the importance of listening in providing responsive care to clients has been described (SmithBattle, Drake, & Diekemper, 1997). Supporting teen mothers is a common role for PHNs, and to listen with care is to pay close attention to the context in which the teen mother is living and to support her by "validating strengths, joys, difficulties, learning, and development" (p. 369). When PHNs are attuned to the teen mother's situation, needs, and strengths, they can maintain a relationship that facilitates effectiveness in the care they provide. Importantly, this care at times might simply mean being silent and listening to the teen mother. In an engaged, caring relationship, PHNs will know when to teach and when not to teach, so that the relationship is sustained and preserved.

It is not easy to be attuned to a client's perspectives, beliefs, fears, desires, and needs, but effective PHNs seek to achieve embodiment, the third theme of the relational ethics framework. Embodiment can appear to be somewhat esoteric (i.e., available only to the enlightened), but it is a useful and understandable concept. Simply, PHNs demonstrate embodiment when they grasp the essence of conversations, not only the mere words but also the intertwined meanings and emotions. In a caring relationship, PHNs need to value authenticity, which requires that they, at times, be willing to be influenced by the relationship as much as the client they are serving.

The fourth element in the relational ethics framework is environment, emphasizing the need for PHNs to be in an environment that encourages them to reflect and work through the moral dilemmas and ethical challenges they are going to encounter when establishing and maintaining caring relationships (Marcellus, 2005). PHNs regularly encounter dilemmas that challenge beliefs, perspectives, and at times, best intentions. In the context of a caring relationship, PHNs use reflection to arrive at the best decision for that moment, recognizing the emotions, needs, and vulnerability of those who are going to be influenced by their decision. For example, how do PHNs report child mistreatment and continue to provide home-visiting services to the family? This is not an uncommon scenario faced by PHNs, and they face numerous similar examples of difficult yet surmountable challenges to maintaining caring relationships with individuals, families, and communities. The list below identifies common reflective questions.

- How was I feeling during this experience?
- What does that experience mean for me?

- How can I use what I've learned from this situation as I move ahead?

- Is there another way I can think about this experience?

- What other things can I learn from this experience?

- How might the outcome have been different if I would have…?

- What other people were affected by my actions or inactions?

The next week, Julie came into the office asking for Susan. Susan was immediately concerned. Julie had pink and black hair, a pierced nose and eyebrow, and she had no children with her. Susan brought Julie into her office to explore her outward changes and what brought her to the office. Julie broke down in tears, saying she had no energy, was not sleeping, and hinted that she was cutting herself. Susan had a moment of inward reflection. How should she respond to reflect how much she cared, yet do her job of protecting Julie and her children? Susan gently explored who was watching the children when Julie was having difficulty functioning, knowing that a 3 year old and 1 year old need constant supervision. Julie's answers were vague. Susan had to tell Julie she was concerned and that if the children were not supervised or cared for, she could end up with child protection involved with her family. This made Julie very upset, and Susan, at that point, realized she needed to do more. Susan put herself in Julie's shoes. She relied on the trust and strength of the relationship she had with Julie to suggest immediately seeing a crisis mental health nurse working for the county. Julie stated she would if Susan felt it would help. Susan connected them within 15 minutes, and Julie and the mental health nurse initiated a plan of safety and follow-up within a couple of days with a mental health specialist. This meeting seemed to give Julie hope and energy. Susan felt like she had done what she needed to do, but she felt sick to her stomach that she had upset Julie with her discussion of safety for the children.

The following Evidence Example provides a glimpse into caring relationships developed with the elderly.

Evidence Example: Care for the Elderly at Home

In a study, the unique role of PHNs in providing care to individuals in their home environments was described (Sundelof, Hansebo, & Ekman, 2004). The purpose of this study was to examine the meaning of caring relationships with the elderly as perceived by the PHNs providing the home-visiting services. Twelve public health nurses in Sweden were interviewed and the transcripts analyzed for consistent themes regarding the caring relationship. The PHNs described the caring relationship in four themes: balancing between being professional and being a private person; understanding presence of today in light of former meetings; feelings of togetherness; and friendship and caring communion founded in the local community. Complicated by the fact that family members often provide the health care services for their loved one, the PHN-client relationship needs to incorporate these family members because, often, the care and the relationship are long-term. In this way, the PHN develops a relationship with (a) the client and (b) the family members/relatives. For these nurses, a caring relationship was most readily experienced in the caring of elderly persons in their homes over long periods of time, and for many, the caring relationship became interwoven with a sense of friendship.

Note: The sense of friendship that the authors describe might be controversial for some, and warrants reflection within the context of what is known and expected in terms of professional boundaries. That said, it is likely that many PHNs can readily share examples of appropriate, caring relationships with clients or families that also have aspects of friendship.

In addition to trust and respect, empathy is foundational to establishing and maintaining a caring relationship. Many people confuse empathy with sympathy, which is problematic, as described by Douglas Chismar (1988). "[B]lurring the distinction between empathy and sympathy has caused us to miss important complexities in human motivation as well as to overlook and fail to develop the unique capacity to empathize" (p. 257). Empathy is the ability to respond to someone else's emotional state by experiencing similar feelings whereas sympathy goes a step further by inherently feeling positive and lasting concern toward the other person (Chismar, 1988). For example, someone might empathize with a stranger after hearing about the loss of his or her child in a car accident and might express emotions of sadness, including crying. That same person, however, might sympathize with a brother who has experienced the same loss, not only expressing emotions of sadness and tears, but continuing to care for and support the brother over time. Also, empathy includes an ability to care while not necessarily agreeing with the perspective of the other person. PHNs employed in jails are often asked how they care for criminals who have committed horrible crimes; empathy enables PHNs in this context to care for and even emotionally mirror the needs of an inmate while not agreeing with or supporting aspects of that individual. Table 9.1 presents distinctions between empathy and sympathy.

Table 9.1   Empathy versus Sympathy

Empathy	Sympathy
Responds to another's perceived emotional state by experiencing feelings of a similar sort	Having a positive regard or a feeling of benevolence for the person
Understands but might not agree with the perspective	Agrees with the viewpoint
Senses what the other is feeling but without "mutuality"	Offers supportive response to the other's situation
Directed toward anyone, including someone you don't necessarily like	Expressed toward those one feels positive about or close to
Usually occurs where there is no prior attachment to the person	Usually occurs in the context of a personal relationship or insider knowledge
Often involuntary experience of feelings similar to someone else	Often voluntary experience of feelings alongside someone else

Source: Adapted from Chismar, 1988

Despite the complex conceptualization of empathy in nursing, a scale was developed that could measure a nurse's level of empathic understanding, or ability to understand a client's emotions, feelings, and perspective (Nagano, 2000). The instrument is designed to measure nurse awareness and actions, and research is ongoing to improve validity and reliability. The 20-item scale includes verbal (e.g., "restates important points in own words and confirms with client") and nonverbal (e.g., "looks at the client with a warm expression") elements that in many ways mirror simple yet effective nursing communication strategies.

Judeen Schulte (2000) conducted an ethnographic study exploring the perspectives of PHNs regarding building relationships with clients. These nurses felt particular actions yielded successes in developing caring relationships because they helped clients feel they could open up and share, including "being a resource, detecting/asking the next questions, and making informed judgments" (p. 7). Often, the nurses were conducting home visits with no particular disease or problem identified beforehand; a caring relationship was essential for the PHNs to accurately assess and intervene with the family. For them, honesty and being direct was important to relationship building, and the nurses described needing to ignore "rude behavior" (2000, p. 7). Schulte (2000) shared comments from a participant that summarize the study well:

> Felicia's words strongly communicate the link between caring and connections: "Public health nursing is more than a job. ... When I'm out there, I care about the people, about what happens to them. I don't think I'd make a really good public health nurse if I didn't care. You get results if they know you care—they're willing to make some change. If they don't think you care at all about them, why should they take a risk for you? I think public health nursing is all about caring about people" (p. 8).

For the PHNs in this study, caring meant listening to "more than what is said" (Schulte, 2000, p. 7), which is consistent with attention in nursing to nonverbal communication and to contextual factors in the family, community, and society environments.

Although much of what has been discussed thus far in this chapter is specific to nursing care for individuals or families, many of the guiding principles for establishing a caring relationship apply to relationships at the community or systems levels. At times it can seem (and be) more challenging simply because usually many more people are involved. (See Chapter 5 on collaboration.) Some literature, however, does describe community-level caring in public health nursing. Consider the importance of caring for communities:

> Nurses must care about what happens to groups of citizens, as well as particular clients. ... Although proponents of "caring" seem to have drawn a distinction between an ethic of justice and an ethic of care, this is bipolar, even antithetical. Building the health of communities requires universal application of the principles of justice. It further requires that nurses care enough about their communities and the individuals in them to do battle in political, social, and economic arenas (Chafey, 1996, p. 15).

Betty Smith-Campbell (1999) developed and tested a caring model for communities (see Figure 9.1) because "nurses collectively care with and for communities" (p. 405). In the model, the foundation of caring actions is the principles discussed earlier in this chapter, including affect and moral imperative. Interaction is not only with an individual but is with the "community," in whatever way the community is defined. Caring actions result not only from the underlying foundation, interactions, and planning, but also from the direct and indirect influences that encompass the community (e.g., economics, policies, politics, and supporting or opposing communities). For example, a parish nurse caring for the congregation will want to plan health promotion activities with an understanding of the neighborhood and other characteristics and influences on those the PHN is serving. If the PHN is in an affluent neighborhood with abundant health care resources, she or he can more easily develop a caring relationship that involves extensive health screenings and referrals to outside resources (e.g., services for high blood pressure, weight management, and stress reduction) than if the PHN is serving a congregation in an impoverished neighborhood with limited health care. It would be unethical and not very caring if the PHN were to proceed with extensive screenings for that congregation without first establishing where they can receive care needed for identified problems. A PHN cannot effectively care for a community unless time is taken to understand and appreciate the complexity of factors in and surrounding the community.

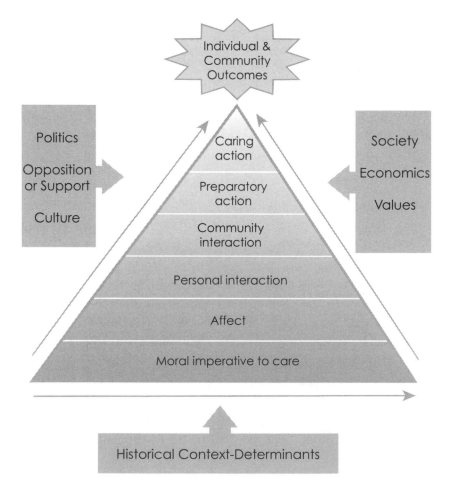

Figure 9.1 Smith-Campbell Caring Community Model (1999, adapted with permission)

Follows Through with Commitments

PHNs cannot be trusted unless they can demonstrate consistency in care for individuals, families, and communities. Clients PHNs are caring for need to know those PHNs are dependable and reliable in addition to being honest, respectful, and trustworthy. Teri Aronowitz (2005) conducted a grounded theory study to examine the ways in which adolescents develop resilience and change risk behaviors amidst environmental stressors in their lives. One of the most important findings from the interviews was that the processes by which the teens felt supported were possible only within the context of a relationship with a "reliable, caring, and competent adult." These youth were able to "envision the future" when they were feeling competent and had higher expectations for their behavior and their future. These feelings and sentiments were not apparent in the absence of a caring relationship with an adult, and notably, with an adult who was reliable.

The study highlights ways in which PHNs can support resiliency among at-risk youth, either by being that reliable caring adult or by supporting development and presence of these characteristics in mentors serving adolescents. At the community level, PHNs can also advocate for strategies that make the community more supportive of at-risk youth (e.g., development of after-school programs, internship experiences, and leadership opportunities).

Maintains Appropriate Boundaries

Boundaries can be very challenging, yet they are so important in establishing and maintaining caring relationships. If the PHNs are too personal and close to a client, they might not garner respect as a professional, but if they are too distant, the PHNs might not gain the trust of a client. Knowing where the right boundary is, and when it should be moved or adjusted, takes time, experience, and practice. New PHNs can benefit from gaining the insights of experienced PHNs, who undoubtedly have numerous positive and negative examples. Refer to Chapter 7 for a discussion of professional boundary issues.

When a PHN works in a community where he or she also lives, it is important that the PHN establish appropriate boundaries when he or she encounters clients in social contexts (Sundelof, Hansebo, & Ekman, 2004). How to best accomplish this comes with experience and the ability to simultaneously achieve closeness and appropriate distance. Setting limits is the responsibility of the nurse, not the client, and this is particularly important when the nurse is caring for someone with whom he or she might have had prior, personal interactions (e.g., such as might often occur in rural communities).

Evidence Example: Caring PHN-Family Relationships

A study was conducted in Manitoba, Canada to describe the relationships among PHNs and families they visited in their homes as part of an early childhood program (Heaman, Chalmers, Woodgate, & Brown, 2007). Twenty-four PHNs and 20 parents were interviewed. All of the nurses had at least a bachelor's degree and on average 14 years of work experience. Both nurses and parents spoke about three phases of the caring relationships: establishing, maintaining, and terminating relationships. It was clear that the best way to end the relationship was to establish a planned exit that occurred over the last few visits. Key characteristics of caring relationships were described, including respect, support, trust, partnership, and for the nurses, appropriate levels of supervision and evaluation. A key finding was the maintenance of professional-client boundaries and the need for the PHNs to affirm the professional nature of the relationship. Study findings emphasized the need for the PHNs to put effort into establishing relationships, not only with the clients, but also with colleagues, such as "home visitors" (e.g., home health aides).

Another element of maintaining boundaries is taking care of yourself to ensure personal safety when you are working as a PHN. Personal safety is important for PHNs, who can often find themselves in vulnerable or potentially harmful situations. This clearly can influence the speed at which a caring relationship is developed, but PHNs should never place themselves at risk for personal harm to advance a caring relationship. Instead, PHNs should creatively explore ways in which relationships can be developed and safety can be maximized. However, note that seeking to be safe does not mean seeking to be comfortable. A home environment might be uncomfortable because of the presence of head lice, cockroaches, or disorder, but the PHN caring for the family needs to work amidst these factors. In doing so, he or she gains respect and trust with the family. If the PHN were to keep the visits short, because of discomfort, it might be difficult to reach the level of a caring relationship that can yield positive, lasting results with the family.

In contrast, a PHN might feel unsafe if criminal activities are observed during a visit (e.g., drug use) or if the neighborhood is known for gang violence (see Table 9.2 for factors influencing safety when conducting home visits). Patricia Fazzone, Linda Barloon, Susan McConnell, & Julie Chitty (2000) conducted a study with PHNs and other home visiting staff and observed that the staff felt risks to their personal safety were high; this finding is consistent with additional research on safety for staff providing care in homes, public settings, and communities (Gellner et al., 1994; Kendra et al., 1996; Schulte et al., 1998). Fazzone and coauthors found that the staff felt some personal characteristics were protective in terms of safety, including "self-confidence, self-reliance, self-motivation, flexibility, 'being comfortable with the unknown,' and self-assurance about their personal judgment" (p. 49).

Table 9.2   Factors Influencing Safety when Conducting Home Visits

Conditions In/Outside the Home	Environmental Conditions	Organizational Factors
• People loitering around the home or street • Known felon in home • Verbal, physical, and sexual aggression • Gangs and gang activity • Police raids and drug busts	• Night travel • Traveling in remote areas • Increase of garage or home-based methamphetamine labs • Domestic, neighborhood violence • Poverty	• Absence or inaccessibility of written policies/procedures • Safety policies not enforced • Safety policies not relevant to home care issues • Staff unfamiliarity with community • Lack or delay of security assistance • Cellular phones not provided for staff

Conditions In/Outside the Home	Environmental Conditions	Organizational Factors
• Weapons and shootings		• Absence of ''call-in'' or ''check-in'' systems
• Garbage, debris		• Lack or minimal administrative support
• Poor lighting or ventilation		• Staff delay or failure in reporting incidents
• Homes in disarray		• Staff not always aware of violent or unsafe history with clients or families
• Pests		

Source: Adapted from Fazzone et al., 2000, p. 47

Generally, when students are assigned a public health nursing clinical experience, the faculty ensures that appropriate safety precautions are taken. Also, most clinical sites review their policies and procedures for safety during orientation with new students. If a student is unsure of what to do or feels concerned about the safety involved in a clinical experience, that student should immediately approach a clinical instructor or preceptor before proceeding. For example, many students do not feel comfortable conducting a home visit alone; although it is becoming more popular to assign students in pairs for home visits, many programs continue to encourage students to conduct a home visit alone. In the case when a student is uncomfortable making a visit alone, that student needs to talk through the decision with a preceptor and clinical instructor. Similarly, students might be involved in planning a community health fair but might not feel comfortable attending the fair during evening hours. Students need to address their concerns with a clinical instructor and determine a plan that both meets learning goals and maintains appropriate levels of safety. Remember, too, that feeling uncomfortable in an unfamiliar environment or climate is not the same as feeling unsafe. In many public health nursing clinical experiences it is common to feel uncomfortable and to learn through reflecting on those feelings and experiences.

Demonstrates Tact and Diplomacy

In a caring, professional relationship, PHNs act in tactful and diplomatic manners. Consistent with ethical standards and expectations, PHNs strive to develop caring relationships without consideration of personal or social characteristics such as income level or social status (Fredriksson & Eriksson, 2006). Effective PHNs are consistent in how they deliver nursing care and services, including the effort they make in seeking and obtaining resources for clients and communities. Beth Crisp and Pam Lister (2004) described how PHNs who were working with families involved in child protection situations made an effort to see all families so that they avoided the possibility that some families would feel stigmatized. Indeed, sometimes families who receive a visit from a social worker feel stigmatized or feel that they are the worst families. When PHNs are addressing sensitive issues with families or communities, acting in a tactful or diplomatic manner enhances the potential for effective impact and enables the PHNs to be viewed as allies (Crisp & Lister, 2004).

When PHNs act in a diplomatic manner, considerate of the opinions, beliefs, ideas, and perspectives of others, they are more likely to be successful in having a caring relationship. Diplomacy takes time and patience, as well as a willingness to listen and truly hear what others are saying. Successful PHNs know this well and protect the time they need to serve individuals, families, and communities in a diplomatic manner. Thomas Gantert (Gantert, McWilliam, Ward-Griffen, & Allen, 2009) found that for both clients and their family members, relationship building is critical to how they perceive the actions of the staff providing care in their home (e.g., PHNs, home health aides). The relationship is not static, but rather fluid, and requires ongoing attention and determination on the part of PHNs. An established caring relationship needs to be maintained, requiring tact, respect, patience, and the ability to perceive/assess the state of the relationship on an ongoing basis. Effective PHNs do not presume that the relationship, once established, is settled and certain. Instead, they regularly take note of the relationship dynamics and make efforts with every interaction to continue to build an optimal caring relationship. This is the environment in which interventions are successful and lasting, as reflected in both client feedback and observed outcomes.

Evidence Example: PHN and Mother Perceptions and Satisfaction

A cross-sectional study was conducted in Ireland to examine the perceptions of nurse-client dyads (n=44) about their relationship, including identified needs and provided services (Mulcahy & McCarthy, 2008). Surveys were administered to nurses and their clients and analyzed for similarities and differences. Important findings included that the nurses and clients showed agreement regarding the client needs that were identified and addressed by the PHN. However, the study observed a difference between the nurses and the clients regarding the match between the "needs" and the "actions" to address the needs. The PHNs felt a close agreement between the needs and responses/actions, whereas among the clients, the agreement was not as close and was not statistically significant. However, with a small sample size the importance of the findings should not be based on the "significant" nature of the statistics but instead should focus on what was found and what might be more carefully examined in future studies. This study demonstrates that the nurses and clients both felt satisfied with the participatory nature of the relationship, perhaps indicating that the PHN had effectively established a caring relationship with her client.

Seeks Assistance when Needed in Managing Relationships

Unquestionably, nurses at all levels of experience bring an inherent desire to care and respond to a moral imperative to do so. However, it is also apparent that relationship skills are honed over time as inexperienced PHNs begin to appreciate the daily struggles of clients' lives and learn to judge what works and what does not work, with increasing refinement (SmithBattle, Diekemper, & Leander, 2004a, p. 9).

Susan was still not sure of the way she handled the situation with Julie, and went to her supervisor. Her supervisor listened to Susan, and together they explored other options for wordage and interventions. Her supervisor shared some of her experiences and supported Susan's desire to see this family more often to monitor the status of the mother's mental health and the interactions with her children. Susan's supervisor reassured Susan that her caring relationship appeared strong and that her actions might have initiated actions by the mother that can improve her quality of life and safety of the family unit.

Skills in developing and maintaining caring relationships are built over time; conscientious PHNs early in their careers will seek the input and guidance of experienced PHNs as they encounter challenges in relationships with clients and communities. Asking busy colleagues to sit and talk through a challenging situation can be difficult, yet positive results can come from doing this. Creative solutions or ideas for addressing a barrier often result from simply talking through the challenge with someone else. More often than not, other PHNs have experienced many similar situations and have a variety of strategies they have used to overcome problems and succeed in developing a caring relationship. Although rare, at times a PHN is unable to establish a caring relationship with a client; in this case, the PHN should bring the matter to a manager as soon as possible so that if necessary, the client can receive care from another PHN. These situations are rare, but can occur. The PHN should not feel ineffective, especially if she or he has made a solid effort toward a caring relationship. Sometimes characteristics or experiences beyond the control of a PHN make it difficult for a client to receive care from that PHN. For example, a student who has recently been sexually abused or assaulted might find it difficult to work with a client who has been sexually abused and needs resources to heal. Similar experiences can create a degree of closeness that makes it difficult for the student, or PHN, to separate herself or himself from the client and provide appropriate nursing care.

 ACTIVITY

What might be your plan of action in a situation such as the one presented in the paragraph above, in which the student has experienced something traumatic and similar to the client being served? In whom should the student confide?

More often than not, PHNs experience caring relationships with clients, families, and communities. And over time, experience is gained with each new client. As SmithBattle Diekemper, and Leander offered, "Cumulative experience provides the foundation for becoming more responsive, for appreciating the strengths as well as the vulnerabilities and suffering of clients, for becoming more open and attentive to clients needs and concerns" (2004a, p. 9). Cumulative experience occurs in each PHN but can also be shared across PHNs, as occurs when cases are reviewed or staff meetings provide time to express challenges and seek input from peers.

The emphasis here on seeking input from peers is not meant to negate the effectiveness of new PHNs. Indeed, new PHNs often bring passion, energy, excitement, and determination to their roles in ways that can inspire and recharge their peers. Also, new PHNs experience much success in identifying and addressing client and community needs, sometimes because their optimism levels are high and matched by willingness to act. This is not to say that experienced PHNs are not willing or optimistic, but rather that they are more likely to "ask first" rather than "act first, apologize later." This new nurse's story about identifying an unmet community need because of a caring relationship she had with a client is inspiring.

There was this gentleman who had really bad toenails. And one of the family members asked if I could trim his toenails. I was like, "Well, I guess I can. I don't know why I can't." [Laughter] So I did, after soaking his feet. And they were really bad. Turns out that after I trimmed them, he stood up and started tap dancing. And this was a really old guy who had tap danced in another life. Well, of course, word got around. They would call, "Is the foot lady there?" [Laughter] It was actually kind of a nightmare. All these people needed nail care. . . . [Eventually] we started a foot clinic and got real podiatrists in (SmithBattle, Diekemper, & Leander, 2004b, p. 98).

Ethical Considerations

Much of public health nursing occurs in the places where people live, recreate, worship, and work. These are very personal settings, and often, PHNs are alone when delivering care. A caring relationship is critical to the success of what PHNs do with the client (e.g., assessment, planning, intervention, and evaluation). Regardless of how simple or complex the care is, PHNs can accomplish much more in the presence of a caring relationship. Amidst many potentially challenging ethical factors, PHNs can act in a way that optimizes empathetic care. Rosalind Ekman Ladd, Lynn Pasquerella, and Sheri Smith (2000) propose ethical ideas for building relationships that are cognizant of "decision-making authority and autonomy, allow the exercise of the nurse's moral rights, and recognize the patient's relationships to significant others" (p. 103). It is interesting that Ladd and coauthors realize both the importance of autonomy among clients and the moral rights of the nurses. This is important, because it emphasizes that PHNs are not expected to simply go along with everything a client expresses to maintain a caring relationship. Instead, effective PHNs use judgment in every situation so that optimal care is delivered, autonomy is encouraged, and morals are respected. At times, this requires PHNs to maneuver between contrasting opinions and preferences among the client and family members or community members. Caring relationships and subsequent interventions are rarely straightforward, but when ethical standards are upheld, the outcomes that are yielded are worth the invested effort.

Susan continues to see Julie and her two children. Julie has received mental health services along with psychological support as she deals with past issues and her newly diagnosed bipolar disease. Julie is stable and appreciates the day Susan made her take stronger action for herself. The issue of safety now is part of the family home visits that they share. Susan continues to be committed to the relationship by empowering this mother, building on her strengths, providing her support through education, and of course, listening. Julie continues to feel that the relationship is beneficial and supportive for her. They both recognize that boundaries must exist in maintaining a caring and ethically strong nurse-family relationship.

Table 9.3   Ethical Action in Establishing Caring Relationships

Ethical Perspective	Application
Rule Ethics (principles)	• In relationships, PHNs must realize the autonomy, and the authority to make decisions, of individuals, families, and communities.
	• Encourage autonomy by asking the primary client what information can be shared with others, including other family members.
	• Encourage shared decision making.
Virtue Ethics (character)	• Respect is critical to successful caring relationships.
	• Act in a manner that encourages a mutually trusting relationship.
	• Be patient with the development of a caring relationship.
Feminist Ethics (reducing oppression)	• Respect is critical to establishing and maintaining a caring relationship.
	• Respect beliefs, perspectives, feelings, opinions, ideas, cultural traditions, and preferences.
	• Recognize that most clients come to the relationship feeling they have little power.
	• Encourage shared power in the relationship by practicing mutuality and empathy.

Key Points

- Caring relationships are core to effective public health nursing.
- Caring relationships can be established with individuals, families, communities, and systems.
- Caring relationships are built on trust, respect, and empathy.
- A caring relationship will not last if PHNs do not follow through on commitments, maintain appropriate boundaries, and demonstrate tact and diplomacy.
- PHNs need to operate in ways that are safe for themselves and others.
- Establishing a caring relationship might require PHNs to step outside of personal comfort zones but should never require PHNs to work in an unsafe setting.

Exercises

Learning Examples for Establishing Caring Relationships

The following learning examples represent some real-life situations in which the PHN has developed a caring relationship and yet experienced challenges in providing care. As you read these examples, consider how you might respond, and what resources you might access to overcome the challenges.

- A PHN is proactive in breast-feeding efforts and is working to increase breast-feeding statistics within the county where she works. After receiving education on the benefits of breast-feeding, the new mother states she wants to formula feed her new infant. The PHN confirms this decision and then assists the mother, in a caring way, to properly feed her infant with formula/bottles.

- The PHN has gone three times to a home for a visit, and the family is not present. The nurse does not take this personally and continues to try and make a connection. The PHN believes that a caring relationship exists and that the visits did not occur because it was "a bad day" for the family. When the PHN finally reaches the family, she immediately states how she has missed seeing their family and asks if everything is okay. She doesn't make them feel guilty and listens. This demonstration of concern reflects caring toward the family. The family had personal issues unrelated to the PHN, and now the PHN can continue to serve this family. Many new PHNs make the mistake that families not at home equate to families not wanting to see them, and they prematurely end the nurse-family relationship.

- PHNs share stories of their experiences in the wake of the devastation of hurricane Katrina. The establishment of caring relationships was essential at all levels of structure; maintaining the infrastructure of public health (systems level), establishing essential services within communities (community level), and of course, caring for families/individuals in need (family/client level). Many resources explore the caring relationships that occurred during and following this natural disaster. One such example can be obtained from the following site: http://www.apha.org/about/news/booksreleases/books1242006.htm.

Reflective Practice

The questions below provide you additional opportunities for reflecting on the challenges a PHN can experience developing or working in a caring relationship with a client.

In the case study presented in this chapter, describe the actions Susan utilizes to develop a caring relationship within each of McNaughton's relationship phases.

As you reflect on this chapter, do you feel that a caring professional relationship can also be a friendship? Why or why not? (See Chapter 7 for discussion on professional boundaries.)

_____

_____

_____

Describe possible differences in development of a caring relationship if the initial visit with the client is at the clinic versus it occurring in their home.

_____

_____

_____

A PHN has been seeing a family for several visits, and then the family is not home at the next planned visit. How might you address this with the family in a caring manner?

_____

_____

_____

You are going on your first PHN family home visit. What aspects of this visit might be uncomfortable for you? How will you deal with these feelings? How are these "uncomfortable aspects" different from "safety issues"?

_____

_____

_____

PHNs value authenticity in caring relationships with their clients. How can PHNs better prepare themselves emotionally to be willing to be influenced by the relationship as much as the client is?

_____

_____

_____

What are some ways trust between PHNs and clients could be threatened?

_____

_____

_____

What can PHNs do if trust is broken with the client and the relationship is no longer caring or therapeutic?

_____

_____

_____

What are possible implications if PHNs find themselves unable to care for a client and they do not address this concern but continue to provide care?

_____

_____

_____

Application of Evidence

1. Identify the steps you take in your current nursing practice to develop effective caring relationships with clients.

2. Describe three resources available to you in public health nursing practice for difficult caring situations.

3. What are some ways a PHN can assess the extent to which her perceptions of the client-nurse relationship are similar to or different from the client's perceptions?

Think, Explore, Do

1. What makes self-awareness such an important part of caring effectively for another?

2. What are some ways a PHN can progress to listening to more than what is said?

3. You are discussing with another PHN student the state teen pregnancy rate and this student states, "Teen mothers are not ready to be parents; it is so sad." How might you respond to share your knowledge of a caring relationship?

4. Describe the relationships that exist in your life, such as those that exist between you and your parents, siblings, peers, and friends. Describe the caring aspects of each of these relationships. Do you need to work harder at maintaining a caring relationship with some versus others?

5. Describe a friend's strengths. Ask this friend to describe her strengths. How do these two perspectives compare? How can you use this knowledge to build a stronger, caring relationship with this friend?

6. Describe a time when your first impression of someone was inaccurate. How did this influence the relationship you had/have with this person?

7. Reflect on the last argument that you had with someone. Would you have said or done something differently after reading this chapter?

COMPETENCY # 8:
Shows Evidence of Commitment to Social Justice, the Greater Good, and the Public Health Principles

By Patricia M. Schoon
with Noreen Kleinfehn-Wald and Vicki Kyarsgaard

Erica is a new public health nurse (PHN) in a large urban county where 40% of the children live in poverty. During Erica's home visit to a young family, the mother stated that the 2- and 3-year-old children had become "slow to get things and were tripping and falling more than usual." A year ago the family had moved from a newer apartment building into a 70-year-old building when her husband lost his job. Erica noticed paint chips on the floor and was concerned that they were from lead-based paint. She advised the mother to have her children's blood lead levels checked. The mother said she did not have health insurance and could not afford a trip to the doctor. Erica told the mother the paint should be replaced, but the mother was concerned the landlord would not listen to her. Erica consulted with her public health nursing supervisor about what else could be done.

ERICA'S NOTEBOOK

> **Competency #8: Shows evidence of commitment to social justice, the greater good, and the public health principles**
>
> • Differentiates between social justice and market justice
>
> • Applies principles of social justice to promote and maintain the health and well-being of populations
>
> • Advocates for the populations for which the PHN is accountable
>
> **Useful Definitions**
>
> *Advocacy:* Actions to ensure that individuals or populations have basic human rights and justice. "Advocacy pleads someone's cause or acts on someone's behalf, with a focus on developing the community, system, individual, or family's capacity to plead their own cause or act on their own behalf" (Minnesota Department of Health [MDH], 2001, p. 263).
>
> *Egalitarianism:* "The degree of equality of opportunity for health made available by the political, social, and economic structures and values of a society" (Smith, Jacobson, & Yiu, 2008, p. 112).
>
> *Equity:* Absence of systematic disparities in health between social groups who have different levels of social advantage and disadvantage (Braveman & Gruskin, 2003, p. 254).

Human Rights: Individual and family rights to live an independent fulfilling healthy life and earn a living wage for food, clothing, housing, and safe environment; self-determination and autonomy.

Just Society: A society based on egalitarianism that has concern for the common good and takes collective actions to meet the needs of all, particularly those who are vulnerable.

Justice: Fairness in how individuals and populations are treated and how decisions are made about sharing resources and burdens based on the belief that there is a collective obligation of society to meet basic needs (Gostin & Powers, 2006, p. 1053).

Social Justice: (Synonym, distributive justice) The concept that individuals have the right to receive resources based on their needs and that a collective social obligation exists to provide for basic human needs including health services (Budetti, 2008).

Market Justice: Personal resources and choices provide the basis for use and distribution of health care services based on concepts of individualism, self-interest, and individual effort; no collective obligation of society or government exists to provide for health care (Budetti, 2008).

Taking Action for What is Right

Professional nurses have a social contract with their clients and the public to ensure that the health care needs of individuals, families, populations, and communities are met in a caring, nonjudgmental, just, and equitable manner. Nurses as professionals and as private citizens are guided by the rule of law that protects basic human rights and by ethical principles that undergird basic human rights and social justice. Justice, for example, is a core principle that provides the foundation and rationale for what is done in public health services.

Nurses in public health are confronted with ethical issues surrounding human rights and social justice on a daily basis. Two aspects of justice shape public health practice goals—advancing human well-being by improving population health and focusing on fair treatment of the disadvantaged by working to reduce health disparities (Gostin & Powers, 2006, p. 1054). As students, you will be challenged and at times conflicted by the decisions you face that require choosing between what seem to be two important and good things. For example, do you make a choice that respects individual rights or emphasizes the collective social good? Do you decide to respect individual autonomy and confidentiality, or do you find it necessary to enforce a public health law? Will you distribute resources based on need, or will you distribute resources equally to all? This chapter will encourage you to consider many of these challenging situations that are regularly encountered by PHNs. This chapter offers ideas and decision-making frameworks that can help prepare you for difficult decisions and the actions that follow.

Evidence Example: Social Justice and Human Rights Issues Identified by Practicing PHNs

A focus group process was used to identify social justice issues resulting in ethical dilemmas that confront staff PHNs on a daily basis. Sixteen nurses working in a suburban-rural county public health agency participated in the focus group. They used storytelling to draw out the social justice issues and human rights principles that were being violated. Four themes with examples emerged from this discussion.

- **Right to self-determination (human right)**—Clients are in need of services, but do not qualify according to the rules and regulations of the existing programs. For example, an elderly person might be in need of personal care attendant services, but does not qualify for medical assistance, so remains at risk for placement in a long-term care facility.

- **Right to a standard of living adequate for the health and well-being of individuals and families (human right)**—The working poor often work in entry-level jobs and have a salary that makes them ineligible for public services, even though their income is not enough to adequately support their families.

- **Autonomy (human right) versus greater good (social justice)**—A client with a communicable disease chooses to break home isolation and exposes many people by going out in public. Or, parents choose not to vaccinate their child, who then becomes ill with pertussis (whooping cough) and exposes an entire classroom of children including one child who is immune-compromised.

- **Inequitable distribution of power, money, and resources (social justice)**—Legal immigrants arriving in the state have received no health examination in their home country and are not provided with a health screening upon arrival in the United States. Other foreigners seeking admission to the country as refugees have a health examination prior to receiving the designation of refugees, and, in addition, have a health screening upon arrival in their county of residence.

All four of these human rights and social justice inequities had negative health status outcomes for the individuals, families, and populations involved. (Kleinfehn-Wald, 2010)

Differentiates between Social Justice and Market Justice

PHNs use principles of social justice to determine community health priorities, identify the populations they serve, and guide how they allocate resources based on client need such as the timing and frequency of home visits. Social justice dictates that health services are allocated equitably based on individual need rather than allocated equally regardless of need. Advocates of social justice believe that the government has a role to play in the provision of and assurance of basic health services to its citizens. Advocates of market justice believe that individuals and the private sectors are best prepared to meet the healthcare needs of private citizens. Social justice requires that the government be responsible and accountable for the health and well-being of its citizens. Market justice requires that individuals be responsible for their own health and well-being. See Table 10.1 for a comparison of market and social justice in health care.

Table 10.1   Comparison of Value Structure

MARKET JUSTICE	SOCIAL JUSTICE
People are entitled only to those valued ends such as status, income, and happiness that they acquire by individual efforts, actions, or abilities.	**People in society receive benefits by belonging to a community and the burdens and benefits of society should be fairly and equitably distributed.**

Human Rights

• Individual rights	• Common good
• Individualism	• Member of community
• Autonomy	• Collective
• Personal freedom and responsibility	• Responsibility to community

Approach

• Short-term thinking and actions	• Long-term thinking
• Science-based	• Human actions
• Treatment	• Prevention
• Local perspective	• Global perspective

Goals and Priorities

• Profit motive	• Quality of life
• Bottom line	• Stewardship of the future
• Cost effective	• Recognition of "hidden costs"

Rights of Ownership & Allocation of Resources

• People deserve what they earn	• People have rights by belonging to the community
• Private business has the right to earn money	• Private business has an obligation to the community at large

Role of Government

• Mistrust in government, especially big government	• Trust in government to do the right thing
• Individuals are responsible for themselves	• Government is responsible to and for its citizens
• Government infringes on individual rights	• Government has an obligation to protect citizens
• Local control of plans and actions	• Federal control of overall plans and some actions
• Government is inefficient	• Government can be efficient

Source: Modified from Keller, 2010

Working within U.S. Health Care Systems

When PHNs work for governmental agencies, they carry out the social justice goal of protecting and promoting the health of the public to achieve "the greater good." This means that even though PHNs work with individuals and families, they prioritize what they do based on the overarching health priorities of the community. For example, in Minnesota it is the law that all first-time teen moms are offered public health nursing home visits because teen moms and their babies are considered vulnerable and at greater risk than older moms or women who have already borne children. A first-time mom of 20 years of age might not receive the same public health services as a teen mom. PHNs actively seek out individuals and families who are vulnerable because addressing their vulnerability helps strengthen not only the individuals and families but also the community as a whole.

The health care system in the United States is a mix of public, non-profit, and for-profit health care organizations. PHNs work with all of these. Governmental and non-profit health care systems have similar goals based on the "common good" whereas for-profit health care systems have primary goals of profitability and independence. The result is a complex diverse continuum of care in the United States (see Figure 10.1) delivered by organizations with opposing beliefs (social justice and market justice). Federal monies from tax dollars are spent in all three types of health care systems through direct service reimbursement, co-funded programs, or grants. Some individuals and families might receive services from all three types of health care systems concurrently. For example, a person over 65 might belong to a non-profit HMO, receive home-care services from a for-profit home-care agency, and receive reimbursement for health care expenses from Medicare.

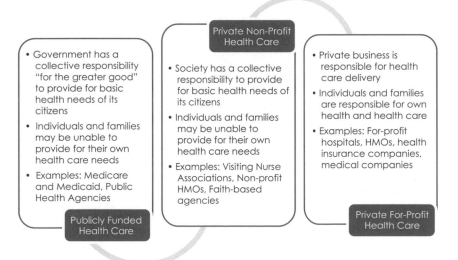

Figure 10.1 Mix of U.S. health care systems and health care resources

Individuals and families do not have equal access to these health care systems. Health care disparities (i.e., lack of equitable access to health care resources) and health status disparities (i.e., differing levels of health based on a complex tangle of health determinants) are in part the result of this unequal access.

Government programs also differ in providing access to health care services. For example, Medicare and Medicaid have different enrollment criteria and serve different populations (see Table 10.2). PHNs must be able to understand the differences between social and market justice as well as the differences in government programs to effectively assist vulnerable individuals, families, and populations in accessing the health care they need.

Table 10.2   Comparison of Medicare and Medicaid

Medicare	Medicaid
Medicare Program is based on concept of equality and referred to as an Entitlement Program.	Medicaid Program is based on concept of equity and is referred to as an Eligibility Program.
All U.S. citizens 65 and over are eligible for the same benefits.	U.S. citizens under 65 who are chronically ill or disabled and unable to work, and children and adults who meet income guidelines, are eligible for benefits.

Erica returned to the family and drew blood from the children. Environmental Health staff visited the family's apartment to determine if the paint and paint chips were lead-based. Two weeks later, Erica, her PHN supervisor, and the Environmental Health staff met to review their findings. Both children had increased blood lead levels, and a significant amount of lead-based paint was found throughout the apartment. Erica arranged for the mother and children to be seen in the county public health clinic. Chelation therapy was recommended for the children, but the county did not provide that service. Lead abatement was recommended for the entire apartment building, but the owner said he could not afford it.

Applies Principles of Social Justice to Promote and Maintain the Health and Well-Being of Populations

The principles of social justice that are key to the health and well being of populations include:

- Collective social responsibility for community members
- Responsibility of government to ensure the basic human rights and health care needs of its citizens
- Allocation of health care resources based on need
- Protection of the rights of individuals and families to live safe, healthy, and fulfilling lives

Social justice dilemmas are part of the everyday lives of nurses. What is different for PHNs is that they often have to confront and resolve these dilemmas when they are out in the community by themselves. In an acute care setting, ethics committees can usually assist in resolving ethical issues related to autonomy, rights to self-determination, rights to refuse treatment, and rights to a safe and comfortable death. In the home and community setting, PHNs are often practicing alone, although they consult with other health team members when faced with challenging situations. Sometimes ethical decisions related to social justice and human rights need to be made during a home visit, such as placing a client who is not taking his anti-viral TB medications on Directly Observed Therapy (DOT), reporting an unsafe "garbage" home to the county sanitarian, or contacting animal control about a client's pet that has just bitten a young child. Sometimes PHNs carry out advocacy interventions by themselves, and sometimes they are part of a group advocating for change. Whether alone or working with others, PHNs need to be aware of client rights so that they can resolve ethical dilemmas and challenges in a way that encourages that health needs are met.

Social Justice and Human Rights

Nurses are obligated by the American Nurses Association Code of Ethics to provide fair and equal treatment that respects the "inherent dignity, worth, and uniqueness of every individual, unrestricted by considerations of social or economic status, personal attributes, or the nature of the health problem" (ANA, 2001, p. 7). Respect for human rights is a basic tenet of ethical nursing practice (ANA, 2010a; ANA, 2010b). Health care is viewed as a basic right for all individuals by the International Council of Nurses (ICN, 2006). Nurses have a responsibility to safeguard client rights at all times and in all places and are held accountable for both their actions and inactions. PHNs ensure their clients' human rights in many ways. For example, PHNs might choose to have a translator present when they provide health education and counseling to a woman who cannot speak English. PHNs might support the right of their client to begin hospice care at home even though her children want her to be hospitalized for another round of chemotherapy. A pregnant teen might ask her PHN not to inform her mother that she is pregnant. The PHN honors that request, even though as the mother of a teen, she knows she would want to know if her daughter was pregnant.

The core human rights on which most nations agree have been summarized in a document ratified by the United Nations (1948; see the following paragraph). These human rights, especially those emphasizing access to living conditions that encourage health, guide much of what is done by PHNs. However, sometimes advocating for the human rights of individuals and concurrently advocating for social justice for vulnerable individuals, families, or populations result in conflict. For example, laws that require reporting specific communicable diseases (e.g., sexually transmitted infections) are consistent with principles of social justice in meeting "the public good." However, mandated reporting violates the autonomy and anonymity of individuals and might interfere with the level of trust in a nurse-client relationship. Nurses have ethical responsibilities to protect the rights of individuals and to protect the health and welfare of the community. Consequently, some decisions require that nurses provide an ethical rationale for whether they choose to protect the individual or the community when protecting both simultaneously is not possible. For example, when a mentally ill client with a history of violent aggressive behavior is not taking his medications and is becoming delusional, PHNs might have to call the police to transport the client to the hospital against his will. The nurse's action in this case is based on a decision to give priority to the health and safety of the public rather to the rights of autonomy and self-determination of the client.

Selected Human Rights from the Universal Declaration of Human Rights, United Nations

In 1948 the United Nations published *The Universal Declaration of Human Rights* with 30 articles enumerating the basic human rights. The Preamble states "Whereas inherent recognition of the inherent dignity and of the equal and inalienable rights of all members of the human family is the foundation of freedom, justice, and peace in the world … a common understanding of these rights and freedoms is of the greatest importance." Articles 1 and 25 provide an international standard for health as a basic human right. Article 25 also speaks to many of the social determinants of health that have both societal and individual origins.

Article 1. All human beings are born free and equal in dignity and rights. They are endowed with reason and conscience and should act towards one another in a spirit of brotherhood.

Article 25. (1) Everyone has the right to a standard of living adequate for the health and well-being of himself and of his family, including food, clothing, housing, and medical care and necessary social services, and the right to security in the event of unemployment, sickness, disability, widowhood, old age or other lack of livelihood in circumstances beyond his control. (2) Motherhood and childhood are entitled to special care and assistance. All children, whether born in or out of wedlock, shall enjoy the same social protection.

The Commission on the Social Determinants of Health, established by the World Health Organization in 2005, has generated specific recommendations for health care in the 21st century that are based on the universal human rights. The Commission recommends that health promotion continue to be a primary focus of world health priorities and activities. Instead of focusing on individual health behaviors, they emphasize that the focus should be on creating the conditions in which health and well-being can flourish (Baum, Gollust, Goold, & Jacobson, 2007). The Commission made three recommendations for action that are supported by social justice imperatives:

1. Improving daily living conditions in which people are born, grow, live, work, and age

2. Tackling the inequitable distribution of power, money, and resources

3. Measuring and understanding the problem of health inequities and assessing the impact of action (Baum et al., 2007)

 ACTIVITY
Brainstorm specific actions a PHN might take based on the Commission's recommendations. Consider programs and activities you have already observed in your public health nursing clinical experiences.

Evidence Example: Safe Motherhood Initiative

Though maternal and infant mortality declined significantly in developed countries in the 19th and first half of the 20th century, it did not change in undeveloped countries. The international Safe Motherhood Initiative, launched in 1987, focused on improving infant and maternal health in developing countries. Not until 1994 did the UN International Conference on Human Rights declare the right of women to go through pregnancy and childbirth safely. This was the beginning of the movement to view maternal mortality as a human rights issue and a public health concern. Ten years after the Safe Motherhood Initiative was launched, a study of outcomes found that very little had changed. In 2008 it was estimated that 536,000 women die annually from pregnancy-related causes and that an estimated 4 million babies die during the first 4 weeks of life, of which 3 million die in the first week. Women in resource-poor countries have a 1 in 16 risk of dying of pregnancy-related causes compared to women in countries with good resources where the risk is 1 in 4800. Although life-saving and injury treatment exists for women who are pregnant and birthing, many women do not have access to these services. This lack of access is a major human rights issue that must be addressed through government policy, legislation, and service delivery (Gruskin et al., 2008).

Erica knows that the human rights of the families in the apartment complex are at risk because of their exposure to lead-based paint and inability to change their living situation because of poverty and lack of affordable and safe housing. She knows that the human rights of the children cannot be met if they cannot receive the medical care they need. Realizing the human rights of the apartment owner are in conflict with the social justice rights of the apartment residents, Erica tries to find just solutions. Erica wonders if the Affordable Health Care for America Act passed in March 2010 will provide medical care for the children with high lead levels. She reviewed the components of the Act. Some of the provisions of the Affordable Health Care for America Act of 2010 that Erica found at www.healthcare. gov are listed in Table 10.3. She knows that not all laws that are passed are enacted or funded but hopes these provisions will be implemented as she thinks they can benefit children and families.

Government's Response—Health Care Reform

An important step toward ensuring access to health care in the United States in the 21st century is the passage of federal legislation that mandates certain health care rights. Certainly legislative efforts are not a "cure" to inequities in health care access, but they can provide the impetus that is needed to encourage creative strategies and solutions. For example, the 2010 Affordable Health Care for America Act requires that health insurance providers cover children with pre-existing conditions; prior to this legislation, children could be denied health insurance coverage because of asthma, diabetes, or other pre-existing conditions. PHNs are supportive of legislation that encourages improved access to health care for vulnerable and underserved populations. While changing political climates may or may not result in continued support of the 2010 Affordable Health Care for America Act, the bill itself is a good example of legislative efforts taken to achieve a social justice goal. Table 10.3 reflects key components of the legislation passed in 2010.

Table 10.3   Key Provisions of Affordable Care Act of 2010 that Benefit Children and Families

New Consumer Protections
- Children with pre-existing conditions cannot be denied coverage

- Eliminates lifetime coverage limits; provides free preventive care

- Provides access to insurance to uninsured Americans with pre-existing conditions

- Allows states to cover more people on Medicaid

- Improves health care quality and efficiency, including the Children's Health Insurance Program (CHIP), thus making care available for more children

- Prohibits discrimination based on gender or pre-existing conditions

Improving Quality and Reducing Costs
- Requires use of electronic health care records to reduce costs, improve communication, and reduce errors

- Links payments to quality outcomes

- Makes care more affordable by providing tax credits to middle-income families

Increasing Access to Affordable and Culturally Competent Care
- Expands coverage for young adults

- Strengthens community health centers

- Increases workforce diversity

- Supports community health workers

- Expands access to Medicaid

Holding Insurance Companies Accountable
- Strives to bring down costs of health care premiums

- Makes insurance companies accountable for rate hikes

U. S. Department of Health and Human Services, 2010

> *Erica referred the family to a social worker to apply for the state Medicaid program and CHIP services. She thinks funding is available for medical treatment for the children through these programs. Erica also referred the apartment building owner to a state program that provides financial assistance for lead abatement. The apartment owner was relieved to know that he could get financial assistance for lead abatement to provide a safer environment for his tenants.*

Addressing Population Health Determinants

Poor health in populations has multiple complex causes including poverty, poor housing, inadequate education, unsafe environments, and other social and physical environmental factors. Individuals and families can only change health determinants that are related to their own biological, behavioral, and life circumstances. They generally cannot change the health determinants that are societal in nature (i.e., convenient clinic location). Health determinants that are societal in nature are called social determinants of health. Health determinants and social determinants of health either increase risk (i.e., risk factors) or reduce risk (i.e., protective factors). Table 10.4 illustrates the diverse risk factors confronting a young family at risk for elevated blood lead levels.

Table 10.4   Selected Health and Social Determinants for Increased Blood Lead Levels in Children

Risk Factors		
Individual/Family Level	**Community Level**	**Systems Level**
• Exposure to lead-based paint in home	• Older substandard housing with lead-based paint	• Lack of affordable private or public health insurance
• Developmental stage and age of children	• Lack of safe affordable housing	• Limited access to affordable health care
• Children's liver and kidneys unable to excrete excess lead	• High poverty level	• Local businesses are laying off workers and not hiring new workers
• Family cannot afford safe housing	• Fewer medical clinics accepting Medical Assistance clients	
• Lack of medical insurance		

ACTIVITY

If you were a PHN, what actions would you take to reduce or eliminate any of these risk factors?

Key social determinants of health that influence access to health care resources and affect health and well-being include the following:

- Neighborhood living conditions (poverty or crime levels, housing quality)
- Employment opportunities
- Community development
- Prevailing norms, customs, and processes
- Social cohesion
- Civic engagement

Addressing Population Health Disparities

Health disparities are differences in health outcomes between individuals, families, populations, and communities that result in some people having a lower level of health and wellness than others. They are most common among vulnerable populations—those who are oppressed, marginalized, disenfranchised, or underserved and, therefore, at greater risk for disease, disability, and premature death. PHNs work to eliminate and weaken the health determinants that lead to health disparities. See Table 10.5 for examples of health disparities, health inequalities, and health inequities in populations.

Table 10.5   Differentiating between Health Disparities, Health Inequalities, and Health Inequities

Health Disparities are population-specific differences in health and disease (incidence and prevalence), health outcomes, or access to care that place some populations at greater risk than others.	African-American men have lower smoking prevalence rates than white male smokers but have higher lung cancer mortality rates (Jones, Waters, Oka, & McGhee, 2010).
Health Inequalities are differences in rates of disease and health outcomes among different populations as a result of their different social positions, their ability to control their life circumstances, and their ability to participate in mainstream society. Deprivation of rights of one population is relative to the rights held by another population. Health inequalities reflect the level of deprivation of one group versus another group.	A study of shelter-based foster youth in Baltimore found that only 10.7% had documented up-to-date immunizations, only 1.2% had a documented PPD (Mantoux testing for tuberculosis) application and reading, and 13.1% had a significant delay in recommended follow-up to care. Center staff members were not aware of many of the foster youth's health needs. This study demonstrated that shelter-based foster youth had significantly less access to health care than non-shelter-based foster youth (Ensign, 2001).
Health Inequities are systematic disparities in health and in the major social determinants of health between diverse populations with different social positions (i.e., race, class, and advantages or disadvantages such as wealth, power, and prestige.)	An African-American baby is 2.5 times more likely to die before his or her first birthday than a white baby. In 2000, 83,500 more African Americans died than would have died if African Americans had not experienced differences in the social determinants of health and reduced access to health care services for centuries (Satcher & Higginbotham, 2008).

PHNs spend most of their time working with individuals and families to modify their health determinants (i.e., reduce their risk factors and strengthen their protective factors) and empower them to manage their own health care needs. PHNs are interested in reducing health disparities among populations as well. To do this, PHNs must understand the multiple causes or health determinants that influence health status of populations. Individuals and families within populations that experience health disparities suffer consequences even if their personal behaviors and biological/genetic factors encourage health. Thus,

PHNs must advocate for change in the societal causes of population health disparities by working at the community and systems levels of practice. Working with individuals and families to help them change their own behaviors and risk factors cannot by itself eliminate health disparities at the population level.

In a perfect world, health resources would be infinite, and everyone would receive all of the health care they need. Unfortunately, this is not the case, and much of the time we cannot even agree on health care that is needed. A comparison of selected death rates and incidence of disease (Table 10.6) illustrates some of the major health disparities in the United States.

Table 10.6   Comparison of Selected Health Status Disparities by Race and Ethnicity

Infant Death Rate	Twice as high among African Americans, American Indians, and Alaskan Natives as among whites
Heart Disease Death Rates	African-American rate is 40% higher than for whites
Cancer Death Rate	African-American rate is 30% higher than for whites
HIV/AIDS Death Rate	African-American rate is seven times that for whites
Incidence of TB	Hispanics are 11% of population but account for 20% of new cases
Diabetes Death Rates	Hispanic rate is twice as high as that for non-Hispanic whites

Office of Minority Health and Health Disparities, 2010

A comparison of life expectancy in the United States illustrates both health disparities and health inequities. For example, the gap in life expectancy between the rich and the poor and those with more education versus those with less education is widening (Congressional Budget Office, 2008). The gender and racial gaps in life expectancy continue to persist (see Figure 10.2). Though gaps in life expectancy might be partially explained by lifestyle decisions and biological factors, societal factors also play a role. Those who are poor or live in poor neighborhoods have less access to healthy food and healthcare compared to those who live in higher-income neighborhoods and have higher incomes. White neighborhoods have four times as many grocery stores as Black and Latino neighborhoods, and 80% of billboards in African American neighborhoods are advertising tobacco or liquor (Unnatural Causes, 2010).

Erica received a phone call from the mother of the children with high lead levels. She had been able to enroll her children in a state-run health care plan and is looking for a medical clinic on a bus line. The clinic she found is no longer taking patients on government assistance. Erica knows there are not many medical clinics in the mother's neighborhood and cannot think of one on a bus line. She checks the county's database on medical clinics and the metropolitan transportation agency website to find out about bus service routes. She contacts the American Red Cross and faith-based and charitable organizations in the neighborhood for transportation assistance. These searches take an entire afternoon, but Erica is successful in finding a clinic that accepts people on government assistance and a local church that has a volunteer transportation program. Erica asks her supervisor how to code these hours on her time sheet as she is not providing direct nursing care. Her supervisor tells Erica that she is carrying out the nursing interventions of Advocacy and Case Management by finding resources that can help her client become more self-sufficient.

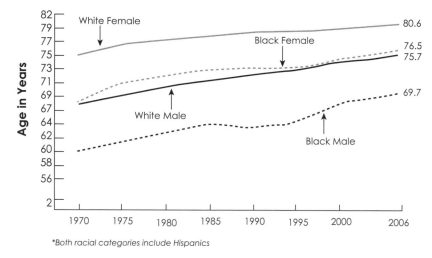

*Both racial categories include Hispanics

Figure 10.2 Life expectancy at birth, by race* and sex, 1970-2006
Health Resources and Service Administration, 2009

Erica's efforts are based on her knowledge of health determinants called protective factors that mitigate or reduce risk factors that negatively impact health. The protective factors for Erica's client family are listed in Table 10.7.

Table 10.7 Health Determinants that Reduce Risk of Elevated Blood Lead Levels

Protective Factors		
Individual/Family Level	**Community Level**	**Systems Level**
• Mother's health-seeking behaviors (observes children's behaviors and seeks help) and acceptance of public health resources including PHN	• Taxpayer funding of public health department	• Public health nursing services
	• Community volunteer resources for transportation	• Environmental health services
• Children healthy except for increased lead levels	• Faith-based resources	• Availability of Medicaid and CHIP funds for health care for children and poor families without insurance
• Apartment owner concerned about health of tenants and willing to apply for funding for lead abatement	• Availability of lead abatement programs reflects community environmental health priority and concern for children	• Clinic willing to admit patients on governmental assistance

Advocates for the Populations for which the PHN Is Accountable

Advocacy is a primary role and responsibility of nursing. Some see advocacy as the fundamental basis of nursing (Curtin, 1979; Gadow, 1999; MacDonald, 2006). Public health nursing includes advocacy as a standard for practice (ANA, 2007; see Standard 16 below). PHNs are often in positions that require them to advocate on behalf of populations that do not currently have the capacity to provide for or manage their own health care needs. In order to foster self-determination, facilitate empowerment, and promote self-advocacy, nurses need to create an atmosphere that supports and respects the rights of the populations they advocate for (Mallik, 1997). We do this by partnering with populations experiencing health disparities. Partnering involves a strengths-based approach in which PHNs first identify the strengths and resources of the population and community and then collaborate with the populations and community to plan and implement effective community and system-wide intervention strategies. In other words, PHNs build capacity among vulnerable populations and their communities.

> **Standard 16. Advocacy, Public Health Nursing—Scope and Standards of Practice**
>
> The PHN advocates to protect the health, safety, and rights of the population.
>
> *Measurement Criteria:*
>
> The PHN:
>
> - Incorporates the identified needs of the population in policy development and program planning
>
> - Integrates advocacy into the implementation of policies, programs, and services for the population
>
> - Evaluates the effectiveness of advocating for the population when assessing the expected outcomes
>
>   - Includes confidentiality, ethical, legal, privacy, and professional guidelines in policy development and other issues
>
>   - Demonstrates skill in advocating before providers and stakeholders on behalf of the population
>
>   - Strives to resolve conflicting expectations from populations, providers, and other stakeholders to ensure the safety and to guard for the best interest of the population and to preserve the professional integrity of the nurse (ANA. 2007, p. 40)

To advocate effectively, PHNs need to understand the context of people's lives, including their race, culture, and ethnicity and what makes them vulnerable. For example, many of the new immigrant groups in the United States are vulnerable populations. Advocacy for populations that are ethnically different than your own, such as new immigrants, requires compassion and an understanding of the group's culture (Pacquiao, 2008). This is true for other vulnerable groups, such as the homeless. Many myths and misunderstandings exist about people who appear different. As one nursing student said after working in a homeless shelter, "I didn't realize that they would be just like me, only homeless."

Evidence Example: Who Are the Vulnerable?

The term "vulnerable populations" refers to social groups with increased relative risk (i.e., exposure to risk factors) or susceptibility to health-related problems. This vulnerability is evidenced in higher comparative mortality rates, lower life expectancy, reduced access to care, and diminished quality of life. Vulnerable populations are often discriminated against, marginalized and disenfranchised from mainstream society, contributing to their lower social status and lack of power in personal, social, and political relationships (Center for Vulnerable Populations Research, 2010).

Two research studies funded by the Center for Vulnerable Populations Research (CVPR) involved studying low-income women with depression. One study found the impact of the environment, particularly poverty and violence, was a significant cause of depression in older women living in poverty (Kiger in CVPR, 2008). Another study found that mothers living with postpartum depression experienced lengthy episodes of depression and that there were "multiple confounding factors and social stressors surrounding their condition" (Abrams in CVPR, 2008). An effective family-centered intervention approach included health education on the symptoms of postpartum depression and information on referral sources, including those for mental health.

Erica reflected on the positive health outcome for the two children with increased lead levels and the lead abatement of the apartment building that is scheduled for next month. She remembered she had been in a hurry on the home visit and was impatient when the mother started talking about her children rather than responding to the questions Erica was asking. Luckily, Erica managed to focus on the mother's concerns rather than her own. She knows that if she had not taken the time to listen carefully, she might have missed the mother's comments about the children's symptoms and might not have noticed the paint chips. Erica renews her commitment to listen to clients tell her what their priorities and needs are. She decides she will be more observant when assessing the homes and neighborhoods of children in her caseload. Erica knows that collecting data and reporting her findings are the first steps in advocating for change.

Evidence Example: National Association of School Nurses: Speaking Up for Children

The National Association of School Nurses (NASN) advocates for child health and the resources needed to promote health and safety among school children. School nurses are aware of the significant number of children coming to school with preventable physical and mental health conditions. School nurses work hard to obtain the needed health and social services for these children. But they know that they cannot solve the problem of inadequate resources by working one nurse, one child at a time. NASN has a history of lobbying for school health resources to meet the needs of children. To more effectively lobby at the national level, NASN moved its headquarters to

Washington D.C. in 2005. The NASN Annual Conference in 2005 brought hundreds of school nurses to Washington D.C.; prepared them for lobbying efforts; and provided opportunities for the nurses to meet with their elected representatives to talk with them about child and school health issues, explain the role of the school nurse, and discuss the positive impact school nurses have on child health. The NASN 2007 policy agenda, *Capital Investment for Children*, was an effort to secure a place at the national policy-making table for school nurses so that they could provide the voice for children with unmet health needs. NASN continues its efforts to work with national, state, and local officials to achieve their goal of achieving a ratio of school nurses to students in each school that can adequately meet the health needs of school children (Denehy, 2007).

Advocacy at the Individual/Family Level of Practice

Nurses advocate for individuals and families by safeguarding their autonomy, acting on their behalf, and championing social justice in the provision of health care (Bu & Jezewski, 2006). Advocacy is aimed at building the capacity of individuals or families to manage their own health care needs. PHNs recognize the inequalities that exist within social determinants of health and challenge the status quo to change the social environment. They enter into the practice of "critical caring" when they recognize health disparities in individuals and families and work to change the context of people's lives to improve their health (Falk-Rafael, 2005a).

When PHNs advocate for individuals and families, they often do so from within a trusting relationship (MacDonald, 2006). This is particularly true for PHNs who work closely with individuals and families over extended periods of time because the time is necessary to build trust. For example, nurses working with abused children or women often become aware of the abusive situation when they are providing trustworthy care for common physical health conditions. A trusting relationship makes it possible for the clients to disclose very personal information about abuse, and then the nurses can effectively intervene and advocate for safety (Hughes, 2010; Vanderburg, Wright, Boston, & Zimmerman, 2010).

Advocacy at the Community and Systems Levels of Practice

Caring and a passionate commitment to social justice drive PHNs to practice active advocacy to create social change and improve well-being. Advocacy at the community and systems levels often translates into efforts such as coalition building, community organizing, collaboration, and policy development (see Table 10.8). Most beginning nurses are much more interested in direct care of individuals and families than in developing policies. Both are important, though. Nurses participate in systems-level activities to address inequalities and barriers in health care that impede the health of populations.

Table 10.8 Public Health Nursing Interventions at the Community and Systems Levels of Practice that Support Advocacy

Coalition building promotes and develops alliances among organizations or constituencies for a common purpose. It builds linkages, solves problems, and/or enhances local leadership to address health concerns (MDH, 2001, p. 211). The process by which parties (individuals, organizations, or groups) come together to form a temporary alliance or union to work together for a common purpose and to enhance each other's capacity for mutual benefit and common purpose (ANA, 2007, p. 41).	A group of diverse organizations in South Carolina formed a coalition to eliminate racial and ethnic health disparities in six priority areas: cardiovascular disease, diabetes, infant mortality, breast and cervical cancer, HIV/AIDS, and child and adult immunizations. A 2-year evaluation of the outcomes of the diabetes coalition, REACH 2010, demonstrated a significant reduction in some diabetes-related disparities. The coalitions continue to work on their goals of eliminating health disparities (Jenkins, et al., 2004).
Community organizing helps community groups identify common problems or goals, mobilize resources, and develop and implement strategies for reaching the goals they collectively have set (MDH, 2001, p. 235).	A community action model was used in California to increase the capacity of the community to address the social health determinants of tobacco-related health disparities. The community was able to take action to develop local policies to eliminate or weaken the social health determinants of smoking (Lavery et al., 2005).
Collaboration commits two or more persons or organizations to achieving a common goal through enhancing the capacity of one or more of them to promote and protect health (MDH, 2001, p. 177).	PHNs in Alberta, Canada, concerned about the incidence of postpartum depression initiated a demonstration project in which they collaborated with a group of obstetricians and a group of midwives to have pregnant women referred to PHNs for psychosocial screening, health education, referral, and follow-up. Of the 150 women assessed, 37% had a history of postpartum depression, and 33% had a family history of depression. They accessed 93 services. Of the 75 women who participated in the program evaluation, 68% reported that the PHN intervention was helpful. The outcomes were so positive that the collaborative program was continued (Strass & Billay, 2008).
Policy development places health issues on decision-makers' agenda. Acquires a plan of resolution and determines needed resources. Policy development results in laws, rules, and regulations, ordinances, and policies.	Barriers that limit access to health care in the uninsured elderly population were explored in this journal article in a special health policy feature. The barriers were identified and analyzed. Key barriers were lack of transportation, lack of insurance, complexity of the health care system, poverty, lack of family support, culture, communication, and race and ethnicity. Recommendations made included

Policy enforcement compels others to comply with the laws, rules, regulations, ordinances, and policies created in conjunction with Policy Development (MDH, 2001, p. 313)

improving health insurance coverage, use of case management model of care, outreach services, improving transportation, and cultural competency and communication. Many of these recommendations were directed toward needed changes in federal health care policy (Horton & Johnson, 2010).

Erica has been with the county public health agency for a year. She is committed to social justice and wants to improve her ability to advocate for vulnerable individuals and families. She wants to be able to support agency initiatives to improve population health in her community. Erica has noticed that agency nurses in management positions frequently carry out community organizing, coalition building, and policy development interventions. Sometimes she supported these agency initiatives. Erica makes a list of the opportunities she participated in and the opportunities she has missed (see Table 10.9).

Table 10.9 Erica's List of Agency Initiatives

Opportunities Taken	Opportunities Missed
Brief conversation with a county health board member. Told a brief client story about a teenage mom that supported the existence of a Healthy Families Collaborative. (Coalition Building)	In the past legislative session during a debate on a ruling regarding preservatives in vaccines, I could have written a personal letter to my legislator. (Policy Development)
Articulated several "talking points" from the state department of health policy on vaccines and autism at the early childhood meeting for parents to motivate parents to encourage other parents to have their children vaccinated. (Community Organizing)	Did not attend a meeting organized by city hall regarding hiking and biking trails in my community. I could have been a voice for obesity prevention in my community. (Community Organizing)
Led a focus group with Cambodian immigrants on cultural competency in services for the elderly in their community. Provided a summary report to the Cambodian community and service providers. (Collaboration)	Missed an opportunity for PHN team case study discussion to identify unmet health needs among their case loads. I could have learned how my case load was similar to or different from other PHN case loads and how this influences our decision-making and priority-setting processes. (Collaboration)

Opportunities Taken	Opportunities Missed
Represented the agency on a task force organized by the state health department to develop guidelines on blood lead and healthy housing. (Policy Development)	Missed a meeting with a senior coalition to lobby county commissioners to extend green light walking time to allow seniors to walk across streets safely. I could have learned more about this health risk for the elderly. (Coalition Building)
Met with the OB nurse manager, Newborn Nursery nurse manager, and the Infection Control nurse at the local hospital to discuss Tdap vaccination of staff as a means to prevent pertussis in newborn infants. (Collaboration)	Did not return a survey regarding vending machine policies in the school district. I could have helped with the data collection process. (Policy Development)

Ethical Application for Social Justice and Public Health Nursing

Public health nurses make ethical decisions on a daily basis. Many ethical decisions are made at the individual level of PHN practice. Using an ethical decision-making framework is helpful.

 ACTIVITY

Consider the following case study: A PHN making a home visit to a recently paroled inmate of the local jail notes on the referral that the man is PPD positive on repeat testing and needs to start antiviral medications for TB. The man has the medication with him, but is not taking it. The PHN considers her options.

Should she start Directly Observed Treatment (DOT)?

Should she notify his physician or parole agent of his noncompliance?

What is the ethical dilemma and how would you resolve it?

Review the ethical principles listed in Table 10.10. Use these ethical principles to resolve the ethical dilemma.

Table 10.10   Ethical Principles and Actions in Advocacy

Ethical Perspectives	Examples
Rule Ethics (principles)	• Public health resources and services are allocated based on need, so they might be distributed unequally.
	• Identify individuals, families, populations, and communities who are vulnerable and experiencing health disparities.
	• Provide public health nursing services to those who are most vulnerable, at greatest health risk, and those who are experiencing health disparities and health inequities.

Virtue Ethics (character)	• Make ethical decisions based on social justice and human rights. • Provide support for individuals, families, populations and communities who advocate for themselves. • Be caring, compassionate, and egalitarian. • Select advocacy goals and actions that are culturally congruent with the racial and ethnic diversity of individuals, families, and populations within the community.
Feminist Ethics (reducing oppression)	• Advocate for the health and well-being of individuals, families, populations, and communities. • Include and partner with clients in priority setting, goal setting, and advocacy actions. • Empower clients to manage their own health care needs. • Work to increase capacity of individuals, families, populations, and communities to manage their health care needs. • Take actions to address social injustice at all levels of public health nursing practice.

Table based on work by Volbrecht, 2002, and Racher, 2007

Key Points

- Social justice serves as the foundation for public health nursing.

- Social justice states that individuals have the right to receive resources based on need.

- PHNs must be able to work in partnership with health care systems based on either market justice or social justice.

- Population health disparities and health inequities persist in the United States and worldwide.

- Nurses are responsible for providing health care as a basic human right.

- PHNs advocate for health equity and justice for individuals, families, populations, and communities at all three levels of practice—individual/family, community, and systems.

- PHNs advocate for vulnerable individuals, families, populations, and communities.

- Key public health nursing advocacy interventions include coalition building, collaboration, community organizing, and policy development and enforcement.

Exercises

Learning Examples for Social Justice: The Story of Edna Dell Weinel, PHN

One's first experience working with people who have been systematically disenfranchised can be a powerful learning experience. It reshapes one's view of the world. Read to the story of one public health nursing leader.

Edna Dell Weinel, was a PHN whose career included positions as a former executive director (1980–1991) of the Family Care Center, a federally funded neighborhood health center in St. Louis, Missouri; a county PHN; a state maternal-child nursing consultant; and a public health nursing educator. She was a leader in public health nursing in the 20th century and held leadership positions in the American Public Health Association. Edna Dell had this to say about her first experience with poverty as a new PHN with the Visiting Nurse Association of St. Louis.

> It was also my first understanding of poverty. I had a district, 20th Street to the Mississippi River, and at one point of the river there was an area that was called Hooverville, where people . . . had houses that were put together with found wood, just desperately poor people, and when the river came up very high, it kind of went behind Hooverville. This meant I had to get to Hooverville by boat. (Kalnins, 2008, p. 195)

This early experience helped to shape Edna Dell Weinel's career. Her career was dominated by four themes: to work to one's highest level of skill; to provide care with a social conscience; to develop effective team relationships; and to become skilled in the strategic use of power and influence for the health of the community (p. 199).

ACTIVITY

Keep track of your stories and listen to the stories of your classmates. These stories and experiences can transform the way you think and act as a practitioner of caring and just nursing care.

What themes emerge about social justice from your stories?

What have you learned about your nursing practice?

Advocating for Justice in the Digital Age

Today's students are very comfortable as members of the "digital age." So, using digital technology for advocacy activities to promote health fits student interests and expertise. Suggested activities include the following:

- *Friending and Social Networking*—Use websites such as Facebook and MySpace to promote social justice issues and advocacy activities. Link to other participants' pages or create your own page with a health promotion and advocacy theme.

- *Real-Time Communications*—Use blast or mailing list e-mail for advocacy alerts; use Twitter for advocacy alerts, press conferences, mobilizing people for demonstrations, increasing awareness of a specific health issue through a planned advocacy campaign.

- *Advocacy Channel*—Develop portals for reporting the news and educating the public on health issues (i.e., website, blog, Twitter, YouTube, BlogTalkRadio, photographs and videos, widgets; Galer-Unti, 2010)

ACTIVITY

What digital technology have you used to share information with your classmates?

Which of the above suggestions might you use to share issues of social justice in the future?

Reflective Practice

It is difficult to think about the bigger picture on a daily basis when providing nursing care to vulnerable individuals and families. The annual review period is a good time to compare professional goals with actual practice in order to determine congruence between goals and practice and identify opportunities for professional growth and development.

> *Erica was preparing for her annual review with her supervisor. She decided that one of her goals for the following year will be to begin developing her advocacy skills at the community and systems levels of practice. She felt that her values and perspectives were consistent with social justice and the mission and goals of the county public health agency. She believed she had been effective in advocating for individuals and families like the family with the children with increased blood lead levels. She now understands that she has to intervene at all three levels of practice to create change to improve population health. Erica was ready to work on the ACTIONS!*

Think about your experiences in your public health nursing clinical.

What advocacy actions did you take for individuals or families?

_____

_____

What advocacy actions did you observe your preceptor or other PHNs taking at the community and systems levels of practice?

_____

_____

Think of a health disparity in the population your agency serves. Is there an unmet health need that could be addressed?

_____

_____

If you were going to develop an intervention at the community or systems level of practice for this health need, what would it be? How would you start?

_____

_____

Think about how Erica developed and demonstrated public health nursing advocacy competencies as she worked with the two young children with increased lead levels and their mother, analyzed her own practice, and set a goal to develop additional advocacy competencies. Discuss the following questions with your classmates.

_____

_____

Application of Evidence

1. What values and perspectives did Erica hold that motivated her to act in a socially just manner?

2. What aspects of the situation required Erica to take actions for this family?

3. What ethical conflict between social justice and individual human rights did Erica have to resolve? How did she resolve it?

4. What advocacy actions did Erica take to help the family and owner of the building?

5. Did Erica work alone or was she part of a team? Explain.

6. What were the health outcomes of her actions?

7. What else might Erica do in the future to protect children from environmental hazards?

Think, Explore, Do

1. How will you prepare to work with vulnerable populations in your public health clinical? Consider the following suggestions.

   • Review literature on topics that are related to your clinical (i.e., health disparities, health determinants, social justice, vulnerable populations, globalization, societal decision-making and resource allocation processes, culture, and ethnicity).

- Review health status data on vulnerable populations you will be working with (national, state, local reports).

- Read about and listen to presentations on health care disparities and quality and culture at the Providers Guide to Quality and Culture website at http://erc.msh.org/mainpage.cfm?file=7.0.htm&module=provider&language=English. Take the cultural competency quiz.

- View some of the six online videos on Unnatural Causes – California Newsreel at http://www.unnaturalcauses.org and discuss with your classmates. Consider the advocacy actions you might take if you were an elected official or the CEO of a charitable foundation.

2. How can you take advantage of the learning opportunities available to you during your public health clinical? Consider the following suggestions.

- Participate in a variety of community experiences so you get a broad exposure to the diverse community populations, their health priorities and concerns, their strengths (resilience, support networks, capacity for change, etc.), and their needs.

- Observe an activity where community members partner with health care providers to solve community health problems.

- Identify social justice issues in your public health clinical setting.

- Use nonjudgmental therapeutic listening to understand your client's perspectives, health needs, and health priorities.

- Empower your clients by providing them with information, community resources, and support network.

3. What actions might you take to learn more about and advocate for the vulnerable populations you are working with? Consider the following suggestions.

- Participate in a service-learning activity with an underserved population experiencing health disparities and health inequities.

- Write letters to the editor or to your elected representatives.

- Develop posters or brochures to be used by agency.

- Attend a community meeting and participate in discussions about how to provide services for populations experiencing health disparities.

- Call in to radio programs discussing health concerns and health reform.

- Find bumper stickers that speak to social justice and advocacy and use them.

- Join a peaceful demonstration in your community.

- Join a community action group or student advocacy group working on public health goals for social justice.

- Talk with friends, relatives, other students, colleagues at work, and neighbors about your public health concerns.

4. Think about the advocacy competencies you developed during your public health clinical.

    - What vulnerable populations have you worked with as a student nurse? Explain.

    - How did you know if an individual, family, or population was experiencing a health disparity?

    - How did you explore the causes of the health disparity?

    - What clients did you advocate for as part of your public health clinical?

    - What advocacy interventions did you use in your public health nursing clinical?

    - What worked and what didn't work? What would you do differently in the future?

5. What advocacy competencies would you like to develop in the future? What is the first step? (Based on work by Boutain, 2008; Cohen & Reutter, 2007; Easley & Allen, 2007; and Falk-Rafael, 2005b)

COMPETENCY #9:
Demonstrates Nonjudgmental and Unconditional Acceptance of People Different from Self

By Carolyn M. Garcia
with Christine C. Andres, Patricia A. Henton, and Karen Jorgensen-Royce

Josie is a public health nursing student completing her final clinical hours before graduating. She and a classmate have been volunteering in a school-based clinic. The school nurse has invited Josie to join her on a home visit to check up on a student who has just given birth. Josie uses the GPS on her iPhone to find the apartment; it is located in a part of the city she normally avoids. She carefully locks her car and joins the school nurse in the apartment lobby. The client answers the call, and they are invited upstairs to the apartment. The unfamiliar hallway lighting and smells cause Josie to proceed cautiously. She hopes to focus on what the school nurse accomplishes rather than on her own feelings of discomfort. What are some of the fears or worries Josie might be experiencing in this, or other, situations that are different for her? What are some things that might have helped Josie prepare for the "discomfort" that can often be experienced during home visits? What does Josie need to know or understand to help her work with clients who don't live like she does?

JOSIE'S NOTEBOOK

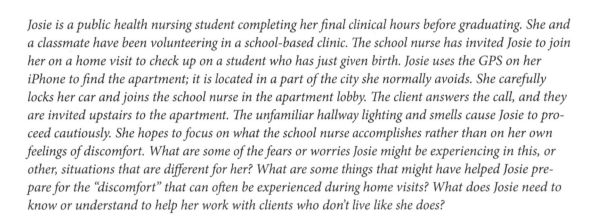

Competency #9: Demonstrates nonjudgmental and unconditional acceptance of people different from self.

- Listening to others in an unbiased manner

- Respecting others' points of view

- Promoting the expression of diverse opinions and perspectives

- Identifying the role of cultural, social, spiritual, religious, and behavioral factors when selecting or designing public health interventions

- Interacting respectfully, sensitively, and effectively with diverse persons

Useful Definitions

Nonjudgmental: "Being open to understanding cultural uniqueness and respect for individuals" (Pasco, Morse, & Olson, 2004, p. 1). A nurse describes being nonjudgmental as she sought to "...establish a ... communion into which I enter having cleansed myself of harmful bias through honest self-reflection; and, in which I exude humility and openness" (Porr, 2005, p. 6).

> *Unconditional:* "A form of respect that involves profoundness of feeling, treasuring, warm regard, [and] solicitous concern" (Dillon, 1992, p. 120).
>
> *Acceptance:* "To consider their patients' culture and incorporate it in care…" (Cioffi, 2003, p. 305) and the "respect of another's individual person and self-defined reality" (Porr, 2005, p. 1).

They Don't Live Like I Do

Public health nursing (PHN) is similar to other areas of nursing when it comes to valuing the ability to deliver nursing care in a nonjudgmental, accepting manner. A public health nurse (PHN) is often in the client's context, such as in the home, and this provides for endless opportunities for a nurse's acceptance of others to be tested, confirmed, or challenged. A PHN might work with a faith community to offer blood pressure screening, which might require the nurse to work alongside others with different values or beliefs. In this chapter we explore the ways in which a PHN can demonstrate nonjudgmental or unconditional acceptance of people. We also provide examples of how PHNs have worked to develop acceptance for individuals, families, and communities across difficult situations. Finally, the chapter concludes with suggestions for assessing your own acceptance of others, and things you might do to develop yourself as a nonjudgmental person, and a nurse.

A nurse can be nonjudgmental and at the same time can disagree with something that is observed or said. This distinction is subtle but important; a nurse should be able to discern whether a behavior is healthy or harmful yet should also be able to make these assessments in a manner that is nonjudgmental. A PHN caring for prison inmates is likely to feel strongly about the crimes that have been committed. This nurse is going to regularly face the challenge to provide nursing care that is equal to the care provided to a nonprisoner, care that is not conditionally based on what the person has done or not done. The nurse's clients and those she or he works alongside can know that the care being provided is nonjudgmental and unconditional when the nurse demonstrates unbiased listening, respect, and openness.

Another example in which PHNs might be confronted with a challenge of being nonjudgmental is when they are providing nursing care to a generation very different from their own. This challenge is often encountered within the context of changing cultural trends. For example, a current cultural trend seen in late adolescence and young adults is expression through the form of body tattooing. Nurses displaced by several decades from this population group might negatively value or view tattooing. Those PHNs have the challenge of trying to "fit" into this generation and to understand the current trends and values and their importance. PHNs can be more successful in building a nonjudgmental, ongoing relationship when they respect possible cultural generational differences. In the case of tattooing, respecting differences might mean not addressing whether or not someone is getting a tattoo, but rather promoting safe tattooing practices.

There are numerous ways in which diversity is reflected. These might include:

- Culture
- Religion

- Socioeconomic position

- Age

- Race

- Physical appearances

- Sexual orientation

- Education level

- Neighborhood

- Geographic region

- Language use

- Immigration status

- Health status

- Beliefs

- Values

Some of the ways that nurses demonstrate nonjudgmental and unconditional public health nursing might include:

- Listening to others in an unbiased manner

- Respecting others' points of view

- Promoting the expression of diverse opinions and perspectives

- Identifying the role of cultural, social, spiritual, religious, and behavioral factors when selecting or designing public health interventions

- Interacting respectfully, sensitively, and effectively with diverse persons (e.g., diverse by culture, socioeconomic position, educational level, race, ethnicity, gender, sexual orientation, religious background, health status, age, and lifestyle preferences)

Listening to Others in an Unbiased Manner

Have you watched yourself in a mirror to observe your nonverbal cues and signals when you are reacting to what someone else is saying? Do you smile? Do you nod cautiously or in positive support for the other person? Do you scowl quickly when something you don't agree with is spoken? Effective listening is a combination of verbal and nonverbal responses to the person with whom you are talking. Listening in an unbiased manner takes effective listening to a higher level because it requires you not only to listen in a way that helps the person who is talking feel they are being heard but also to listen in a manner that expresses acceptance for that person.

As with most communication attributes (refer back to Chapter 8, which is devoted to communication), verbal and nonverbal listening cues can vary by culture, developmental age, and other factors. Therefore, you need to know the clients you are working with and understand what conveys listening and support to them. Don't presume to know. The following are some broad categories that serve as examples of the many ways in which we express listening, support, inattention, or boredom.

NONVERBAL

- Eye Contact (not too little, not too much)

- Facial Expressions (smile, stare, frown, grimace)

- Gestures (head nod, hand motions)

- Intensity (amount of energy you exude to the other person can support or bother)

- Movements and Posture (leaning toward someone indicates interest)

- Space (closeness and proximity to the other person/people)

- Touch (hand on shoulder, hug)

VERBAL

- Supportive Sounds (uh huh, ah)

- Timing and Pace (responding quickly indicates active listening rather than distraction)

- Voice Tone (angry, supportive, authoritarian)

Source: Nonverbal Communication Skills: The Power of Nonverbal Communication and Body Language. (Segal, Smith, & Jaffe, 2006) http://www.helpguide.org/mental/eq6_nonverbal_communication.htm

You need to adequately prepare for interactions with clients and families so that your nonverbal actions are consistent with their culture. For example, in some cultures it is not be appropriate to pat a child on the head, and it is not acceptable to look people of certain cultural groups in the eye.

Respecting Others' Points of View

Are you quick to defend your own views or beliefs? Is it hard for you to listen to someone argue for a value that is not your own? It can be difficult to respect others' points of view when they do not naturally align with your own. However, this skill is critical to being a nonjudgmental nurse. The key is demonstrating respect for another point of view regardless of whether or not you concur. You can express respect verbally and nonverbally. For example, when a PHN visits a mother who has recently delivered her fifth child, the nurse is likely to explore birth control or child spacing plans with the mother. If the mother expresses a view that opposes family planning or use of birth control, the nurse needs to respect that view. One way you can show respect is through offering relevant information in a nonassuming manner and choosing to respect client autonomy for maintaining a different perspective. This respect can be particularly difficult when client, family, or community views are perceived by you to be unhealthy.

Promoting the Expression of Diverse Opinions and Perspectives

Do you seek others' opinions before making a decision? Do you welcome multiple perspectives, or do you find them annoying? Nurses are often in situations that require advocacy for families and communities, and each family and community contains multiple perspectives and opinions. Effective PHNs can assess the situation and intervene in a manner that helps everyone express an opinion. For example, a PHN visiting a family with a hospice client might encounter many opinions from that family about how to best help their loved one go through the dying process. Even though it might be impossible to act upon each opinion, the nurse can assist family members in expressing their perspectives and, ultimately, in coming together to make many difficult decisions.

Identifying the Role of Cultural, Social, Spiritual, Religious, and Behavioral Factors When Selecting or Designing Public Health Interventions

Have you thought about how a nursing action might look different if you are caring for someone with a lot of money or someone with very little? Do you enjoy learning about other cultures? Throughout this book you have been reminded that PHNs consider multiple factors when providing care for individuals, families, and communities. Nonjudgmental PHNs carefully consider those they are serving when specific interventions are being planned. For example, when PHNs implement a child obesity prevention program, they need to consider the cultural perceptions that might impede or support the program. For example, a recent refugee population might view additional weight on a child as a positive, healthy attribute because they are comparing this to the poverty and malnourishment experienced by many children in their home country. Sociocultural expectations can also influence the success of PHN interventions if PHNs are not proactive. For example, in some recent immigrant communities, some leaders are regularly consulted by community members about numerous issues. Effective PHNs assess the extent to which these cultural patterns exist within a community and act in accordance with the sociocultural standards to gain entry and to intervene. Similarly, PHNs, including those who serve as parish nurses, carefully consider the religious or spiritual implications for certain interventions. For example, PHNs might need to schedule a health promotion intervention around certain holidays or celebrations so that attendance and involvement is optimal.

Interacting Respectfully, Sensitively, and Effectively with Diverse Persons

Are you comfortable having a conversation with an individual who is homeless? Do you enjoy learning about cultures different from your own? Do you believe you are deserving of good things, maybe more so than other people? Do you see the person serving you in a store or a restaurant, or do you see through them? Ultimately, your success as a PHN depends on your ability to establish a meaningful relationship with the individual, family, or community you are serving. You can't establish that relationship unless you can interact with diverse people in a nonjudgmental and accepting manner. You are going to find it easier to be nonjudgmental toward some people more so than toward others. You need to engage in learning activities or reflective exercises to help you recognize and address preconceived stereotypes you might have about certain groups of people. Certainly, your worldview provides, in essence, a cultural filter for how you view and interact with others. Over time and with experience you are going to learn more about yourself, including your reactions to those who are different from you. You might find that you are very accepting toward certain people and communities whereas with others you struggle to feel nonjudgmental. Becoming nonjudgmental is a process, and it takes time. Practically, you can begin to implement behaviors helpful to you in your development toward being a nonjudgmental and accepting nurse: being respectful to everyone, interacting in a sensitive responsive manner (rather than an overbearing, assuming one), and developing effective communication (verbal and nonverbal) skills. You can practice these behaviors in a variety of settings, and begin to learn about the environments, situations, or moods that make being accepting more difficult for you. Most important is your being willing to learn, reflecting on personal behavior and thinking, and attempting new skills that enhance your acceptance of others.

In the 1970s the language about being nonjudgmental might not have been as sophisticated as it is in the 21st century. However, the principles are timeless, and what was explored in 1970 with stigma and judgments toward African Americans, the poor, and college students is relevant to nurses today, with populations ranging from those in poverty to ethnic minority groups to adolescent parents. Below are steps to becoming nonjudgmental; remember, "becoming nonjudgmental is hard work and a life time process" (Goldsborough, 1970, p. 2340).

1. Recognize judgmental feelings. (Becoming nonjudgmental begins with openness to yourself, even though it might be painful to acknowledge judgmental feelings.)

2. Accept your judgmental feelings for what they are. (Without acceptance, you aren't able to move toward changing the feelings.)

3. Explore the origin of the judgmental feeling, maybe with a friend or colleague. (Where did this come from?)

4. Take steps to change. (Realize that there will always be another person, another judgment to work through over the course of your life and nursing.)

Adapted from a classic article titled "On Becoming Nonjudgmental," Goldsborough, 1970

 ## ACTIVITY

Have you ever experienced someone acting judgmental toward you? How did you feel? How did you react?

What could that person have done to express their opinion or beliefs in a nonjudgmental manner?

Do you believe that a person can change from being judgmental and become nonjudgmental? How do you think this happens? How can you encourage this process in your life and in the lives of those around you?

Josie and the PHN enter the apartment and find they are in a cheery, well-decorated, but modest home for the teen, her newborn daughter, and the teen's mother. Josie continues to absorb the surroundings as she hears the school nurse ask the teen about her baby and her healing body. She is surprised the apartment is so clean and organized. She considers her reaction and tunes out the conversation. "Why am I surprised this apartment is so nice? Do I expect that if you are poor, you are dirty or unkempt? Where is this opinion coming from? Did my facial expressions portray discomfort when I walked through the door?" Josie reflects on her reaction and compares it to that of the PHN, who appears to be at ease and enjoying her interaction with the new mom and baby. At this point in the visit, Josie is questioning her reaction and the judgments her thoughts revealed. This reflection is critical to growing toward an unconditional acceptance of others. It is an example of mindful nursing practice, which is simply being aware, present, and in the moment with those you are serving or caring for.

Evidence-Based Practice for Acceptance of Others in Public Health Nursing Individual

Much of the research supporting the need for PHNs to be nonjudgmental and accepting when working with individuals, families, or communities focuses heavily on relationship building. This makes sense because, in essence, when a nurse is nonjudgmental and accepting, the client-nurse relationship is likely to be positive and healthy, which leads to more successful interventions and more meaningful interactions for everyone. The Evidence Example below demonstrates positive results experienced by public health nurses working with new moms.

Evidence Example: Nurse-Mother Relationship ... What Moms Want and Nurses Can Offer

In a qualitative study, moms and nurses were interviewed to understand how the nurses engage the mothers in a way that is empowering so that the mothers more effectively bear and raise children (Aston, Meagher-Stewart, Sheppard-Lemoine, Vukic, & Chircop, 2006). In this study, the interaction between the PHN and the mother were observed during a home visit with a new mom (baby born 2–3 weeks prior). Following that observation, the mother and PHN were each interviewed by the researcher to talk about how the home visit had gone. From this information, key themes in the relationship were identified, many of which are directly relevant to the PHN's ability to be accepting and nonjudgmental. For example, the mothers identified key attributes of the PHNs that made them feel comfortable, at ease, and positive toward the nurse. These attributes included being "full of confidence….gentle…quiet…" (Aston et al., 2006, p. 63). The nurses also talked about the importance of their actions in encouraging the moms to feel comfortable and competent, including "respect, trust, listening, confidence, and communication" (p. 63). At a time when women feel incredibly vulnerable and incompetent, these nurses were able to express acceptance in a way that facilitated feelings of confidence in the new moms.

Few scenarios can demonstrate the challenges a PHN might face in providing nonjudgmental and accepting nursing care better than poverty. Caroline Porr (2005) is a PHN who reflected on her interactions with clients in poverty, and specifically challenged herself to answer the following, "By all accounts I was thorough, or was I? I certainly 'dealt with' Karen and her family in scrupulous fashion but did I adequately 'dwell with' Karen; that is, did I understand her lived experience as a lone parent enduring the margins of society due to poverty?" (p. 190). Poverty is something every PHN is going to experience and be exposed to when serving individuals and families in a variety of contexts (e.g., home visits, case management, case finding).

How PHNs respond to a family in poverty influences the relationship and, subsequently, the outcomes of the care provided. PHNs might, without thinking, consider the poverty as more central to the problems and solutions than the individual or family living in poverty perceives. PHNs then need to seek to understand how the experience of poverty is perceived by the individual or family. After this understanding is gained, PHNs can then effectively support and accept the individual or family. Rather than focusing simply on the reason the PHNs are there (e.g., home visit to provide education), a nonjudgmental and accepting PHN can dig deeper and appreciate the person simply for who that person is, not in the narrow context of their situation (e.g., poverty). As Porr concludes, "I had once thought that client assessment and intervention were sufficient until I became curious about who is the Other sitting across from me. It was then that I realized that I did not know this mother and thus could never appreciate the uniqueness of her human existence and of her experiences in the world" (Porr, 2005, p. 194).

The following Evidence Example describes the development of a quantitative tool that could be used by clients to assess the level of empathy they perceive from the nurse caring for them. This is quite different from a qualitative approach, in which open-ended questions might be used to learn the perspectives of the client.

Evidence Example: Quantitatively Assessing Empathy

A scale was developed to assess the level of empathic understanding a nurse has demonstrated (Nagano, 2000). Although the scale is intended to provide an opportunity for a client to give feedback about a nurse, it can also be useful in self-reflection by the nurse regarding verbal and nonverbal behaviors. Examples on this scale include the following:

"The [nurse] summarizes the client's emotions or feelings by saying 'it seems that you are feeling this...'

The [nurse] looks at the client with a warm expression (eyes, facial expression).

The [nurse]'s voice and rate of speaking are calm, slow, and relaxed.

The [nurse] faces the client and shows interest in the client" (p. 26–27).

Community

Culture is an area in which many nurses are regularly faced with opportunities or challenges to be nonjudgmental and unconditionally accepting. Realizing that every nurse has a distinct cultural background is fundamentally important when engaging with diverse communities in health promotion or disease prevention activities. In nursing much time is spent examining culture in the context of providing care.

What exactly is "culture"? Broadly defined, culture is "learned, shared and transmitted beliefs, norms and life practices of a particular group that guides thinking, decisions and actions in patterned ways" (Leininger, 1978). This definition presents some challenges, because any cultural group, or community, always has a range of "patterned ways" that are not necessarily consistently similar. So on the one hand culture might cause a community to share some behaviors or norms that are distinct from other groups, but on the other hand, culture is colorful and inherently diverse, which requires commitment and time to gain understanding. An effective PHN working with communities understands that effective work with a community begins with investment of time and of oneself.

For example, a PHN might have opportunities to promote the health of individuals and families who are part of a religious community. Often the support of religious leaders can foster trust of the PHN among the community members. However, if the leaders are not supportive of specific PHN priorities, this situation can create challenges, especially if the religious leaders are primary decision-makers, and members don't have high levels of autonomy. The PHN in that case needs to respectfully and carefully work with the religious leaders to achieve mutual goals related to health promotion or disease prevention.

The culture of the poor, or those in economic poverty, provides an example of how PHNs rise to provide respectful, quality care amid differences. Public health nursing research on providing care to the poor can be traced back to the first year that the *Public Health Nursing* journal was published! A multidimensional model of poverty has been developed that considers individual/group and environmental factors influencing the person experiencing poverty (Pesznecker, 1984). In this model, a person in poverty is cared for with careful consideration of how that person is dealing with his or her specific situation, and how he or she is feeling (e.g., depressed, powerless, incapable).

ACTIVITY

As a new PHN, you need to learn to carefully reflect on why people might be reacting the way they are when you are trying to intervene. What are they going through? How are they handling it?

How can you determine if the response you are receiving, when it is cautious or unwelcoming, is because of the situation and not necessarily specific to you?

Consider how you might incorporate strategies into your practice that send a message to those you are serving which gives them confidence you come open-minded and open-handed.

Certainly, PHNs are in a work environment that values nursing efficiency. Yet many of the cultural groups PHNs serve have overarching values that conflict with efficiency. For example, in the culture of generational poverty, time is valued differently than the middle class culture. Poverty often necessitates that people view present (i.e., in the moment) time as most important and make decisions based on immediate feeling or survival, whereas those in stable economic situations often value future time as most important, and decisions are made with more consideration of future ramifications (Payne, DeVol, & Smith, 2001). A PHN that has a clear understanding of this distinction is going to allow some flexibility in scheduling visits or appointments. You might view an efficient nurse as one that has planned the week well with full days of scheduled, often back-to-back, appointments. This efficiency might be challenged as the week unfolds and the nurse finds several of the clients are not home at their scheduled visit times. How can the nurse incorporate and respect the time value for this poverty culture and still implement effective nursing interventions? The nurse might incorporate some time each week for same-day home visits, or might have a time each week that families can "drop in" for an in- office visit. This aspect of scheduling can be very distressing to new PHNs, as many view the behavior as a sign of disrespect or a lack of desire to see the nurse. This perspective often changes with a deeper appreciation, understanding, and acceptance of the unique value of time for each person.

Systems

At the systems level, demonstrating acceptance of others is most often reflected in policy or program level strategies. Policies that support interpreter services for those who do not speak English well are an ideal example. Much research has been done to show that the quality of health care is better when interpreters are available for Limited English Proficiency (LEP) persons. The following Evidence Example summarizes recent studies on interpreter services and health care quality.

Evidence Example: Interpreter Services and Health Care Quality

In a broad critical review of literature about interpreter services and health care quality, many studies were identified that showed when needed interpreter services were not provided, the quality of that health care was low and not ideal (Flores, 2005). The review also clarified the importance of using trained professional interpreters, rather than informal interpreters such as friends or family members. The evidence exists to support systems-level policies that require professional interpreter services. When these services are provided, clients are more likely to receive better quality care and are likely to feel respected, and accepted, for who they are. Pam Garrett (2009) has proposed a model for an interpreter service policy that can serve as a guide for health care organizations needed to implement such a policy. These types of models can be useful when organizations are not sure where to begin in creating a policy.

The use of cultural brokers, or community health workers, in providing health education, outreach, support, and resources to others in their community is another example of systems realizing the need to provide culturally relevant care and outreach (Mack, Uken, & Powers, 2006; O'Brien, Squires, Bixby, & Larson, 2009). Although many responsibilities need to be carried out by a PHN, others can be appropriately delegated to a paraprofessional such as a community health worker. In many situations, a community health worker can be an important liaison for families new to a complex United States health care system. You need to note, though, that PHNs can serve diverse cultural groups and can effectively care for those who are different from them. This is the essence of this competency, namely, realizing that PHNs need to develop acceptance of others, which can go far in reaching clients and communities. Policies that support unconditional PHN care, and approaches such as using community health workers when appropriate, can promote optimal delivery of nursing care.

The following example illustrates the impact that can be made when a policy does not exist to support particular activities and when a policy is changed without considering the impact to others. In a community that has a large population of African immigrant families, Personal Care Attendants (PCAs) were providing care for men who lived alone. As part of their home care, the PCAs were cooking meals because the men had no knowledge or experience preparing meals. The law changed with respect to PCAs' scope of practice, limiting them from preparing meals for these clients. No organizational policy was in place to support this informal job duty the PCAs had been performing. As a result of this change, the community had to generate creative options to address the gap in care. Although the community did come up with alternative solutions (e.g., cooking classes for the men, a home meal delivery service), in the short term the men lost valuable care and services because a reimbursement law changed.

Broadly, you also need to recognize the societal practices, values, and standards that influence the delivery of public health nursing care in an accepting manner. Society is always changing, and with these changes come challenges or solutions that support or impede what you are trying to do. For example, many "groups" in the United States have endured societal oppression that directly and indirectly influences how they receive services such as public health nursing care. Being respectful of where people have been or come from, and what they have experienced in the past, or recently, is imperative to being a successful PHN. Even if you are a very accepting person, you are going to have barriers to overcome if you are providing care to someone who has experienced discrimination or judgments from a person who looks or acts in ways that are similar to you. You need to maintain awareness of the societal climate, federal and state policies, and local sentiments within which you are working as a PHN. When you do this, your care is going to be attuned, aware, and ideally, effective and meaningful.

Intra-Agency

Finally, public health nurses must also demonstrate acceptance of each other, and of colleagues in the workplace. This can be difficult but is critical as workforce diversity expands in health care, nursing, and public health. Co-workers might experience differences in work ethics, differences in time management, and differences in opinion concerning how a nursing procedure should be done. Experiences in practice, or in the field, certainly contribute to opinions as to how things should be done in PHN practice, and it is not uncommon for two experienced nurses to differ in their opinions about what should be done or not done. These differences represent another reason why evidence-based practice is so important to guide practice, because with growing bodies of evidence, some of these disagreements can be minimized.

Some studies addressing health care work environments have relevant research findings. For example, although conducted with nursing assistants, not PHNs, an important study was conducted examining organizational respect and emotional exhaustion, or burnout (Ramarajan, Barsade, & Burack, 2008). Organizational respect was measured using statements such as "staff members respect each other," "cultural diversity of staff is valued," and "staff members are treated with dignity." Not surprisingly, when nursing assistants reported higher levels of organizational respect at time one, when they were re-surveyed at time two, they were less likely to report feeling emotional exhaustion than their colleagues who reported feeling that organizational respect levels were low. PHNs need a work environment that respects and values them. This respect is very important because without it, a nurse might be less satisfied with work, might be more emotionally exhausted, and might choose to leave public health nursing. Because the need for PHNs is so great across the United States, workplace environments need to be supportive and accepting. If you feel judged by coworkers, consider the following strategies:

- Get support from other co-workers

- Talk to someone about your feelings and the actions you should take (co-worker, friend, manager)

- Confront the person making you feel this way. Explore with that person why the differences exist (are you from different generations, cultures, experiences?)

- Approach human resources staff for assistance

Similarly, new PHNs need to be in an environment that supports their learning and growing in new roles and experiences. Experienced nurses might find it difficult to adapt to the next generation of PHNs, but the effort needs to be made to understand each other and to grow together. In this way, the public health nursing workforce can remain strong and can express acceptance to one another, and to clients being served. Following are techniques to gain trust.

Individual level: Find a commonality with which you can connect to the individual or family

- Respect client's time schedule and availability. For example, clearly state your intended length of visit at the time you set the appointment, or upon arrival, so that you provide an opportunity for the client to make any necessary adjustments. This builds trust through mutual investment in the commitment.

- Respect the client's "home rules" that might be different than your own, such as shoe removal, where to park, or what door to use to enter home. If you are not sure, ask.

- Whether seeing a specific client or an entire family, include and interact with additional family members present at the home visit. By this inclusion, you can develop a trusting atmosphere that expresses an understanding that they function within the context of their family unit.

- Ask easy, open-ended questions on the telephone or at initial home visits with a genuine interest, allowing the client/family to share information. This action is essential to developing a trusting, non-judgmental relationship.

- Initially, focus on positive aspects and strengths of the client or family unit. Until a trusting relationship is established, interventions are going to be less effective when they lack emphasis of assets and focus solely on problems to be addressed or fixed.

- Ask if you can share information prior to providing it. This allows respect and trust to develop.

- Utilize basic language, avoiding medical or technical language/terms.

- Avoid use of a laptop in the home if it is apparent that the clients/family do not trust that data won't be shared (because of prior experiences they might have had).

Community Level: Find a fit with their goals (e.g., working with churches)

- Invest time in building professional relationships with key community members and in understanding the goals and missions of other community agencies that are serving the community. This can lead to the establishment of trusting collaborative efforts in serving community population segments.

- Be honest and provide accurate, consistent messaging to the community about health-related situations that might arise (e.g., a pertussis outbreak).

Systems Level: Ensure that policies are accepting and do not ostracize

- Implement policies and programs that meet the needs of the population being served. For example, if women utilizing the Women, Infants and Children (WIC) program, a supplemental nutrition program, are surveyed in the community and 25% indicate that they could only come to the office to receive their food vouchers between 4 and 6 p.m., it would be appropriate to have some evening hours available and to establish a policy supporting this within the agency. This act displays openness and acceptance to the needs of this WIC population segment.

- Use community-based participatory research methods so that communities have an opportunity to participate in planning, implementation, and evaluation of interventions or policies.

Intra-agency: Show acceptance of co-workers within and across disciplines

- Openly share and discuss evidence-based nursing practice in a nonthreatening way that encourages group reflection. This approach can lead to a more unified nursing force that has a basis of mutual respect and trust in research and essentially in each other's nursing practice.

- Engage in reflective supervision and/or reflective practice groups. This process goes beyond reflection and journaling and has become increasingly popular in evidence-based home visiting protocols/models. Simply, reflective supervision provides a PHN with feedback she can use to examine the patterns she might be using in caring for her clients and to readjust caring patterns that are not optimal.

Ethical Application

Feminist and virtue ethics provide excellent principles with which to examine this competency. Feminist ethics emphasizes that actions not be oppressing to others. In this competency, we talk a lot about accepting others, and not being judgmental. As you respect the clients you are working with, you demonstrate acceptance, and you do not oppress. Similarly, virtue ethics emphasizes tolerance and justice as two leading principles. When you are tolerant of others' experiences, beliefs, or perspectives, you are achieving this competency and acting as an ethical nurse. Finally, when you act in a just manner, you express to the other person that they have worth and dignity. Imagine the positive influence you, the PHN, can have in the diverse lives and communities you serve when you ethically provide care. This positive influence might come from something as simple as maintaining appropriate confidentiality, facilitating a nonjudgmental environment in a home visit or a community screening event, and expressing acceptance in verbal and nonverbal ways. In the case study in this chapter you have observed Josie address many preconceptions regarding the client she was visiting. You have noticed how easy it can be to make judgments and how challenging it can be to provide nursing care in a nonjudgmental manner. Yet, when nursing care is nonjudgmental, it is much more likely to be effective and to promote lasting change (see Table 11.2).

Table 11.2   Ethical Action in Providing Nonjudgmental and Unconditional Care

Ethical Perspective	Application
Rule Ethics (principles)	• Nonjudgmental public health nursing should simultaneously encourage beneficence or promote the good of families and communities. • Encourage autonomy by listening respectfully and showing respect for the opinions of those being cared for, in verbal and nonverbal ways.
Virtue Ethics (character)	• Be respectful in actions and words. • Be persistent in showing tolerance and creatively promoting health. • Be accepting and aware of how responses and actions can promote or discourage those being served.
Feminist Ethics (reducing oppression)	• Conduct assessment in a manner that appreciates strengths while also identifying areas for intervention. • Respect everyone. • Advocate for individuals and community groups who might have less power because they are regularly judged (e.g., homeless youth).

Key Points

- Even the most experienced PHN can struggle with being nonjudgmental and accepting of people.

- People and communities can be different from each other on multiple levels: social, economic, geographic, religious, behavioral, age, ethnicity, race, or sexual orientation.

- Acting in a nonjudgmental manner does not mean that a PHN is accepting of everything.

- PHNs can increase the potential for program or intervention success by carefully examining the key cultural or social beliefs or practices within a community.

- Reflecting on your own reactions toward those who are different from you is a critical starting point toward achieving this competency.

- Remember that policies can promote acceptance or judgment of people or groups and they should be made with input from diverse stakeholders.

Exercises

Learning Examples for Strategies to Increase Acceptance of Others

This is one of those competency areas that is not so easily translated into a set of experiences or exercises that can assure you develop into a more accepting person, or nurse. However, you can undertake some experiences that are likely to encourage reflection on how you react in an uncomfortable or unfamiliar setting or among people who differ in beliefs, culture, or behaviors. Becoming culturally competent, or proficient, is a lifelong learning process, but you can start by gaining appreciation of diverse cultures, learning about other health practices, and being meaningful in your desire to increase your competent care of others. For some, being culturally competent is possible only when you can be a cultural broker, which includes language fluency and deep cultural understanding. Though many nurses might not be "competent" in that way, they can be culturally respectful and responsive. Most important is your willingness to evaluate yourself with respect to how nonjudgmental or accepting you are and, based on that evaluation, to identify things you might do to enhance acceptance. The following are examples to help increase the acceptance of others.

- Engage in self-reflection via journaling or simple thought, because "this is an opportunity … to expose my biases" (Porr, 2005, p. 192).

- Example journal questions: "What do I believe contributes to my own health status?" "How am I different from other students, family members, neighbors?" "How am I similar?" "When I felt uncomfortable in a recent experience in the community, why did I feel that way?" "How have I been made to feel comfortable in a group or with someone different from myself?"

- Engage in activities that *develop perceptual* (nurse's ability to make relevant observations) and *conceptual skills* (ability to give meaning to observations). Examples include role-playing and observing and analyzing DVDs of actual family/nurse interactions (Wright & Leahey, 2005, p.184–185). Engaging in these activities allows observation and analysis of interactions that might impede/increase acceptance of others.

- Invest in developing virtues essential to good nursing character. Good nursing character includes virtues such as compassion, integrity, fidelity, courage, justice, mediation, self-confidence, resilience, and practical reasoning (Volbrecht, 2001, p. 102). This development not only increases your acceptance of clients, but the client's acceptance of you.

- Invest time in reading and developing background knowledge pertaining to aspects of the client, population, or system that you are serving as a PHN.

- Consider visiting a setting that is not familiar or comfortable to you and reflectively journal about how you felt and what you experienced (e.g., a religious ceremony, a cultural event, a shelter, or a nursing home).

- Read books that challenge your perspectives and deepen your understanding. Examples include *The Spirit Catches You and You Fall Down* by Anne Fadiman (1998); *Nickel and Dimed* by Barbara Ehrenreich (2002); and *A Thousand Splendid Suns* by Khaled Hosseini (2008).

Reflective Practice

Considering what you have learned in this chapter, identify what Josie might do next to act on her reflections during the home visit and her realization that her preconceived judgments were not only inaccurate but also were not helpful in providing optimal care for the teen and her new baby. After writing your responses to the following three reflective questions, compare the questions and strategies you identify with those noted at the end of the chapter.

What does Josie need to understand about being nonjudgmental and accepting?

_____

_____

What are some additional reflective questions that Josie needs to ask herself, and what information sources might be useful to her in growing more accepting of others?

_____

_____

How will Josie know that her efforts to be increasingly accepting of diverse people and communities are successful?

_____

_____

Application of Evidence

1. What ethical considerations are important to think about in responding to individuals, families, and communities in a nonjudgmental manner?

2. How might you work with colleagues to process judgmental feelings and work toward becoming more nonjudgmental?

Think, Explore, Do

1. What might you ask yourself before you go on a home visit or meet with a client?

2. Where is the neighborhood? Have you been there before? What do you think about it?

3. What is something you can find you have in common with the family you are visiting?

4. Does the policy you are enforcing encourage acceptance of others' beliefs, cultures, etc.?

5. How might you change a policy in your department so that it is nonjudgmental?

6. What resources might you use to learn about a new cultural group you are serving?

7. What are the key issues you need to consider when outreaching to an elder group?

8. What are two things you can do to create a welcoming, accepting physical environment?

9. How might you show that you value another person or community?

10. When designing a health promotion activity for a religious audience, such as cholesterol screening, what are some things you want to consider so that the screening is most successful?

11. How can you show acceptance to your coworkers and interdisciplinary colleagues?

12. When you see someone acting in a judgmental manner, what steps might you take to model acceptance?

COMPETENCY #10:
Incorporates Mental, Physical, Emotional, Social, Spiritual, and Environmental Aspects of Health into Assessment, Planning, Implementation, and Evaluation

12

By Carolyn M. Garcia
with Christine C. Andres, Maureen A. Alms and Pamela Nelson

Maria had just finished her 6-month orientation at a local public health department in the Maternal Child Health division. She received her nursing license just 7 months before, after spending a decade in business management as a supervisor of a large customer service and sales department. Maria was concerned about how she could possibly assess all aspects of health in high-risk populations. That weekend, Maria received a referral from the local hospital involving a child that needed to be seen by a public health nurse (PHN). Maria was excited and nervous about this first case. The only information she received was that the family had a 2 year-old boy that was being released from the hospital after suffering an asthma attack. Newly diagnosed with asthma, the boy and his family needed education and a home assessment.

Maria called the mother and set a time for the visit. While driving to the home, Maria mentally reviewed everything she knew about asthma. She anticipated education would be easy, because she had a son with asthma and was familiar with the disease process and management. Upon arrival at the home, she became slightly uneasy with the multiple dogs and cats roaming the yard. She knocked several times on the trailer door before a man answered and let her inside the home. Maria entered the kitchen, and everyone exchanged introductions. Marcus, the boy with asthma, was quiet in his mother's arms. His brothers, 1 and 5 years of age, were running around the kitchen table, trying to open Maria's nursing bag, jumping on her, and trying to take her pen. It was very chaotic. Maria had to overcome her anxiety, and she realized that completing a nursing assessment was going to be a challenge.

MARIA'S NOTEBOOK

Competency #10: Incorporates mental, physical, emotional, social, spiritual, and environmental aspects of health into assessment, planning, implementation, and evaluation

- Assesses the mental, physical, emotional, social, spiritual, and environmental health of individuals, families, communities, and systems

- Develops intervention plans that consider the mental, physical, emotional, social, spiritual, and environmental health of individuals, families, communities, and systems

- Implements interventions that improve the mental, physical, emotional, social, spiritual, and environmental health of individuals, families, communities, and systems

- Evaluates the impact of public health nursing interventions on the mental, physical, emotional, social, spiritual, and environmental health of individuals, families, communities, and systems

Useful Definitions

Assessment: "Assessment is holistic and conducted with emphasis on fine observation over time in addition to standard tools" (Kemp, Anderson, Travaglia, & Harris, 2005, p. 257).

"Accurate assessment of the state of cultural diversity within health care organizations and service communities is essential for the development of appropriate culturally congruent care" (Schim, Doorenbos, Benkert, & Miller, 2007, p. 106).

Environmental: "Environmental health addresses all the physical, chemical, and biological factors external to a person, and all the related factors impacting behaviors. It encompasses the assessment and control of those environmental factors that can potentially affect health. It is targeted towards preventing disease and creating health-supportive environments. This definition excludes behavior not related to environment, as well as behavior related to the social and cultural environment, and genetics" (World Health Organization; http://www.who.int/topics/environmental_health/en/).

Holistic: " The characteristics of the spiritual self in combination with those of the emotional and physical self respond to situations as a totality" (Labun, 1988, p. 314).

"The interrelationships among the physical, emotional and spiritual aspects of the person.." (Labun, 1988, p. 315).

Intervention: "The nature of intervention described in the generalist nurse competencies is to be reactive to identified problems or requests, based on nursing assessment and nursing priorities" (Kemp, Anderson, Travaglia, & Harris, 2005, p. 256).

Spiritual: "The emerging data surrounding the language of spirituality implies that spirituality has different meanings and interpretation," and "spirituality is very subjective, diverse and complex. Therefore the need to provide individualized care in this area is of paramount importance" (McSherry, Cash, & Ross, 2004, p. 940).

From the Seen to the Unseen

One of the reasons nursing is such an exciting profession is the breadth and depth of nursing practice. Nurses work in so many different arenas and engage in a range of health promotion, intervention, and healing or transition process activities. Public health nursing is no exception, and to an extent, it sets a precedent for the diversity of nursing practice. In public health nursing one can be employed in a local public health department, a manufacturing plant, a school, a church, or a prison. PHNs care for people where they work, recreate, worship, and live. An appreciation for this complexity informs this public health nursing competency. Indeed, competent PHNs can holistically assess numerous aspects of health and then intervene in creative, meaningful ways. In this chapter, we explore the tenth Henry Street Consortium Competency, with particular emphasis given to those aspects of health that can be subtle and perhaps more challenging to consider for a beginning PHN. Rather than overwhelm, we hope this chapter informs and encourages you to consider the range of possibilities in public health nursing as viewed through a holistic lens.

Assessing the Mental, Physical, Emotional, Social, Spiritual, and Environmental Health of Individuals, Families, Communities, and Systems

Assessment gives PHNs an understanding of what is going on, including what might be contributing to or preventing solutions and how the nurse can assist or intervene. In preparation for becoming a nurse, you spend numerous hours learning and practicing assessment. In a clinical assessment for heart disease, nurses might take a blood pressure, measure cholesterol, run a stress test, and take a verbal personal and family history. In PHN assessment, these objective and subjective types of data are also collected, yet the scope is often broader in that PHNs conduct assessments at the community and systems levels. At all levels, the nurses' emphases on objective and subjective data remain similar. PHNs systematically observe, document, and summarize data to support assessment findings. These data are quantitative (e.g., rates of disease, symptom frequency, number of risks, number of assets, costs) and qualitative (e.g., personal experiences of those affected, expressed opinions, photographs that demonstrate risks/assets). Most important is that an assessment is carefully planned and thoroughly implemented so that results are useful and can be acted upon.

At the individual level, examples of direct care assessment include examining a newborn for signs of healthy development, screening a new mother for postpartum depression, and determining the spiritual state of someone recently diagnosed with a terminal cancer. In the home setting, PHNs consider the environment in which a family is living by assessing home safety (e.g., loose rugs that might cause an elder to trip or lead paint flakes a toddler could ingest), and the social environment, such as neighborhood safety (e.g., crime levels) or access to healthy food sources.

Another type of assessment is conducted when individuals are asked how they might be best supported by a PHN. Fifty mothers who had gone through drug dependency court were asked in a study how they could be best supported by a PHN in their treatment and reunification with their children (Somervell, Saylor, & Mao, 2005). In interviews, the mothers suggested they would like PHNs to serve as a bridge of information to them, reporting on the health and well-being of their children while those children were in foster care. This needs assessment provided the PHNs with clarity of what the mothers wanted, and did not want, in services; this knowledge was useful in planning the activities of PHNs working with these mothers.

Family-level assessment expands the individual-level focus to the family unit, which can be large. The family is viewed as an interactional system with its holistic health determined by such factors as family dynamics and relationships, family structure, and family functioning (Friedman, Bowden, & Jones, 2003). This approach is particularly useful when PHNs try to manage a health condition that is somewhat dependent on the family setting. For example, a school nurse might work with a student to manage asthma, but without adequate family assessment, the nurse might miss risk factors in the home that are aggravating the asthma (e.g., smoking family members, dust, presence of rodents). Assessment of family-level risk behaviors can also contribute to a family-level intervention, such as efforts to increase the activity level of all family members to reduce obesity and risks for diabetes. Holistic public health nursing at the family level might use family strengths theory, a theoretical approach that emphasizes building on existing strengths within the family, as a guide to assessment and intervention planning and implementation (Sittner, Hudson, & Defrain, 2007).

Evidence Example: Holistic PHN Care for the Family

The following are some helpful clinical examples of holistic PHN care for the family unit (Sittner, Hudson, & Defrain, 2007, p. 357):

- Consider assessing a family's strengths when planning nursing care for the family.
- Help families cope with stress and crisis effectively by providing consistent information.
- Be sure to listen and work toward establishing a trusting relationship with families.
- Acknowledge the family's individualized spiritual perspective and implement nursing interventions that promote their spiritual needs.
- Help families understand that enjoyable time together during an illness is important.
- Encourage families to be physically close and celebrate occasions.
- Encourage individuals and families to express appreciation and affection for assistance during an illness.
- Help nursing students understand the family strengths perspective.

Maria started with a simple focused assessment of Marcus. He had no temperature and no apparent difficulty breathing. His lung sounds were clear. When she asked about using the nebulizer, the parents asked, "What nebulizer?" Maria called the hospital triage nurse and, after multiple transfers, reached a nurse who discovered the order was never placed but that they would deliver it immediately with arrival expected yet that day. Maria wanted to start addressing some of the asthma triggers present in the environment. The floor was coated with food crumbs, and dishes in the sink had flies hovering over them. The windowless room where the boys slept had three mattresses on the floor with dirty blankets and pillows without coverings. The bathroom had a strong air deodorizer smell; it was also where the parents smoked. Maria started to feel an itchy sensation on her legs and assessed the ankles and legs of the children. They were covered with little red marks, and Marcus's legs felt rough like sandpaper. She mentioned the bites on the children, and the mother stated they have a flea problem but haven't had the money to do anything about it. Maria felt overwhelmed. How do you help a family with so many needs?

Table 12.1 offers an example of a home safety checklist a public health nurse might use in a home visit with an elder person, which would be a different safety checklist from one used with a family with young children, for example.

Table 12.1 Example Home Safety Checklist for an Elder Person

Home Safety Checklist
Living Room and Family Room
1. Can you turn on a light without having to walk into a dark room?
2. Are lamp, extension, or phone cords out of the flow of foot traffic?
3. Are passageways in this room free from objects and clutter (papers, furniture)?
4. Are curtains and furniture at least 36 inches from baseboard heaters or portable heaters?
5. Do your carpets lie flat?
6. Do your small rugs and runners stay put (don't slide or roll up) when you push them with your foot?
Kitchen
7. Are your stove controls easy to see and use?
8. Do you keep loose-fitting clothing, towels, and curtains that might catch fire away from the burners and oven?
9. Can you reach regularly used items without climbing to reach them?
10. Do you have a step stool that is sturdy and in good repair?
Bedrooms
11. Do you have working smoke detectors on the ceiling outside of bedroom doors?
12. Can you turn on a light without having to walk into a dark room?
13. Do you have a lamp or light switch within easy reach of your bed?
14. Is a phone within easy reach of your bed?
15. Is a light left on at night between your bed and the toilet?
16. Are the curtains and furniture at least 36 inches from your baseboard heater or portable heater?

Bathroom

17. Does your shower or tub have a nonskid surface, such as a mat, decals, or abrasive strips?

18. Does the tub/shower have a sturdy grab bar (not just a towel rack)?

19. Is your hot water temperature set to 120° or lower?

20. Does your floor have a nonslip surface or does the rug have a nonskid backing?

21. Can you get on and off the toilet easily?

Stairways

22. Is there a light switch at both the top and bottom of inside stairs?

23. With the light on, can you clearly see the outline of each step as you go down the stairs?

24. Do all stairways have sturdy handrails on both sides?

25. Do handrails run the full length of the stairs, slightly beyond the steps?

26. Are all the steps in good repair (not loose, broken, missing, or worn in places)?

27. Are stair coverings (rugs, treads) in good repair, without holes and not loose, torn, or worn?

Hallways and Passageways

28. Do all small rugs or runners stay put (don't slide or roll up) when you push them with your foot?

29. Do your carpets lie flat?

30. Are all lamp, extension, and phone cords out of the flow of foot traffic?

Front and Back Entrances

31. Do all entrances to your home have outdoor lights?

32. Are walkways to your entry free from cracks and holes?

Throughout Your House

33. Do you have an emergency exit plan in case of fire?

34. Do you have emergency phone numbers listed by your phone?

35. Are there other hazards or unsafe areas in your home not mentioned in this checklist that you are concerned about? If so, what?

Making Your Home Safer

What home safety changes do you want to make?

1.

2.

3.

Provided by: California Department of Aging, Senior Housing Information and Support Center
Adapted from: "Home Safety Checklist Summary"
Developed by: Community and Home Injury Prevention Project for Seniors (CHIPPS)
Sponsored by: Community Health Education Section, San Francisco Department of Public Health
_Located at: http://www.aging.ca.gov/resources/home_housing/Home_Safety_Checklist.pdf_

Community assessment broadens the PHN perspective to consider the health of a group. Remember that community can be defined in many different ways, as a group of people connected by geography, age, ethnicity, spiritual beliefs, or health and risk behaviors. PHNs working with a community need to earnestly examine the strengths and needs in that community before engaging in health promotion or disease prevention activities. For example, a parish nurse might assess the need for a cardiovascular or diabetes screening program and determine the presence of existing resources or gaps in resources in the parish and surrounding community. The PHN in this case is also going to want to know the extent to which a cardiovascular or diabetes screening program might be a priority health concern for parish members. A detailed assessment contributes to increased likelihood of a successful, accepted program.

An occupational PHN might assess the needs and preferences of workers prior to starting a health promotion intervention. This assessment is necessary because without it, the PHN can't have a clear picture of the needs, the problems, and how possible solutions are going to be received. Oxygen delivery truck drivers might benefit from an intervention that teaches them stretching and ways to prevent repetitive motion injuries, but assessment can inform the PHN if the drivers have any interest in such a program. Without interest or some level of motivation, the intervention could be a significant waste of time, energy, and other resources.

PHNs in local public health departments have often undertaken large-scale geographic community assessments, driving through cities and documenting risks (e.g., crime, abandoned buildings, manufacturing plants) and assets (e.g., police, recreation, grocery stores). It is more common in today's environment with constraints on resources (e.g., time, finances) to see PHNs conducting focused or targeted community assessments to inform specific initiatives or activities. However, especially if PHNs are new to a setting, they might conduct a thorough community assessment to drive PHN or agency priorities and goal setting. Often an assessment helps decision makers determine how best to use limited funds and resources by prioritizing the greatest areas of need. The following lists the components of a community health assessment (also see Chapter 3, which is devoted to assessment in public health nursing).

Note that this process is not intended to be linear, and that many aspects of an assessment might be "combined, rearranged, or worked on simultaneously" (MDH, 2007, p. 9).

1. Describe the community.

2. Collect and analyze data and community perspectives.

3. Create public health issue statements.

4. Select local public health department priorities.

5. Summarize who is going to address community health issues.

    Source: MDH, 2007, p. 9

The systems level is often more difficult to understand with respect to the nursing process and public health nursing. If you think about the system being many of the larger, overarching policies and governmental/societal forces that influence health, then it might be easier to grasp this concept of "system." PHNs employed with the local public health department must work within the guidelines of local, state, and federal level policies, rules, and regulations (see Competency #4, Chapter 6). Assessment at the systems level, then, can be useful when PHNs believe that a particular policy or regulation is needed, or needs to be eliminated. An example of this situation is the assessment that took place in states across the United States, resulting in a realized need for indoor anti-smoking regulation. PHNs worked with many colleagues to assess the potential impact of an indoor smoking ban, including the costs, the ethics, and the health implications. Systems-level assessment is complex, yet so important because when policies or laws are made, they have the potential for extensive, long-lasting influence.

PHNs can often contribute to the successes of statewide screening programs. When PHNs are directly involved in assessment, planning, implementation, and evaluation of infant screening programs, they are more likely to be successful (Kemper, Fant, & Clark, 2005). Specifically, PHNs work directly with infants, parents, and families, and this experience is valuable when large-scale efforts are planned. The PHNs are ideally prepared, for example, to develop the screening tools that can be used not only in the home but also in common health care settings, such as clinics (Kemper, Fant, & Clark, 2005). Another example is the Follow Along Program (FAP), a Minnesota statewide screening method for young children that is intended to assure early and continuous screening for health concerns and developmental and behavioral delays. This is a cooperative arrangement between the Minnesota Department of Health, Children with Special Health Needs Sections, and local FAP agencies, which are typically public health agencies. The PHNs use a computerized tracking program to holistically screen all aspects of a child and to work with families as concerns arise to assure appropriate child and family interventions and support. When the early screening data were evaluated in 1999, the counties with an FAP identified many more children who were eligible for early intervention than those counties that did not have an FAP (MDH, 2009).

See Table 12.2 for an example of assessment at the individual, community, and systems levels for primary, secondary, and tertiary interventions strategies.

Table 12.2   Example of Assessment Addressing Adolescent Substance Use

Levels of Assessment and Intervention	Individual	Community	Systems
Primary	Assess risk and protective factors that might influence substance use decision making. School nurses might screen/survey all students to determine which prevention messages might be ideal based on existing beliefs, assets, and risks among peers, families, and neighborhoods.	Assess community-level attitudes and ideas regarding substance use among adolescents. PHNs might partner with local schools, religious institutions, community parks and playground facilities, and health care organizations to conduct focus groups, walk-along interviews, and community assessment to identify key points of intervention—attitudes, behaviors, knowledge, or infrastructure.	Identify the laws and policies that support prevention of substance use among adolescents. PHNs might advocate for stricter penalties for bars selling to underage drinkers if this is a problem in the particular area/city.
Secondary	Assess adolescent substance use behaviors, including risk and protective factors. PHNs might screen a pregnant teen during a home visit to determine substance use behaviors and plan risk reduction intervention.	PHNs might assess substance use behaviors among homeless adolescents to determine incidence and prevalence of drug use and help guide the development of interventions. PHNs might screen homeless youth seeking health care and offer cessation programs for those reporting use.	Assess level of substance use treatment programs available to adolescents in the state. PHNs might work with health insurance providers to ensure that coverage includes adequate time for adolescent participation in a cessation program.

Levels of Assessment and Intervention	Individual	Community	Systems
Tertiary	Assess adolescent's level of willingness to participate in efforts to reduce risk behaviors during pregnancy. PHNs might provide case management and support for pregnant adolescent trying not to use during the pregnancy and explore resources with her that promote self worth, including emotional and spiritual resources.	Partner with community members to assess readiness for change in a community where many adolescents are already using or abusing substances.	Assess the scope of existing resources to serve/treat adolescents who are using/abusing substances. PHNs might collaborate with local community organizations to support or establish treatment centers that can reach and target adolescents.

ACTIVITY

Using the table above, construct a similar table for a new health problem or condition you have discussed in class or observed in clinical.

Develops Intervention Plans That Consider Mental, Physical, Emotional, Social, Spiritual, and Environmental Health

At some point the assessment findings are used to prioritize possible interventions and inform decision making. The next step, then, is to develop an intervention plan for the target individual, family, community, or systems (see Figure 2.1 for this process). PHNs often work with a family, for example, so that together they consider the findings from the assessment and arrive at a plan to address concerns. Sometimes the intervention plans are very narrow and focused, driven by an assessment that obviously leads to a clear problem and solution. Other times, the intervention plans are broad and encompass several goals and strategies to reach those goals. Regardless of whether the intervention plan is narrow or broad, it can and should be holistic and address multiple aspects of an individual, family, community or system.

For example, a PHN might conduct home visits with a newborn and mother for the first few postpartum months. Assessment might indicate healthy newborn development but a risk of postpartum depression. The intervention plan is likely to consider all aspects of health for that mom and baby, yielding a multilayered strategy that might include mom breaks (mental), medication for depression or regular walks outside (physical), friend connections (emotional and social), yoga or meditation (spiritual), and housecleaning help (environmental). In this way, a focused intervention to prevent or minimize postpartum depression encompasses, or has potential to encompass, every aspect of health.

At the community level, the parish nurse might conclude that a cardiovascular screening program is needed and desired. The resulting intervention plan might include a variety of activities that consider varied aspects of health, including stress evaluation (mental), blood pressure or cholesterol measures (physical), stress levels (emotional), relationships (social), prayer practices (spiritual), and access to exercise outlets/recreation (environmental). In this example, the screening program is holistic and will lead to relevant, individualized interventions.

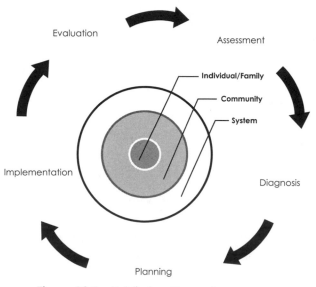

Figure 12.1 Public health nursing process

Maria went back the next day and wanted to review with the family what was important to them and how to prioritize and develop a plan of care. The nurse and parents agreed that managing Marcus's asthma was a top priority. Maria completed hands-on education on utilizing the nebulizer. The flea infestation and environmental asthma triggers were considered important. They planned together how and when they could treat the home to get rid of the fleas, minimize dust, etc. Maria addressed some safety issues, such as having the bedroom with no window and hearing Marcus at night if he was having an asthma attack. The father was appreciative for her help in getting connected to a company that supplies an alarm system that instead of producing noise, flashes lights.

Implements Interventions That Improve Mental, Physical, Emotional, Social, Spiritual, and Environmental Health

After an intervention plan is identified, the PHN needs to identify resources and arrange the logistics (e.g., details) for implementing the plan. This might include collaborating with colleagues, finding community partners, or leveraging financial resources to ensure success. Careful planning is necessary to ensure successful intervention implementation.

In the previous example, the PHN working with the mother and baby can implement the intervention by carefully discussing the approach with the mother. It would be overwhelming to recommend and implement every part of the plan immediately. Instead, the nurse and mother can work together to prioritize parts of the intervention. For example, asthma medication might be a first step, and the PHN can work with the mother's primary care provider to arrange a prescription and ensure insurance coverage is available. The PHN can also explore local resources for the mother, such as a community center offering yoga classes or a nearby babysitting service that has drop-off options for moms who need an urgent break. Depending on financial resources, the PHN might explore housecleaning services or might put the mom in touch with youth willing to do this service for needy families at little to no cost. The PHN does not simply give the mother a list of to-dos. The PHN works with the mother in a thorough and thoughtful manner to appropriately implement the intervention plan and assesses the process and the acceptability to ensure that the mother is not overwhelmed.

A case management intervention, where the PHN intervenes to address many health needs over the course of many visits, has been shown to be effective (see the following Evidence Example).

Evidence Example: PHN Prenatal Care Case Management

A study was conducted evaluating the effectiveness of case management by PHNs for prenatal care, as compared to programs offering limited prenatal assessment and/or referral programs (Ricketts et al., 2005). The PHN prenatal care case management was provided to over 3,500 women. Key findings for the women receiving the prenatal care case management were that many of them decided to reduce risk behaviors that could lead to poorer birth outcomes. For example, mothers who acted on PHN advice to quit smoking during pregnancy or to gain enough weight had fewer low birth weight babies than mothers who did not address these risks. Consistent with case management practices, women who had numerous visits, more than 10, were more likely to reduce their risks than those who received fewer visits. The study demonstrated the particular value of PHN case management in helping to reduce risks during pregnancy and to promote healthy pregnancy outcomes and the well-being of newborns.

At times, PHNs have insights and experience that are also helpful to colleagues working with the family. PHNs are often valuable resources and sources of support to colleagues addressing child protection or abuse concerns with families (Crisp & Green Lister, 2004). The issues surrounding child protection situations are complex and require intention toward understanding multiple factors (e.g., social, emotional, spiritual, and environmental) rather than simply carrying out mandated reporting requirements. (See Competency #4, Chapter 6.) Indeed, PHNs have an important role in helping to link the public health and child welfare systems so that optimal care is provided to the families in an integrated, comprehensive way

(Schneiderman, 2006). When integration occurs, children in the foster care system, for example, can more easily have their health care needs met because PHNs can provide a critical link for the families to the health care system while being aware of the foster care requirements and restrictions. In another example of prenatal care, PHNs conducted a demonstration project in which they assessed each referred pregnant woman to identify psychosocial risks and to increase awareness of local community resources available to her during the pregnancy (Strass & Billay, 2008). The key to the success of this intervention was the effort of the PHNs to assess and consider the diverse psychosocial risks, rather than to focus solely on the physical nature of the pregnancy. Health care providers making the referrals to the PHNs wanted them to continue providing the service, demonstrating support for, and the value of, the PHN intervention.

At the community level, the PHN planning a cardiovascular screening program in her role as a parish nurse needs to organize a team of individuals, depending on how many people will be screened and how frequently the screenings will occur. The nurse arranges the logistics, organizes volunteers, and provides leadership for the Screening program (see Table 12.3). The most successful intervention is one that is carefully planned and considers all the possible influencing factors for success or failure. Key factors include time of day, day of week, conflicting local activities (e.g., holidays, meetings), ease of registration process, adequate trained staff, childcare, refreshments, signs, if multiple events or screenings are in one large room, and privacy, to name a few.

Table 12.3 Setting Up a Screening Clinic

IN ADVANCE

- Assess risk to determine need for screening clinic.
- Identify screeners (e.g., determine if you will use volunteers, paid staff, people from the community or outside of the community). Conduct interviews/application process as needed. Note that screeners might need criminal background or reference checks depending on their activities.
- Train screeners (e.g., screening equipment, process).
- Establish protocol and schedule for screening, referrals, and follow-up.

DAY OF THE EVENT

- Logistics (i.e. details specific to the event that can include things like signage, refreshments and supplies, and the staffing schedule).
- Childcare.
- Clear communication and decision-making structure.
- Plan for adequate, supportive, and thorough follow-up and referrals.

ACTIVITY

Reflect on how you might conduct a holistic screening event in your community.

Identify how you would set up the event and which interventions you would offer to address physical, emotional, and spiritual needs or concerns.

Maria developed a strong relationship with this family, especially the mother and children, over the next year. She spent time following up on past referrals and interventions. Maria monitored the emotional, physical, environmental, and spiritual health of this mother through tough times of multiple housing moves, relationship issues, and a period of homelessness. The mother ended her marriage in a bitter divorce that resulted in many "crises" for this family. Maria helped the mother monitor Marcus's asthma. As Maria continued to monitor the development of the children, she became concerned about the youngest son and helped the mother access local services, including early childhood education and parenting groups.

ACTIVITY

Reflect on the ways in which Maria was providing a holistic case management intervention for this family and the benefits of this strategy as compared to one or two home visits only.

Evaluates the Impact of Public Health Nursing Interventions on Mental, Physical, Emotional, Social, Spiritual, and Environmental Health

As the intervention plan is being implemented, PHNs begin to evaluate the impact it is having on the target individual, family, community, or system. It is true that some outcomes might not be realized in the short term, yet PHNs need to pay careful attention to how the intervention is influencing aspects of health right away. Evaluating the impact of a PHN intervention can be complex. Generally, PHNs need to evaluate the intervention process, such as how it went, whether implementation was successful, and how future interventions could be improved. PHNs also need to focus on the impact of the intervention, the outcomes. Has the intervention contributed to health? How so? PHNs then return to the assessment strategies that identified the need for the intervention to reassess the situation. This return is a good way to see if changes have occurred and to complete a cycle of assessment, intervention, evaluation, and assessment, which can then lead to refined interventions.

Evidence Example: Evidence for Home Visits with Mothers and Children

One of the most exemplary studies evaluating the effectiveness of public health nursing interventions is a randomized controlled trial that measured outcomes of public health nursing visits to 743 mothers and children (Olds et al., 2007). Numerous aspects of health were evaluated over nine years, including the economic, social, physical, and educational health of the mothers, and the physical and educational health of the children. Importantly, children receiving the PHN home visits were less likely to die between birth and 9 years of age and more likely to report higher grade point averages and reading scores than those who did not receive PHN visits. Mothers who received home visits from a PHN were more likely to wait longer to become pregnant with their second child and to maintain longer relationships with their partners, and reported less use of economic assistance (e.g., welfare assistance or food stamps) than mothers who did not receive home visits from a PHN. The findings from this study have informed national initiatives across the United States to implement PHN home visiting programs for at-risk first-time mothers.

A qualitative approach can also be used to evaluate the effectiveness of the nursing process (see the following Evidence Example). In another example of qualitative evaluation, essays written by 62 clients who have received PHN home visits in Alaska to help prevent child abuse and neglect were analyzed (DeMay, 2003). Some clients received "intense" services and about twice as many home visits as those assigned to receive "standard" home visit services. The evaluation, however, was not focused on whether one group showed greater benefits compared to the other, but instead, focused on the extent to which the essays about the PHN visits reflected the PHNs' perspectives about the visits. Interestingly, parents in both groups wrote in their essays about the trusting relationship with their PHN and the importance of a positive relationship with the nurse. It was noted that those receiving more visits (the intense group) wrote much longer essays than those in the other group, possibly reflecting the depth of relationship that can be built when more home visits are involved.

Evidence Example: PHN Home Visits to Elders

A qualitative approach was used to evaluate the impact of PHN home visits to elders after they had been hospitalized (McKeown, 2007). In interviews, the older people shared that the PHNs helped meet many, but not all, of the needs they experienced following hospitalization (e.g., access to services, social aspects, and home environment safety). In this study, it appears that only one home visit is provided, which certainly could be important in interpreting the findings specific to unmet needs. The study is helpful in that it shows the importance of evaluating PHN services to (a) identify what has been successful and (b) what is lacking or could be strengthened. It is very likely that with increased visits and support, these older adults would have shared different experiences in their interviews.

At the community level, a child obesity surveillance program implemented in numerous Canadian public health clinics with over 7,000 participants was evaluated (Flynn et al., 2005). In addition to outcomes such as rates of childhood obesity, parent satisfaction was evaluated because the authors of this study felt that one measure of their success was the extent to which the parents participating in the surveillance program were content with their experience. PHNs administered the obesity surveillance program with families, and among those who completed the evaluation survey about the program, over 98% indicated they were "very happy" or "happy" with the information received. The confidence of the PHNs in conducting obesity screening, providing education, and making referrals for follow-up was also assessed in questions posed to the PHNs who participated in the screening pilot project. This assessment is important because the success of any nursing intervention is in part dependent not only on the nurse's abilities but also on his/her confidence in those abilities. Study results indicated that after participating in this screening program, the PHNs had increased confidence in their abilities to screen children accurately for weight and obesity risks and to provide parents with information they could use to improve the health of their children.

An evaluation of services delivered via a PHN sexual health clinic also yielded valuable information about the PHN's role and successes. Surveys and semi-structured interviews were conducted with 166 at-risk young people who had visited the clinic to learn their perspectives of the services they received from the PHN (Hayter, 2005). In the interviews, participants reported they had confidence in the PHNs' ability to provide services in a confidential manner. Other abilities and attributes of the PHNs were assessed via the survey, and the majority indicated they felt comfortable talking with the PHNs (84%) and that the PHNs were good listeners (over 90%). These findings led to conclusions that PHNs were successfully delivering sexual health care to at-risk, marginalized young people in a manner that was acceptable and welcoming to the youth. The data were important because they informed program planning about how to staff and continue the sexual health clinic.

These types of evaluations, including not only the participants but also the PHNs delivering the interventions, require more time and economic resources, yet they yield more holistic information that can be useful in determining whether or not an intervention is effective and efficient. In today's world, interventions need to be cost-effective and efficient (i.e., with respect to staffing), or they will not be sustained over time. Evaluations that include data to justify the value and efficiency of an intervention are critical.

> *Time passed. Maria had not seen this family for a while since they had moved out of the county. She received a phone call from the mother updating her on her situation, including that she and her boyfriend were expecting a baby. Maria asked about how Marcus was doing with his asthma. His mother stated he had not had any episodes for 6 months and took his medication every day. They discussed the development and successes of all the children. The mother called again prior to the birth of her baby to tell Maria she was being induced the following day at a local hospital. Maria stated she might be able to stop by and see her and her new baby. The mother was very excited. Maria entered the hospital room and was greeted by the mother nursing her new baby of only a couple of hours. No concerns or crises arose at this visit. Maria left with tears in her eyes. This was the beginning of a new "family," and they would be residing in another county. Therefore, Maria had to accept that she could no longer serve this family she had become part of for the past 3 years. She reflected on the journey from that first flea-infested day to the sharing of this birth. Maria had addressed many physical, emotional, environmental, and spiritual issues with this family.*

Ethical Considerations

PHNs must conduct assessment, planning, implementation, and evaluation in an ethical manner. PHNs should engage with individuals, communities, and systems in ways that demonstrate respect, willingness to listen and learn, and desire to come alongside rather than dictate or demand. The way in which an assessment is conducted directly informs the type of intervention that is developed and implemented; if the assessment focuses only on problems or risks, the intervention might not build on existing strengths or assets. This can lead to dependency rather than autonomy or capacity building. Instead, PHNs need their assessments to be holistic, focused on strengths and weaknesses, assets and risks. Interventions should not be dictated but should be collaboratively designed, with input from those who are receiving the intervention. This collaboration should enhance the potential that the intervention will be welcomed, or adhered to, which will increase likelihood of success. PHNs will find evaluation of the impact an intervention has made most useful when that evaluation is thorough and includes multiple sources of data. When PHNs take care to make sure the PHN process is holistic and inclusive, they gather the ingredients for successful health promotion and disease prevention. And when ethical ideals are adhered to, the PHN is doing what is needed to yield healthy, sustainable outcomes. See Table 12.4 for application of ethical perspectives to using the holistic nursing process.

Table 12.4 Ethical Action in Holistic Assessment, Intervention, Planning, and Evaluation

Ethical Perspective	Application
Rule Ethics (principles)	• The goal of a holistic PHN process should be beneficence or promoting good (improvement in health status). • Encourage autonomy by ensuring that those being affected, including children, have input in determining interventions to improve health.
Virtue Ethics (character)	• Be respectful when conducting an assessment and carrying out an intervention. • Be persistent in obtaining what is needed to successfully intervene based on what the assessment reveals. • Be patient when it takes time for an intervention to bear fruit, or for it to be acceptable to those it is for (e.g., a family or a community).
Feminist Ethics (reducing oppression)	• Ensure that assessment includes strengths and assets, not only the risks, problems, or challenges. • Respect everyone. • Emphasize strengths and assets when developing an intervention. • Advocate for individuals and community groups who have less power. • Evaluate using qualitative and quantitative approaches that consider the broad ways in which an intervention has, or has not, been effective.

Key Points

- The process of assessment, planning, intervention, and evaluation is a cycle.

- Thorough assessment is critical to the success of the other nursing process phases.

- Assessment should include consideration of mental, physical, emotional, social, spiritual, and environmental assets and risks.

- Successful interventions build on strengths and are implemented with the collaboration and support of those being served.

- Evaluation of interventions should be planned before the intervention is initiated.

- Thorough evaluation should include qualitative and quantitative strategies.

- PHNs are uniquely positioned to collaborate with many different agencies in promoting the health and well-being of individuals/families, communities, and systems.

Exercises

Learning Examples for Effective Assessment, Intervention, Planning, and Evaluation Strategies

You can find many examples of PHNs undertaking activities for individuals and communities that reflect obvious consideration of not only physical needs and concerns but also emotional, social, environmental, and spiritual needs and concerns. These examples should encourage you to consider the ways in which you can thoroughly and holistically promote the health and well- being of those you serve in public health settings. The following are learning examples for holistic assessment, planning, intervention, and evaluation.

Environmental Health (Hayes, Davis, & Miranda, 2006)

- Nursing students and students from an environmental education program collaborated to conduct walkthrough assessments of a local community.

- Student teams presented their assessment that integrated concepts of environmental health to their class and health policy representatives.

Vision Problems Among Children (http://www.trihealth.com/aus/nws/nws_parishnurse.aspx)

- Parish nurses and school nurses worked together to screen children in Catholic schools for vision problems, leading to quicker identification of problems and subsequent in-depth eye examinations.

Bioterrorism Planning (Mondy, Cardenas, & Avila, 2003)

- PHNs have a critical valuable role in the planning, implementation, and evaluation of bioterrorism drills and activities.

- PHNs facilitate important collaboration of diverse disciplines mutually concerned with prevention of bioterrorism.

Reflective Practice

Conducting a blood pressure screening clinic in a church with a Spanish-speaking congregation takes careful and thoughtful planning. Parish nurses need to carefully conduct an assessment that considers the extent to which the congregation needs and is ready for screening activities. They also have to thoughtfully address many logistical aspects. Realizing that holistic assessment, planning, implementation, and evaluation processes are complex, consider how you might answer the following questions.

What might Maria need to consider in planning a health promotion activity in the neighborhood near the family she has been visiting?

Where might Maria go to find out if the needs she is observing in one family are common to others in the neighborhood?

_____

_____

Who would be potentially valuable partners to Maria when she decides a health promotion/ nutrition screening fair might be of benefit to the neighborhood?

_____

_____

How will Maria know if the health promotion fair has been successful?

_____

_____

What will Maria want to know from this health fair before she undertakes another one?

_____

_____

How might Maria self-reflect on the process to realize the holistic nature of the screening and to encourage even more effective public health nursing in her future work?

_____

_____

 Application of Evidence

1. When a PHN conducts a neighborhood needs assessment, where will she find data and who might she want to speak with about the community?

2. To enhance the potential for the nutrition health fair to be successful, who are the people/agencies a PHN will want to partner with in planning, implementation, and evaluation of the fair and its outcomes?

3. What are the differences in home safety checklists that a PHN might provide to a family with young children, a family with adolescents, or a family with elders?

4. What are some qualitative and quantitative ways to assess the successes of PHN programs or interventions?

Think, Explore, Do

1. Why is assessment necessary before you intervene with a family?

2. What data might you collect as part of an assessment of community violence?

3. How might you create a safety checklist so that it is attractive and accessible to families with a hard-of-hearing child? What would you include? Would it be paper or electronic?

4. If you are planning a community health screening event, how will you get the word out so that you have a successful, well-attended event?

5. When might you use an interview to evaluate the success of a health screening event instead of surveys? (Hint: Consider levels of education, population being served, languages spoken, etc.)

COMPETENCY #11:
Demonstrates Leadership in Public Health Nursing with Communities, Systems, Individuals, and Families

13

By Patricia M. Schoon and Marjorie A. Schaffer
with Bonnie Brueshoff, Maureen A. Alms and Vicki Kyarsgaard

Jose is with the Elders at Home Program for his public health nursing clinical. He is assigned to Mr. and Mrs. Santos, a couple in their 70s struggling to manage their health care needs and stay in their home in an older inner city neighborhood. Mrs. Santos provides primary assistance for her husband, who has advanced chronic obstructive pulmonary disease (COPD). After a recent hospitalization, Mr. Santos received home care services from a home care nurse, respiratory therapist, occupational therapist, and a home health aide. These services were reimbursed by Medicare because Mr. Santos met the criteria of potential for rehabilitation and progress toward independent living. All went well. Then a 60-day health assessment resulted in a determination that Mr. Santos was no longer eligible for home care services. He was referred to the county public health Elders at Home Program but was resisting a home visit. Jose wonders, "I am just a student nurse. What can I do?" Jose sighs, "Well, it looks like my preceptor has handed me a challenge I can't avoid. Isn't there a chapter we are supposed to read on leadership in public health nursing?"

JOSE'S NOTEBOOK

Competency #11: Demonstrates leadership in public health nursing with communities, systems, individuals, and families

- Seeks learning opportunities

- Works independently; autonomous in practice

- Willing to work in an unstructured environment; tolerates ambiguity

- Seeks consultation and support

- Takes initiative; is a self-starter

- Adapts to change

- Is willing and able to respond to population needs

- Demonstrates flexibility

- Contributes to team efforts

- Prioritizes and organizes workload, time, materials, and resource

Useful Definitions

Leadership: The art of Influencing, motivating, and leading others to achieve shared goals.

Advocacy-based Leadership: Ethical leadership based on principles of social justice that focus on improving the health and well-being of others.

Clinical Leadership: Leadership by an expert nurse who provides direct care, works effectively with health care team, and strives to improve the quality of care (Stanley, 2006; Stanley, 2008).

Organizational Leadership: Leadership directed at carrying out the mission and goals of an organization; can be formal or informal.

Servant Leadership: Leadership that starts with serving others and leads when it is the best way to serve others; responds to a call to leadership (Swearingen & Liberman, 2004).

Shared Leadership: Leadership initiatives shared by a team working together to achieve common goals (Avolio, Walumbwa, & Weber, 2009).

Transactional Leadership: Leadership that focuses on immediate needs; meets day-to-day functional needs of organization.

Leading Through Relationships

You are starting your public health nursing at the individual/family level of practice. This is where entry-level public health nurses (PHNs) often begin to develop their skills and understanding of the role of the PHN. Nursing leadership begins with the nurse-patient relationship in clinical practice; so does public health nursing leadership. Nursing leadership is advocacy-based, as is nursing practice. In other words, you begin to *lead* when you identify an unmet client need and take the *lead* in advocating for your client with others. In doing so, you are demonstrating advocacy-based leadership. When you move beyond the nurse-client relationship and advocate within the health care system or community for changes in attitudes, beliefs, knowledge, actions, and resources that will help meet your client's needs, you are practicing *leadership*. You do not have to be in a formal position of authority such as a supervisor or manager to be a leader. You are already an emerging leader. So what are these leadership skills and behaviors that you are already practicing? How can you develop your nursing leadership as you progress in your career? In this chapter we guide you in understanding PHN leadership roles and functions with each level of practice: individuals and families, communities, and systems.

> *Margaret, Jose's public health nursing preceptor, said to Jose, "I hope you like a challenge because this couple has lots of them. You are going to have to 'think outside of the box' to keep Mr. and Mrs. Santos in their own home. You really are going to have to use all of your communication, advocacy, and leadership skills to work successfully with this family."*

> *Jose wonders, "Do I have any leadership skills? I thought that came later after 5 to 10 years of practice."*

What Are Foundational Leadership Skills for Becoming a Public Health Nursing Leader?

As someone new to public health nursing, you might find thinking about the skills needed for leadership in public health nursing practice daunting. Remember that all good nursing leaders start at the beginning with becoming competent in their practice specialty and then as they develop confidence as an expert practitioner, they build a repertoire of leadership skills. The Henry Street Consortium generated a set of leadership skills (see the following list) that a beginning public health nurse needs for building his or her expertise through learning experiences and establishing a foundation for leadership in public health nursing.

- Seeks learning opportunities

- Works independently; autonomous in practice

- Willing to work in an unstructured environment; tolerates ambiguity

- Seeks consultation and support

- Takes initiative; is a self-starter

- Adapts to change

- Is willing and able to respond to population needs

- Demonstrates flexibility

- Contributes to team efforts

- Prioritizes and organizes workload, time, materials and resources

Seeks Learning Opportunities

An effective way to build your expertise is to identify and capitalize on learning opportunities that are consistent with your professional goals. The first step is to determine specific goals for your own professional development. In public health nursing you find myriad learning opportunities. Initially, you can strive to see the big picture of public health nursing—look beyond the individual to understand community and systems processes. Then match your interests and goals for self-development to the learning possibilities in your clinical setting. You are likely to find that preceptors and mentors in public health nursing will be happy to work with you to organize a desired learning experience. For example, if you are working with new moms who are breast-feeding, you might want to spend some time with a lactation consultant. Or, you might want to know more about food safety and would like to spend a day with the public health staff person who conducts restaurant inspections.

Works Independently; Autonomous in Practice

In many other clinical areas of practice, you might have encountered a hierarchy in being given an assignment and have experienced frequent supervision in completing your assignment. In public health, you are often out and about in the community on your own. Of course, students and new PHNs experience supervision of their work, but often the faculty member and PHN supervisor are not in the same space or immediately available. Although PHNs collaborate, they also make many independent decisions (sometimes based on established programs or protocol), especially when they are the only PHN in the setting (home, school, or occupational health setting). Autonomy in practice means that PHNs make decisions based on their own expertise within the framework of ethical and professional standards or practice. You might want to attend a PHN team meeting to observe how PHNs share experiences and to get suggestions about dealing with complex family situations.

Willing to Work in an Unstructured Environment; Tolerates Ambiguity

PHNs practice in settings where people live, learn, and work. The priorities in these settings are often not health or health care. For example, a family might be struggling to get enough to eat and not immediately worried about treating lice their child picked up at school. The school nurse is focused on making sure the lice outbreak at the school stops and recommends treatment. The family might not be able to purchase the lice treatment. This situation creates a challenge the nurse needs to sensitively work through. The challenge for many PHNs is collaborating to integrate health goals into the focus of the setting, whether that setting is in education, at work, or in a family living situation. Sometimes the goals of others are not clear or consistent with the goals of PHNs. PHNs learn to be in ambiguous situations while working to determine individual, family, and community goals. The PHN suggests health-oriented goals but ultimately works within the structure of each setting to accomplish goals that are mutually determined or sometimes rejected. Talk with your preceptors about the challenges they have confronted.

Seeks Consultation and Support

Seeking consultation and support is essential in a practice area where role models are often not physically present. Seeking consultation from others contributes to reflective practice. By reflecting on your experiences with expert practitioners, you can experience both validation of your thinking and actions and learn about more effective approaches to your work. When making a joint visit with your preceptor, you might want to discuss with her or him before the visit the teaching approach you think would be effective with a specific client.

Takes Initiative; Is a Self-Starter

As a PHN, you are responsible for organizing your own schedule. Many activities in public health nursing involve long-term planning, especially when building partnerships and coalitions that focus on community and systems change. This means that PHNs anticipate the steps needed to engage others in the change process. As you are learning the skills needed for public health nursing practice, you can be proactive in identifying ways to prepare for clinical experiences. Do you need to do background reading? Do you need to identify specific objectives to guide your preparation? What questions do you need to ask?

Adapts to Change

The settings where people live, work, and learn undergo constant changes. Bioterrorism and pandemic flu become threats. Hurricanes, flooding, and tornadoes endanger communities. Aging populations increase in communities. Communities decline in population or grow in the percentage of ethnic minority populations. Families experience change, communities and systems change, and the norms of health behavior change as well. Adapting to change is a constant in public health nursing practice. As someone new to public health nursing, you need to change your frame of thinking to a public health model in contrast to the medical model (Competency #4, Chapter 6).

Is Willing and Able to Respond to Population Needs

Healthy People 2020 priorities are based on the most recently identified health goals for the United States (U. S. Department of Health and Human Services, 2010). PHNs and local health departments must adapt to these changes if they are to be relevant in the interventions selected to improve population health.

Review the health data and health disparities data for your community. Ask your preceptor how the public health or community agency is responding to those needs. Identify a priority that you would like to work on as a student or a volunteer in your community.

Demonstrates Flexibility

Being flexible is consistent with adapting to change. However, flexibility is also required in situations where families or other professionals oppose change. Such situations can hinder goals for improved health or health care. Sometimes being flexible means being patient and waiting while encouraging others to make a change. Examples are working with a family to access a resource for meeting a health need or working with a community to create more open space for recreational use to increase physical activity.

Contributes to Team Efforts

Collaboration (Competency #3, Chapter 5) is essential to the practice of public health nursing. Public health initiatives and change cannot be accomplished by one person. PHNs need to cultivate skills that make them effective team leaders and team players. Listening, being open, valuing the contributions of others, and identifying a common vision and goals are all important when bringing others together to improve public health. Many public health learning experiences include collaborating with your peers on a health promotion project for the community. Use this experience to work on your team-building skills.

Prioritizes and Organizes Workload, Time, Materials, and Resources

Public health nursing can be overwhelming because so many areas exist in which nurses could spend time and energy for improving population health. Similarly, as someone new to public health nursing, you might be overwhelmed by what you need to do to prepare for public health nursing clinical or your workday. Sometimes the feeling of being overwhelmed can lead to inaction. Learning time management skills at the beginning of your public health nursing experience can serve you well. Make a plan for what you need to do, gather the information you need, and seek out needed resources. You can always modify your plan as you evaluate how well your plan is working. You can also share your plan with your preceptor or mentor who can help your reflect on your organization and preparation for your learning experiences. You might be asking yourself why these skills are important in public health nursing. How do you think these skills contribute to leadership? If you are interviewing for a nursing position, how might your interviewer respond to your self-assessment that you are flexible and organize your time well?

Leadership for the Entry-Level Public Health Nurse

So, what would be helpful to you at this point in your nursing career? You can begin answering this question by taking a brief look at nursing leadership in general and the leadership competencies expected of staff level PHNs. Leadership involves influencing others to achieve specific goals (Morrison, Jones, & Fuller, 1997). Nursing leadership can be formal or informal. In other words, nurses can demonstrate leadership at all levels of nursing practice from novice to expert and as staff nurses, clinical experts, nursing specialists, supervisors, managers, educators, or administrators. Leadership is a process, not a role. Much of the research on leadership in the literature looks at the leadership roles of managers; however, leadership styles and strategies can be used by all nurses. Leadership is an expected competency for PHNs, regardless of their position (Quad Council, 2004; American Nurses Association, 2007). The following text provides an overview of the ANA leadership standard for public health nursing.

ANA Public Health Nursing Scope and Standards of Practice

Standard 15. Leadership

The public health nurse provides leadership in nursing and public health.

Measurement Criteria:

The public health nurse:

Engages in multi-sector team development and coalition building including other professionals, the population, and stakeholders.

Promotes healthy community and work environments at local, regional, national, and international levels.

Articulates the mission, goals, action plan, and outcome measures of nursing and public health programs and services to other professionals and the population.

Advocates for opportunities for continuous, lifelong learning for self and others.

Teaches peers, stakeholders, and others in the population to succeed through mentoring and other strategies.

Exhibits creativity and flexibility through times of change.

Fosters a culture where systems are monitored and evaluated to improve the quality of policies, programs, and services for populations.

Coordinates programs and services across various community settings and among the multi-sector team.

Serves in leadership roles in the work setting, in the community, and with the population.

Promotes advancement of public health and nursing through participation in professional organizations.

Functions as a public health team leader in emergency preparedness and response situations, delegating tasks as delineated in standardized protocols (ANA, 2007, p. 38).

Some public health agencies include leadership development in their annual performance appraisals (Kalb et al., 2006). You might be expected to demonstrate the leadership skills you have developed after you have been in public health nursing for a year or so. See the following Evidence Example.

Evidence Example: Performance Appraisal Tool for Public Health-Seattle & King County (Washington) Component #8: Leadership/Systems Thinking – PHN Field Nurse

- Provides leadership and acts as a liaison with other community agencies and professionals, advocates on behalf of vulnerable individuals and populations, and participates in assessing and evaluating health care services to ensure that people are informed of available programs and services and are assisted in the utilization of those services

- Demonstrates support of the public health mission to protect and promote the health of all residents through implementing primary prevention strategies that prevent health problems from starting, spreading, or progressing

- Delegates and supervises tasks assigned to paraprofessional staff

- Participates in department and possibly community emergency response training and drills in support of disaster preparedness

- Participates in research and demonstration projects that seek to improve the health of communities and determine new ways to address health issues

- Participates in program development, implementation, coordination, and support

- Participates in quality management activities using quality improvement and evaluation approaches

- Performs in a manner consistent with site/organizational productivity goals

- Assumes responsibility for own professional development by pursuing education, participating in professional committees and work groups, and contributing to a work environment where continual improvements in practice are pursued

- Encourages use of community resources in support of public health practice

- Aligns practice with overall organizational goals

Note: Other performance appraisal components in this tool also include leadership development: Component #2. Policy development/program planning; Component #6. Partnership and collaboration (Kalb et al., 2006).

New PHNs need to be able to carry out entry-level leadership competencies. Initially their leadership will be tied to their daily clinical practice with individuals and families. However, depending on the size and nature of the agency, they might soon become involved in leadership activities at the community and systems levels of practice. This chapter discusses leadership styles and skills that you will be developing as students and those appropriate for entry-level practice.

Leadership is authentic influence that creates value (Cashman, 2008, p. 24). Leadership comprises the following:

- **Authenticity:** Awareness that openly faces strengths, vulnerabilities, and development challenges

- **Influence:** Communication that is meaningful and connects with others to remind both self and others of what is genuinely important

- **Value Creation:** Passion and aspiration to serve multiple constituencies: team, self, family, organization, community, and world

Jose has just completed his first visit to Mr. and Mrs. Santos. Mrs. Santos is experiencing caregiver stress and Mr. Santos is becoming less and less active. He loves to smoke even though he has a portable oxygen tank in his bedroom. The Santos' don't want nurses and social workers coming in and telling them what to do. They are afraid of strangers. Jose tells them he will make a joint visit with the social worker and introduce them to her. He is going to take the initiative to find the resources Mr. and Mrs. Santos need to live independently in their own home.

Clinical Leadership

Working in the community is challenging because of the diversity, uncertainty, and constant change you experience in an environment that is not within your control. As one student said, "The patients aren't lined up nicely in their beds all in a row down the hall." In home settings children are running around, animals abound, and the sounds of the television and people coming and going are often disconcerting. Older or disabled adults might like their slippery throw rugs on the floor and might want to have their favorite snacks available even though they are not on their prescribed diet. You might find homes without heat in the winter and homes without refrigerators in the summer. Some people live alone, and others live with a myriad of relatives and friends. You never know what to expect when you knock on the door. But you need to be ready for both the expected and unexpected. One student several years ago was in the process of changing a catheter for a paraplegic man when the man's cat jumped on the bed. What was the student to do? Her sterile field was about to be compromised. She was wearing her only pair of sterile gloves and her equipment was laid out on the bed. She thought for a moment. Then, very calmly, she asked the man if he would hold his cat while she changed his catheter—this student responded with flexibility, creativity, adaptability to a changing environment, and comfort with making decisions autonomously. She was demonstrating clinical leadership. As you develop the ability to practice nursing in the community, whether in a home, school, clinic, faith-based organization, or other type of community agency, you will be developing your leadership skill set.

Clinical leadership has an evidence base. Clinical leaders are recognized for their expertise, their approachability, and their ability to be effective communicators (Stanley, 2006; Stanley, 2008). By using their expertise and values and beliefs, they are empowered to do what is necessary on a daily basis and to role model effective care and communication to others. They are able to motivate and empower others. Think about how you feel as you become comfortable working in the community and in people's homes. Do you share your successes with your classmates and give them helpful suggestions? If you do, you are on your way to becoming an effective clinical leader.

Evidence Example: Characteristics of Clinical Leadership

In a qualitative research study based on grounded theory, David Stanley (2006) interviewed nurses and supervisors to identify clinical leaders and their characteristics. Clinical leadership characteristics included the following:

Clinical competence: Competent and credible in a specific clinical area

Clinical knowledge: Linked to clinical competence and expertise; knowing how teams work and having knowledge of relationships

Effective communicator: Have listening skills and the ability to explain things to others; have the ability to influence and lead by virtue of their opinions

Decision maker: The ability to make decisions about a "whole host of issues" including clinical decisions

Empowerment/motivator: Enthusiastic about what they are doing, empowered and able to empower and inspire others

Openness/approachable: Approachability is key to effective leadership, not being controlling or dictatorial

Role model: Models effective care, having their "values on show"

Visible: Present in clinical environment

(Stanley, 2006, p. 109)

Jose made a joint visit with the social worker. Mr. and Mrs. Santos are committed to living in this home that they worked so hard to purchase and maintain. It is obvious that home maintenance is poor. Stacks of old papers litter the house, they lack working smoke detectors, and they have minimal food stored in the cupboards or refrigerator. The kitchen sink is not draining properly, and the washer and dryer are not working. The social worker offered to help the couple apply for assistance for home repairs and for Meals On Wheels. Jose was glad he could share the care needs with the social worker. He felt they would be more effective in helping Mr. and Mrs. Santos by working as a team.

Sharing Organizational Leadership

When team members work together to achieve common goals, they are practicing shared leadership (Avolio et al., 2009). PHNs work in teams to more effectively meet the health needs of their communities. Shared leadership refers to the concept of being an effective team member: sharing responsibilities; mutually organizing the work of the team; maintaining team communications; taking the initiative to try a new approach if something isn't working; supporting team members; providing positive feedback; and allocating resources equitably. When leadership is shared, PHNs have more time and energy to care for their clients.

The day-to-day work of the organization needs to be done. This means two things: carrying out the mission and goals of the organization and carrying out the priority work of the organization. For staff nurses that means managing their caseload of clients on a daily basis, setting priorities based on the changing needs of their clients, and being willing to take on tasks that need to be done. Organizational leaders are often called transactional leaders; they are goal-oriented, focused on getting things done, and are not afraid to take the lead among team members or classmates when tasks need to be organized and responsibilities need to be assigned.

An example of how nursing students effectively practiced shared leadership occurred during a clinical at a homeless shelter. Public health nursing students conducted a monthly foot care clinic from September through May each year. During a 3-hour clinic, 6 to 8 students usually provided foot care to 20 to 45 clients. The instructor and homeless shelter staff oriented the students to the shelter and the foot-care clinic. Then the instructor turned the clinic over to the students to manage. The students determined how to arrange the clinic space, how to allocate the foot care supplies, and who would carry out the different clinic roles (i.e., recruitment and registration of the clients; assigning the clients to different students for their foot care; keeping each workspace stocked with supplies; providing hospitality; documenting client assessments and services given; and following up on clients after they received care to make sure all of their priority health needs were met). The instructor noticed that when she turned over the management of the clinic to the students, they were much more engaged and took more responsibility for the clinic and their clients. Every group of students organized their clinic a little differently. Each month, they shared responsibility, freedom to be creative and practice autonomously. Mutual contributions to team efforts always led to a successful clinic. Because of their ability to prioritize what needed to be done and organize their workload effectively, students managed to take the time to provide a therapeutic encounter with each client who visited the clinic. As one man said after he spent an hour with one of the students who listened patiently to his story, "This has been the best day of my life."

> *Jose makes a second co-visit with the social worker. They talk to Mr. and Mrs. Santos about their health care needs. Mr. Santos is on oxygen therapy. Mrs. Santos states that she knows her husband should stop smoking and that she turns off his oxygen when he does smoke. Mr. Santos cannot care for his personal needs. Mrs. Santos says that she is uncomfortable assisting him with hygiene and that he has not had a good bath or shower for several weeks. Mrs. Santos is becoming very stressed and showing signs of depression. No one has contacted Mr. and Mrs. Santos about home maintenance. Jose decides he needs to prioritize. The social worker starts the application process for a home health aide to assist Mrs. Santos with Mr. Santos' personal needs. Jose is going to follow up on the*

home maintenance referral and also work with Mr. Santos on a safe smoking program. He will focus on Mrs. Santos's stress and possible depression on the next visit.

What Does Leadership Mean in Public Health Nursing Practice?

PHNs spend their daily lives in the community and deal with social determinants of health and the impact of these determinants on health outcomes with individuals, families, populations, and communities. They know that they must go outside of the health care system to promote and protect the health of their clients. The use of leadership is crucial to successful efforts. PHNs carry out leadership at the individual/family, community, and systems levels whether in the home, in the multidisciplinary public health team, in the community, or within diverse systems such as government, health care organizations, schools, home-care agencies, prisons, faith-based communities, and homeless shelters. They use many leadership strategies and interventions such as collective social action, persuasion, influencing, role-modeling, coalition building, networking, social marketing, and collaboration. Effective PHNs demonstrate passionate commitment, risk-taking, and personal bravery.

> Public health nurses practice at that intersection where societal attitudes, government policies, and people's lives meet. Such privilege creates a moral imperative not only to attend to the health needs of the public but also, like Nightingale, to work to change the societal conditions contributing to poor health (Falk-Rafael, 2005, p. 219).

Advocacy-Based Leadership

Advocacy-based leadership is foundational in public health nursing. Advocating for clients whether those clients are individuals, families, populations, or communities is part of the social justice mission of public health nursing. Though all nurses advocate for the unmet needs of their individual clients, PHNs have a responsibility to advocate for the health of the public, to care about what is causing the health disparities in their communities, and to take actions to improve the health status of the individuals, families, populations, and communities. This means that PHNs need to be aware of emerging health needs and connect the patterns of health disparities they observe among their individual clients. Sometimes advocacy-based leadership is an unconscious response to an unmet health care need. The following Evidence Example illustrates this form of leadership from the perspective of a public health nursing student from a school of nursing in the Henry Street Consortium.

Evidence Example: Student Initiative Demonstrates Leadership and Improves Population Health

A student nurse completed her leadership clinical in an inner city school with a 95% poverty rate among its students. She developed a dental screening program for the third grade as her leadership project. After screening all of the children, she found that almost all of them had dental disease such as decay, bleeding gums, abscess, and missing or broken teeth. Almost none of them had received dental care in the last year and few owned a toothbrush. All of the children were given a toothbrush, toothpaste, and were taught how to brush their teeth. The nursing student then decided to screen all of the children in the elementary school. She managed to screen about 90% of the children. She prepared a report showing the need for dental care in almost all of the children screened, sent home referrals to all parents, and included information on local dental clinics that provided care for low-income patients. The principal used the report to obtain a grant to put a dental clinic in the school. Within a few years, dental clinics were established in elementary schools located in high poverty neighborhoods throughout the school district.

Source: Schoon, 2010

From Advocate to Servant

Advocacy-based leadership leads to servant leadership. While you are practicing advocacy-based leadership, observe the actions of your preceptors and other PHN staff and management. You will probably notice that many of them have a passion for public health nursing. They have a mission to carry out. Part of their mission is to promote and protect the health of the public. Another part of their mission is to prepare future PHNs for the population needs of the 21st century. As servant leaders, your PHN preceptors are primarily interested in serving the common good. They take on leadership roles and responsibilities to achieve social justice and to serve others (Swearingen & Liberman, 2004). Helping people grow and reach their goals is primary. Mentoring, modeling, and nurturing are key leadership strategies. Collaboration and cautious use of power are both important (Robinson, 2009). Effective characteristics and attributes of servant leadership are listed in Table 13.1 (Russell & Stone, 2002). You might want to think about which of these characteristics and attributes you observe in your preceptors. Think about which of these characteristics and attributes you already have. You can enhance your skill set by working with preceptors who model servant leadership.

Table 13.1   Most Important Characteristics and Attributes of Servant Leadership

9 Most Effective Characteristics	10 Accompanying Attributes
• Vision	• Communication
• Honesty	• Credibility
• Integrity	• Competence
• Trust	• Stewardship
• Service	• Visibility
• Modeling	• Influence
• Pioneering	• Persuasion
• Appreciation of others	• Listening
• Empowerment	• Encouragement
	• Teaching and delegation

Source: Russell and Stone, 2002

Jose returns for a fourth visit to Mr. and Mrs. Santos. Mrs. Santos is crying and wringing her hands. Jose asks Mrs. Santos if she would be willing to see a mental health case worker. She refuses. He remembers that the local Latino Catholic church has a pastoral ministry home visiting program. He wonders if Mrs. Santos would allow the pastoral minister to visit her. Mrs. Santos agrees to let Jose contact the church. Jose is pleased he thought "outside of the box." He is really stretching himself to try to find ways to help Mr. and Mrs. Santos. He is going to be their advocate.

Leadership in Action

As a nursing student or nurse who is new to public health nursing, you will likely look to practicing PHNs to provide an example of leadership actions. Keep in mind that your focus is on the development of beginning leadership skills, as well as a having a vision for growing as a leader. The study in the following Evidence Example (Zilembo & Monterosso, 2008) explored nursing students' views of important leadership qualities observed in their preceptors for their clinical learning experiences. This study is not specific to public health nursing preceptors but does address the leadership strategies that nursing students valued in their preceptors who helped to guide their learning in clinical experiences.

Evidence Example: Nursing Students' Perceptions of Desirable Leadership Qualities in Nurse Preceptors

Melanie Zilembo and Leanne Monterosso (2008) conducted a mixed-methods study to explore Australian nursing student (n = 23) perceptions of what leadership qualities in their preceptors contributed to a positive clinical learning experience. First, the researchers developed a quality-of-leadership survey based on leadership qualities identified in the literature. Participants completed the survey and responded to four open-ended questions, which the researchers analyzed for main themes. Out of 23 leadership qualities, the top 12 qualities (selected by 20 or more of the 23 respondents) were as follows: purposeful, clinically competent, supportive, motivating, approachable, consistent, organized, effective at communication, confidence inspiring, a critical thinker, one who sets goals and targets, and passionate.

The four major themes identified by the researchers were as follows: 1) interpersonal communication, 2) continuity of preceptor, 3) integration of theory and practice, and 4) psychomotor proficiency. These themes give clues to what leadership actions on the part of preceptors are meaningful for nursing students. Preceptors with effective interpersonal communication are likely to be perceived as more supportive and approachable by nursing students, which can enhance the quality of their learning experiences. Students viewed working with a greater number of preceptors as confusing or starting over. Consistency in working with the same preceptor provides an opportunity for developing a relationship that is supportive and inspires confidence in learning. Theory and practice become integrated for the student through real-world learning experiences that also give time for reflection. The fourth theme in this study primarily addresses increasing confidence in performing technical skills. The parallel for public health nursing is the development of skills for addressing the health needs of populations such as community assessment and analysis of population data. Students will likely gain confidence and competence as they work with preceptors who are leaders in public health nursing.

ACTIVITY

What leadership qualities have you observed in your preceptor, nursing faculty, or expert public health nurses?

How do these leadership qualities contribute to effective public health nursing practice?

What leadership qualities would you like to purposefully develop?

What are some ways or strategies you could use to develop these leadership qualities?

Jose makes a fifth visit to Mr. and Mrs. Santos. He notices that Mr. Santos is still smoking in the same room as his oxygen tank. Jose is concerned about the safety issues and the possible neglect of a vulnerable adult. He wants to honor the couple's independence and wishes, but understands that his professional responsibility requires him to report the potential for harm to this vulnerable adult. Jose consults with Margaret, his preceptor. She says she will make a joint visit with Jose the next day to see if there is anything else they can do. During the visit the next day, Jose observes Margaret's approach to Mr. Santos. Margaret and Mr. and Mrs. Santos set up a smoking schedule for Mr. Santos that allows him to smoke while on the front porch. Mr. Santos will use his oxygen before and after each smoke but not during his smoking session. Jose is impressed with Margaret's skill in working with Mr. Santos. He is going to use her technique during his next visit.

How Does Organizational Leadership Support Public Health Nursing Practice?

PHNs practice within an organization, which might be a local or state health department or non-profit organization. The leadership culture of the organization in which the PHN works determines the support available for effective public health nursing practice. The culture of support for achieving public health nursing practice goals must permeate the entire organization as demonstrated in Figure 13.1. Nurses at all levels within the organization must take responsibility and leadership for carrying out the work of public health nursing practice.

As you consider possibilities for a public health nursing position, ask questions to determine the type of support the organization provides to help you learn and accomplish expectations for practice. What orientation to public health nursing programs and activities is provided? Is a preceptor or mentor available to you to help you reflect on and guide your work? Do evaluations also focus on your development as a PHN?

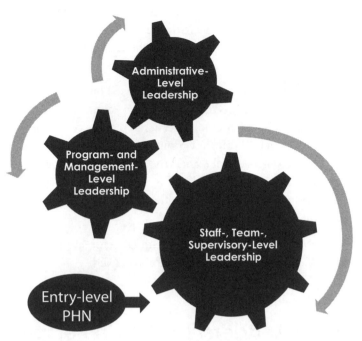

Figure 13.1   Organizational culture of support for public health nursing practice

Evidence Example: Organizational Attributes that Support Public Health Nursing Practice

A Canadian study (Underwood et al., 2009; Meagher-Stewart et al., 2010) identified effective leadership as an organizational attribute that supports public health nursing practice. Their study analyzed survey data from over 13,000 community nurses across Canada and data from 23 focus groups of PHNs and policymakers. Focus group participants identified organizational factors needed for effective public health nursing practice: government policy that supports public health, supportive organizational culture, and good management practices.

All the groups said visionary, empowering and motivational leadership figured in public health nurses practicing their full scope of competencies. When effective leadership permeates organizations, everyone feels empowered and motivated to be effective in their roles. Leadership must respect, trust, and value public health. (Underwood et al., 2009, p. I-7)

What Are Leadership Expectations for Entry-Level Public Health Nurses?

Leadership needs change depending on the situation of the organization and of the community. Also different nurses bring different leadership abilities to their work. Diverse styles of leadership are necessary to get the work of public health nursing accomplished. PHNs select leadership strategies and interventions based on what is most effective. Flexibility, a willingness and openness to develop new skills, and the courage to practice your new skills in the public arena are the key to your success in developing new leadership skills. Consider what a public health nursing director (Brueshoff, 2010) has to say about leadership and starting public health nurses.

> **Leadership for Entry-Level Public Health Nurses.** Based on the PHN population-based practice focus in public health, a new PHN needs to demonstrate clinical leadership for the work with individuals and families while also providing leadership at the community level. This leadership might be as a participant or a lead role on various committees such as a family service collaborative, early intervention, or other school teams. The PHN must also be a leader in doing community outreach and group education. The "client" in public health is often the community, and having skills to lead groups, coalitions, and committees is essential to achieve the goals of improving the health of the population.

> —Bonnie Brueshoff, MSN, RN, PHN, Public Health Director and Robert Wood Johnson Executive Nurse Fellow (2006–2009), Dakota County Public Health

Putting Entry-Level Leadership Skills in Perspective

PHNs practice at three levels: individual/family, community, and systems. So you need the ability to practice leadership at all three levels. Figure 13.2 illustrates how you can practice entry-level leadership.

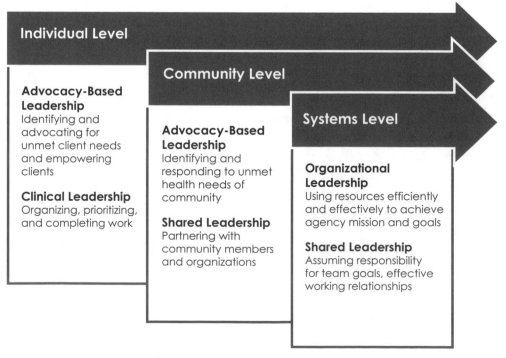

Figure 13.2   Entry-level leadership at three levels of practice

Developing Leadership at the Community Level of Practice

As leaders, PHNs aim to be change agents to reduce the social conditions that contribute to poor health (health disparities). Power to influence is gained through developing alliances (coalition building) with individuals and groups who have influential power. Florence Nightingale made alliances with politicians, journalists, philosophers, scientists, and influential thinkers and writers that contributed to her understanding of the public health issues of her time but also helped her to bring about change for improving the health of populations (Falk-Rafael, 2005). PHNs need to move from behind the scenes to put forward strategies that can make a difference for the health of populations. This means increasing one's knowledge about the sociopolitical environment, increasing self-confidence, and developing political advocacy skills to bear witness to the effects of policy decision on the lives of the people (Mason, Backer, & Georges, 1991; Falk-Rafael, 2005).

Evidence Example: Bringing About Social Change to Reduce Child Poverty

Benita Cohen and Linda Reutter (2007) reviewed literature from Canada, the United States, and the United Kingdom, as well as the professional standards and competencies for nursing practice in Canada. Based on their review, the authors recommended using Clare Blackburn's (1992) framework for working with families living in poverty. Blackburn conceptualized three broad roles, which can be carried out at all levels of practice: 1) *monitoring*—collecting and analyzing information to determine the impact of poverty on families, 2) *alleviating and preventing*—helping families to avoid, reduce, and counteract the impact of poverty, and 3) *bringing about social change*—working with organizations and the government to create policy that reduces or eliminates poverty.

PHNs can bring about social change through initiating public discussion on effects of poverty and the contribution of policy decisions to creating poverty. Actions include putting poverty on the agenda of professional organizations and using the media to increase awareness. PHNs can use the data from their monitoring activities to inform other professionals, organizations, and the public about how poverty contributes to health disparities. Partnership skills for collective action (Competency #3, Chapter 5) are essential in bringing about change through advocacy action.

Though public health can identify and study the impact of these health determinants, it cannot solve problems such as poverty, housing, unemployment, and an unsafe environment. Public health can, however, call attention to these problems and get them on the policy agenda and into the public discourse. Public health can also study the causes and results of these health determinants and examine the effectiveness of social and collective responses to these problems. And it can help to mobilize public will and coordinate actions of the public and private health care, education, and business sectors.

Several authors suggest innovative approaches to leading change in communities and systems. Karen Hill (2008) identifies lessons learned for leading change in public health nursing practice. Laura Nissen, Daniel Merrigan, and M. Katherine Kraft (2005) provide additional lessons learned from leadership initiatives for community and systems change that are applicable to public health nursing practice. Their recommendations are outlined in the following list.

- Define the roles and responsibilities for stakeholders involved in leading the change.

- Seek input from all who will experience the change.

- Be present "at the table." "Interpersonal and political skills and personal presence are essential during periods of change" (Hill, 2008, p. 460).

- Look for traditional as well as nontraditional partners, including funding sources.

- Consider the big picture.

- Collaborate with others to create a positive vision of the future and choose strategies to work toward that vision.

- Remember that leadership is about relationships every day.

- Engage in self-examination and self-correction.

- Consistently integrate evidence-based approaches.

- Be hopeful but realistic when planning change.

Sources: Hill, 2008; Nissen, Merrigan, & Kraft, 2005

You might have noticed that Jose is practicing many of the entry-level leadership competencies in his role as Mr. and Mrs. Santos' PHN. Leadership is integrated into many of the activities that PHNs and student nurses carry out. Table 13.2 has examples of activities listed in a clinical menu for students used by one of the public health agencies in the Henry Street Consortium.

Table 13.2 Entry-Level PHN Leadership Activities for Novice PHNs and Students

PHN Intervention	Example
<u>Advocacy</u> Advocacy pleads someone's cause or acts on someone's behalf, with a focus on developing the community, system, individual, or family's capacity to plead their own cause or act on their own behalf (Minnesota Department of Health, 2001, p. 263).	Observing/participating in a town meeting designed to address or change a determinant of health Advocate for parenting classes at a conference center in an apartment complex (community level)
<u>Policy Development</u> Policy development places health issues on decision-makers' agendas, acquires a plan of resolution, and determines needed resources. Policy development results in laws, rules and regulations, ordinances, and policies (p. 313).	Working with schools/worksites to change vending and fundraiser policies to healthy food choices (systems level)

PHN Intervention	Example
Policy Enforcement Policy enforcement compels others to comply with the laws, rules, regulations, ordinances, and policies created in conjunction with Policy Development (p. 313).	Responding to concerns/complaints about smoking in restricted areas based on Freedom to Breathe Act (community level)
Surveillance Surveillance describes and monitors health events through ongoing and systematic collection, analysis, and interpretations of health data for the purpose of planning, implementing, and evaluating public health interventions (p.13).	Attending or participating in immunization registry meetings (systems level) Locating unlicensed daycare providers and providing teaching on home safety (individual level)
Coalition Building Coalition building promotes and develops alliances among organizations or constituencies for a common purpose. It builds linkages, solves problems, or enhances local leadership to address health concerns (p. 211).	Recruiting and inviting family daycare providers to join the childhood obesity prevention committee (community level)
Community Organizing Community organizing helps community groups identify common problems or goals, mobilize resources, and develop and implement strategies for reaching the goals they collectively have set (p. 235).	Participating/helping plan youth program such as smoking or alcohol use prevention (community level) Helping/coordinating a bioterrorism table top exercise (systems level)
Disease and Health Event Investigation Disease and other health event investigation systematically gathers and analyzes data regarding threats (bioterrorism, chemical or other hazardous waste spills, or natural disasters) to the health of populations, ascertains the source of the threat, identifies cases and others at risk, and determines control measures (p. 29).	Following up on reports of pertussis cases; communicating with MDH, clinics, and area schools about the outbreak and doing case investigation (individual and systems levels) Meeting with clinics and hospitals regarding prenatal Hepatitis B Program (systems level) Working with veterinarians, meat packers, and hunting associations on chronic wasting disease (systems level)
Case Management Case management optimizes self-care capabilities of individuals and families and the capacity of systems and communities to coordinate and provide services (p. 93).	Participating in Student Attendance Review Board (SARB) meeting within a school (systems level)
Collaboration Collaboration commits two or more persons or organizations to achieving a common goal through enhancing the capacity of one or more of them to promote and protect health (p. 177).	Participating in meetings to observe the collaborative process, decision making and problem solving in groups (e.g., children's mental health, early childhood family education) (systems level)

PHN Intervention	Example
Consultation Consultation seeks information and generates optional solutions to perceived problems or issues through interactive problem-solving with a community, system, family, or individual. The community, system, family, or individual selects and acts on the option best meeting the circumstances (p. 165).	Working with child day care centers, adult day care centers, and battered women's shelters to establish standards and criteria for prevention of infectious disease (systems level)
Social Marketing Social marketing utilizes commercial marketing principles and technologies for programs designed to influence the knowledge, attitudes, values, beliefs, behaviors, and practices of the population of interest (285).	Designing messages and materials on "how to make a healthy home" that PHNs can use on home visits to help families deal with asthma (systems level)

Source: Brueshoff, 2010; Dakota County Public Health, 2004; Henry Street Consortium, 2004; MDH, 2001

Jose has almost completed his public health nursing clinical. He is going to attend a Nurses Day on the Hill event at his state capitol. He wants to talk with his senator and representative about the need for funding programs to help people like Mr. and Mrs. Santos stay in their own homes. He asked Mr. and Mrs. Santos if it would be okay with them if he shared their story. He knows that real-life stories are more effective than statistical data. Jose attended Nurses Day on the Hill and talked with his senator and representative. He was surprised at how receptive they were to him and that they treated him as an expert! Over 1,000 nurses were at the event. Jose was surprised that so many nurses and students took the time to attend. He felt proud to be part of such a large group that advocated for the health needs of the community. He realized that nursing is more than just working a shift. Jose knows that if he is going to make a difference, he needs to advocate for his clients at both the systems and community levels of practice.

Participating in the Political Process

PHNs often participate in the policy development and enforcement process. This requires an understanding of how the political process works and the critical points in moving forward. Taking the time to understand the policy-making process is essential if you want to advocate for vulnerable populations with your elected officials (e.g., legislators, mayor, city council, county commissioners, school board). After you understand how laws, regulations, and ordinances are made, you can be more confident about participating in the process. Your knowledge of health care and the health needs of your community make you an expert in the eyes of elected officials. Development of a trust relationship with your legislators can help you in influencing health policy development (Deschaine & Schaffer, 2003).

Nurses need to be involved in the political process from the electoral process to the legislative audit process (see Figure 13.3). Jose decides to review some basic civics on the political process and think about what he might do to advocate for older adults who need assistance to stay in their homes. See Table 13.3 for examples of what Jose could do.

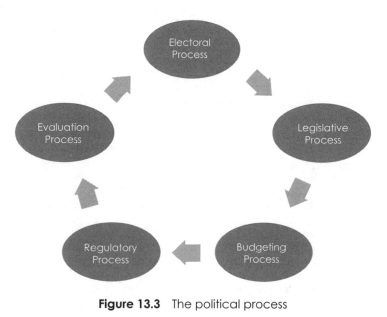

Figure 13.3 The political process

Table 13.3 Political Process—What Could Jose Do?

Electoral Process
Candidate selection, endorsement and support in the primary and general elections.

Jose can do phone calling, door-knocking, mailings; he can put up yard signs, donate money, attend rallies and other campaign activities for candidates who support his political agenda for keeping older adults in their homes. He can participate in candidate screening through his local nurses' association.

Legislative Process
Writing, introducing, holding hearings, passing the bill, and enabling legislation for funding. Both houses of Congress (one or two at state level) must pass the bill, and the bill must then be signed by the governor.

Jose can contact his legislators about bills he wants them to support that provide funding for stay-at-home programs. He can write letters and e-mails or go to the Hill for a face-to-face meeting. He can attend hearings on the bill. Jose can also testify at conference hearings. He can write letters to the editor of the local newspaper; post online blogs; and call in to radio programs.

Budgeting Process
The omnibus reconciliation bill at the end of each legislative session provides enabling funding. A government department is given "budget authority" or the right to implement the legislation and allocate the funding.

Jose can lobby for funding of the bill. He can find out which state agency has budget authority to enact and fund the legislation. He can provide testimony on the best way to fund programs and discuss who is going to benefit.

Regulatory Process

The department with budget authority prior to implementation of legislation holds hearings to determine the rules and regulations that need to accompany the bill.

Jose can attend hearings about the rules and regulations that are going to enable the bill to be implemented and monitored for cost, quality, and access. He can ask to be put on an e-mail mailing list for notice of meetings and actions taken.

Evaluation Process

The legislature has a 2-year budget cycle. Every program funded and implemented has to be evaluated and a report sent to the legislative auditor's office. The evaluation of the success of the project is a significant factor in determining if a program is continued or renewed.

Jose can download a copy of the report and meet with his legislator's staff person and/or the "budget authority" agency to discuss the evaluation and make recommendations for continuation or modification of the program.

The American Public Health Association (2010) has identified ten key points of advocacy that might be helpful to you as you think about approaching your legislators.

1. Get to know legislators well—their districts and constituencies, voting records, personal schedules, opinions, expertise and interests. Be sure to have a good understanding of the legislator and his/her concerns, priorities, and perspectives.

2. Acquaint yourself with the staff members for the legislators, committees, and resource officials with whom you will be working. These people are essential sources of information and have significant influence in some instances in the development of policy.

3. Identify fellow advocates and partners in the public health community to better understand the process, monitor legislation, and assess strengths and weaknesses. Finding common ground on an issue sometimes brings together strange bedfellows but makes for a stronger coalition.

4. Identify the groups and other legislators with whom you may need to negotiate for changes in legislation. Do not dismiss anyone because of previous disagreements or because you lack a history of working together. Yesterday's opponent may be today's ally.

5. Foster and strengthen relationships with allies and work with legislators who are flexible and tend to keep an open mind. Don't allow anyone to consider you a bitter enemy because you disagree.

6. Be honest, straightforward, and realistic when working with legislators and their staff. Don't make promises you cannot keep. Never lie or mislead a legislator about the importance of an issue, the opposition's position or strength, or other matters.

7. Be polite, remember names, and thank those who help you—both in the legislature and in the public health advocacy community.

8. Learn the legislative process and understand it well. Keep on top of the issues and be aware of controversial and contentious areas.

9. Be brief, clear, accurate, persuasive, timely, persistent, grateful, and polite when presenting your position and communicating what you need/want from the legislator or staff member.

10. Be sure to follow up with legislators and their staff. If you offer your assistance or promise to provide additional information, do so in a timely and professional manner. Be a reliable resource for them today and in the future.

Ethical Considerations

In addition to considering the impact of decisions on the health of individuals, families, communities, and systems, public health nursing leaders must also consider how decisions affect PHNs and other public health staff. Nursing leaders can apply ethical perspectives to guide decisions that affect their teamwork and leadership activities (see Table 13.4).

Jose called the social worker to report on how he and his preceptor had resolved the unsafe smoking situation with Mr. Santos. The social worker remained concerned and felt that Mr. Santos should be reported to county social services as a vulnerable adult. Jose felt that Mr. Santos should be allowed time to try the new approach. He advocated for the social worker to wait awhile to see how Mr. Santos was doing.

ACTIVITY

What ethical perspectives might Jose use in explaining this viewpoint to the social worker?

Table 13.4   Ethical Action in Public Health Nursing Leadership

Ethical Perspective	Application
Rule Ethics (principles)	• Make leadership decisions that promote good and prevent harm to families, communities, organizations, and public health workers.
	• Consider what leadership actions promote justice in the community and among public health staff members.
Virtue Ethics (character)	• Be a servant leader by valuing serving others through leadership actions.
	• Be a leader who establishes caring relationships as a foundation for leadership actions.
	• Be a leader who values both the success of the organization and the well being of public health staff members.
	• Be flexible.
	• Value the contributions of all team members.

Ethical Perspective	Application
Feminist Ethics (reducing oppression)	• Make decisions by including all populations groups who will receive services. • Use a team approach vs. a hierarchical approach to prioritizing public health strategies.

Table based on work by Volbrecht, 2002, and Racher, 2007

Key Points

- Leadership is a process of development. You can begin building your leadership skills through your clinical and work experiences.

- Leadership in public health includes leadership at all three levels of practice: individual/family, communities, and systems.

- Leadership theories that are particularly relevant for entry-level public health nursing practice include advocacy-based leadership, clinical leadership, organizational leadership, and servant leadership.

- Leadership in public health nursing involves leading social change to reduce health disparities.

- Advocacy and policy development are interventions that nurse leaders use in collaboration with other influential organizations and persons to bring about change.

- PHNs can influence all steps of the political decision-making process by using evidence and practice expertise.

- Leadership in public health nursing can be demonstrated while using many of the public health interventions.

Exercises

Learning Examples for Leadership

There is a concept called "glocal" which means think global, act local. That is a good way to look at your leadership development as a nursing student and when you begin your professional nursing practice. Select an issue you feel strongly about. Maybe it is limited access to needed services for vulnerable individuals and families or environmental health issues or drinking and driving. Maybe you like working in teams and taking on the leadership role. Whatever you are passionate about, that is where you start your leadership development. Consider the following examples of student actions in which they chose to take the leadership initiative. What might you do?

Acting on a Suspicion of Child Abuse

A student nurse was carrying out health screening in an elementary school. She noticed that one young girl did not respond to questions, avoided eye contact, and flinched when she was touched. The student nurse conferred with her instructor and then took her concern about the child, including possibility of abuse, to the school principal.

Nurses Day on the Hill

Nursing students went to the state capitol to participate in an event sponsored by their state nurses association. Each student selected a health advocacy topic of interest, researched information about the topic, and prepared a one-minute speech to present to a legislator that included a story about real people. Students visited with their elected representatives providing both verbal and written information. They also participated in a rally in the capitol rotunda for safe patient care.

Infection Control Interventions with a Daycare

A team of student nurses was working with a daycare staff to help them develop their disaster management plan. The students noticed that there were no infection control policies and procedures in place. They took their concerns to the daycare director and proposed an intervention plan. The students taught the staff the basics of infection control and universal precautions. They also taught a hand-washing class to the preschoolers.

Groundwater Contamination in a Rural Community

Students working with a public health agency were asked to gather information about groundwater contamination by census track in a specific community. The students gathered the information and presented their results by creating a colorful map with different levels of groundwater contamination by census track. They also prepared a binder with the scientific data that supported the map and discussed the impact of the groundwater contamination on populations. The map and binder were so well done that county environmental health staff used them both in testifying at the state legislature.

Source: Schoon, 2010

Reflective Practice

The focus of public health is primary prevention. We seek to promote population health and protect community members from accidents, injury, disease, and disability. Focusing on primary prevention requires a paradigm shift from illness care to wellness care and from focusing on changing the health behaviors of individuals and families to changing the health determinants and social determinants of health at the societal level.

Read the following story and reflect upon upstream and downstream thinking.

> Two people were walking by a river. Suddenly, they observed babies floating down the river. They ran to the river to pull out as many babies as they could possibly reach. One of the rescuers yelled, "I'm going upstream to find out how these babies are getting into the river." This rescuer climbed the pathway up the side of the river, found where the babies were being thrown in the river, and immediately stopped more babies from

being thrown into the water. This is upstream thinking and action in contrast to down-stream action. Falk-Rafael (2005) explained how downstream approaches that are aimed at meeting the needs of individuals and families must be paired with upstream approaches that aim to change power in societal relationships and structures to give voice to those with poor health and social disadvantages.

Think about the difference between upstream and downstream approaches when working with pregnant and parenting teens. Though PHNs need to work with the young families to provide health teaching and connect them with needed health and social services, the strategies are downstream in focus, because nothing is being done to change the population health disparities often experienced by the young families who experience adolescent pregnancy. Upstream policies involve changing the societal conditions that result in poorer health and economic outcomes for this population. Examples of upstream policies are inclusive education for young mothers in the school system, universal health care, and the availability of "living wage" jobs.

Think of a health disparity you would like to see changed.

_____

_____

How would you use upstream thinking to achieve your goal?

_____

_____

Application of Evidence

1. What examples of public health nursing leadership do you see at the individual, community and systems levels in the agency where you have had your clinical experience?

2. Identify three leadership characteristics you have read about in this chapter that you would like to develop for your future nursing practice.

3. Give an example of how a PHN can use each of the following leadership strategies in improving the health status of a population group.

   - Advocacy-based leadership
   - Clinical leadership
   - Organizational leadership
   - Servant leadership

Think, Explore, Do

1. How can you practice an advocacy-based leadership intervention? For example, write a letter to the editor of your local newspaper about a public health issue in your community. Clearly state the problem, its causes, and make recommendations for what you would like to see happen.

2. Develop goals for your leadership development in public health nursing. Complete the following table.

Your Plan for Developing Foundational Leadership Behaviors in Public Health Nursing

Leadership Behavior	My learning goal and learning activities
Seeks learning opportunities	
Works independently; autonomous in practice	
Willing to work in an unstructured environment; tolerates ambiguity	
Seeks consultation and support	
Takes initiative; is a self-starter	
Adapts to change	
Is willing and able to respond to population needs	
Demonstrates flexibility	
Contributes to team efforts	
Prioritizes and organizes workload, time, materials, and resources	

3. How would you rate yourself on the following scale of foundational leadership behaviors?

   - Which foundational leadership behaviors do you always do?

   - Which foundational leadership behaviors do you need to develop or try to do more frequently?

   - How will these behaviors contribute to becoming a successful public health nursing leader?

Leadership Component	Always 3	Sometimes 2	Rarely 1
Seeks learning opportunities			
Works independently; autonomous in practice			
Willing to work in an unstructured environment; tolerates ambiguity			
Seeks consultation and support			
Takes initiative; is a self-starter			
Adapts to change			
Is willing and able to respond to population needs			
Demonstrates flexibility			
Contributes to team efforts			
Prioritizes and organizes workload, time, materials, and resources			

PUTTING IT ALL TOGETHER:
What It Means To Be a Public Health Nurse

By Marjorie A. Schaffer

14

This is the beginning of your story as a public health nurse (PHN). The chapters in this book have given you a foundation in the Henry Street Consortium entry-level population-based public health nursing competencies. These competencies emphasize the knowledge, skills, and attitudes needed to be an effective PHN. What are your next steps for developing your expertise in public health nursing?

What Do You Need to Know?

When PHNs and educators created the Henry Street Consortium competencies, they also generated a basic public health nursing knowledge base as a foundation for public health nursing practice. In smaller local health departments, PHNs need a broader knowledge base so that they are competent to provide services in many areas of public health. In larger public health agencies, PHNs might need more in-depth knowledge and expertise in specific areas of public health, such as following up on a population who has drug-resistant tuberculosis or working with schools and community agencies to prevent teen pregnancy. Keep in mind that PHNs also work in many organizations other than official public health agencies, such as in schools, in occupational health positions in corporations, and in non-profit organizations that value and need the expertise of PHNs. Following is a list of basic public health nursing knowledge areas for population-based practice.

- Antepartum/postpartum
- Chemical health issues and behaviors
- Chronic disease prevention and management
- Death and dying
- Disaster and bioterrorism response
- Disease prevention and control
- Environmental health and safety
- Family development

- Family planning

- Health determinants

- Health informatics

- Health promotion for all ages

- Human growth and development

- Human sexuality

- Immunizations across the lifespan

- Injury prevention

- Medication administration/management

- Mental health

- Nutrition

- Parenting

- Social and market justice

- Technical nursing skills

- Violence prevention

Many nursing students worry about being knowledgeable in medication administration and technical nursing skills as they seek their first employment as a nurse. Nurses new to public health nursing might feel similarly less prepared in public health knowledge areas that are essential to successful public health nursing practice. Look carefully at your position description to determine if you have an adequate knowledge base and skill set to perform the job responsibilities. Seek a mentor and establish a plan for strengthening your knowledge base and skill set.

ACTIVITY

Think about the basic knowledge base required for effective public health nursing practice.

Analyze your strengths in basic public health nursing knowledge.

What knowledge areas do you need to strengthen? Consider your intended area of practice. If you are in a new public health nursing position, analyze the knowledge base you need for effective public health nursing practice in your setting and focus area.

What strategies can you use to strengthen needed knowledge areas?

Who Do You Need to Be?

Henry Street Consortium members also identified personal characteristics that contribute to effective public health nursing practice. You can also consider the following characteristics as character virtues that can enhance your ability to be successful and committed to public health nursing.

- Adaptability
- Caring
- Compassion
- Confidence
- Courage
- Creativity
- Flexibility
- Hard work
- Humor

- Independence
- Leadership qualities
- Lifelong learning attitude
- Passion
- Persistence
- Positive attitude
- Resourcefulness
- Risk taking
- Self-care

ACTIVITY

Consider the following questions as you review the table of personal characteristics/virtues that enhance your public health nursing practice.

Why are these characteristics important for effective public health nursing practice?

Which of these characteristics have you observed in expert PHNs? Give a specific example of how you see the characteristic exemplified in the practice of the expert PHN.

How do you see these characteristics contributing to the accomplishment of the competencies (see Table 14.1 for competencies)?

How do you think your personal characteristics/virtues match with the kind of PHN you would like to be?

Table 14.1   Entry-Level Population-Based Public Health Nursing Competencies

1. Applies the public health nursing process to communities, systems, individuals, and families
2. Utilizes basic epidemiological principles (the incidence, distribution, and control of disease in a population) in public health nursing practice
3. Utilizes collaboration to achieve public health goals
4. Works within the responsibility and authority of the governmental public health system
5. Practices public health nursing within the auspices of the Nurse Practice Act
6. Effectively communicates with communities, systems, individuals, families, and colleagues

7. Establishes and maintains caring relationships with communities, systems, individuals, and families
8. Shows evidence of commitment to social justice, the greater good, and the public health principles
9. Demonstrates nonjudgmental and unconditional acceptance of people different from self
10. Incorporates mental, physical, emotional, social, spiritual, and environmental aspects of health into assessment, planning, implementation, and evaluation
11. Demonstrates leadership in public health nursing with communities, systems, individuals and families

What Can You Learn from the Stories of Public Health Nurses and Nursing Students?

You can learn about what PHNs do by reflecting on their stories from practice, which illustrate the competencies and many of the concepts and ideas presented in this book. The following stories represent public health nursing from the viewpoints of both students and practicing PHNs. The stories are evidence at Level V based on the Johns Hopkins Nursing Evidence-Based Practice Model presented Chapter 2. They are stories of experience from practice. The student stories represent the process and experiences encountered in becoming a PHN. The PHN stories represent expert practice in public health nursing and reflect the PHNs' commitment to the populations they serve.

Nursing Student Stories

As you reflect on the meaning of the stories, think about how you are learning to be a health nurse. Use the following questions to guide your reflection about the three student stories.

1. What competencies is the student working on developing?
2. Which public health interventions are being used by the student and preceptor in this story?
3. Which public health nursing Cornerstones are expressed by the student?
4. Which personal characteristics would it be helpful to have or develop to carry out this public health nursing practice example?

Student Story #1

School children comprise a population at high risk for infection and transmitting infectious organisms. In terms of epidemiology, the "chain of infection" is the process by which pathogens are transmitted from the environment to a host, invade the host, and cause infection. Breaking the chain of infection at any point prevents the spread of infection. Hand washing is the most effective mechanism to break the chain and prevent the spread of infection. Two of my classmates and I taught three sessions on hand washing to first graders. A curriculum and resource program had provided us with a hand-washing kit that consisted of a 3-minute video of a young boy explaining and demonstrating how to correctly wash one's hands to remove as many germs as possible, several bottles of "GloGerm Potion" that makes invisible germs glow a bright white under a black light, a black light, and a bunch of "Germbusters!" stickers.

As each session began, we did a few minutes' worth of very basic health teaching about how germs can cause illness, are everywhere, especially on our hands, and that by washing our hands well and often we can prevent spreading germs and stay healthy. After our short presentation we helped the children practice correct hand washing with the GloGerm product. This gave me a nice chance to do some one-on-one teaching and interaction with a few children who were somewhat timid or shy and see them respond positively and come out of their shell. The kids absolutely loved the presentation and our "magic potion!"

This experience shows growth in my ability to communicate effectively and work with others to complete a task. Good communication and organization were required between me and my classmates to work out our own teaching time to learn about the hand-washing kit, to pick up and return the kit, and to put together a good presentation. It was also necessary to communicate with first graders and to understand child development to teach health concepts at their developmental level and not speak over their heads. I believe any one of us could have done the job alone, but it was much more enjoyable to share the work and to be a part of a team than to do it alone. Being a team player is something I, a loner by nature, need to work on. I learned that I am likable and competent, work well with others and really enjoy it, and showed I am responsible for carrying my share of this clinical assignment. This teaching experience was FUN and also gave me more confidence in my nursing knowledge and teaching skills. In looking back, I see that I have become more spontaneous and flexible and can laugh more as I spend more time in real-world settings as opposed to the nursing lab or classroom. This experience of working with others and the necessity of good communication were most useful to me and will help me to continue improving in those areas. This teaching experience will serve as a positive example in times when I feel less than confident in my abilities.

Source: Competency Portfolio, Senior Nursing Student

Student Story #2

My preceptor and I went out to a home to carry out a developmental assessment on a two-year old suspected of being developmentally delayed. My preceptor had a very friendly, informal, yet professional demeanor, which I believe is a very beneficial and important asset to have and develop; she explained what the assessment consisted of and what actions would ensue following the assessment, as well as the other areas of specialty services that might be involved. During the assessment, my preceptor was very warm and casual, but one could see that she was observing our young client very carefully. She observed him in a way that was not distressing to the mother. After, my preceptor and I discussed the results and the process she uses when collecting and processing data within the realm of public health nursing. She stated that working within public health really exposes one in a community. For example, it is not uncommon to run into clients at the grocery store or in various other establishments around the area, and one has to face the questions, *"Do I say hello? Do I ask how things are going? Do they recognize me?"* I asked her how she deals with these simple, yet complex questions. She remarked that a nurse needs to be very sensitive and prepared for these issues, *"We are in their lives and homes and must be respectful."* She stated she leaves it up to the client to make the initial contact and allows them to lead the direction of the conversation. She also made it clear how important confidentiality is because at times a PHN visits one family member and the other members are unaware, so even confidentiality within families is instituted and is mandated by HIPAA.

I became more aware of the importance of having guidelines, such as the Nurse Practice Act to help us provide effective and competent care. My preceptor was an excellent example and resource that I can look back and reflect on when I begin my career as a nurse. The Nurse Practice Act encompasses nurses in all fields; however, the means by which it is carried out is customized to each specialty field. For example, independent nursing functions, in reference to public health nursing, differ from delegated medical functions nurses carry out in the hospitals. Independent functions consist of education, teaching, and providing information to clients and not doing skilled nursing care such as wound care or giving injections that would be done in the hospital. Also, boundaries are harder to manage in public health nursing than within the hospital. It is the client who "runs" the show and is in charge, not the nurse; one must be extra cautious when exchanging information in the field. I feel I will be more adequately prepared and aware of when and how to set boundaries and how to deal with a situation where I might not want to reveal as much to a client that they might want or expect.

Source: Competency Portfolio, Senior Nursing Student

Student Story #3

I worked with my preceptor in a breast and cervical cancer screening program. Part of the screening consisted of checking total (fasting) cholesterol and blood glucose levels. I did a finger stick to draw up a drop of blood into a little plastic case that fit into a machine that would give us the cholesterol and glucose results in about 5 minutes. After we had the results, I entered the data into a computer program created by the Centers for Disease Control and Prevention that analyzes and creates a bar graph and written description of the results that is very easy for the average non-medical person to understand and learn from. It also generates a "Diagnostic Referral" form if any test result is too high. This form can then be faxed to a health care provider immediately with no other data needing to be added. When I had printed out the report, I went over it in great detail with my client, asking her to stop me if she needed greater clarification or had any other questions. She was able to verbalize a general understanding of her results. The computer program had created a referral form for her to be evaluated by a physician because of high cholesterol, and she requested my preceptor to set up an appointment for her. My preceptor will follow up on the woman in 2 weeks to see if she has kept the doctor appointment and if she wants to be involved in the lifestyle interventions and counseling services that are also offered at the clinic.

I learned how to use new-to-me technology in both the blood testing and data entry experience, and I learned so much about the community resources available for this (my) age group. More important to my nursing practice was the review of cholesterol and glucose normal values and the opportunity to do some teaching with my client in which I had to use good communication and listening skills to facilitate her learning. I noticed afterward that I had picked up some of my preceptor's mannerisms in talking with clients—nonverbal communication skills such as leaning forward toward the client. I also learned that I often get in a rush when I'm talking about something I understand but the person I'm talking to doesn't, and that I need to slow down. I have become more aware of my interpersonal behaviors, and this will help make me a better nurse in the future.

Source: Competency Portfolio, Senior Nursing Student

Public Health Nurse Stories

As you read the expert PHNs' stories, use the following questions for reflection.

1. What are the specific activities that illustrate community and systems level interventions? Which Public Health Intervention Wheel interventions are being used by the PHN?

2. What makes the interventions program population-based?

3. What Cornerstones of Public Health Nursing are reflected in the PHN's story?

4. Which competencies are emphasized in the PHN story?

PHN Story #1

I work with pregnant and parenting teens at an alternative high school program that provides educational options for teens whose lives don't fit the traditional school day. Our program includes teens from a variety of cultures and backgrounds. The program currently has eight young women who will deliver their babies during the school year. This year we also have four young fathers enrolled. The program has an onsite child care center, so these students bring their children to school with them and can visit their children during the school day. Another PHN and I share this assignment. We teach weekly prenatal classes in conjunction with the life skills class that all our students are required to take for graduation. Each student spends time working in the child care rooms, both in their own child's room and the next age group's room. We have the opportunity to discuss growth and development and health care and to role-model parent-child interactions. We also work with each student to look at family planning options for him or her and are very proud of a program we started called "The Pregnancy Free Club." This is a voluntary "club" that allows each student to have private time with a PHN to talk about how to use birth control correctly and look at barriers that prevent the student from effectively using birth control. Peer support has also become an unexpected part of this program, making it easier and more acceptable for the students to talk about their birth control choice or their choice of abstinence. Our program currently has a repeat pregnancy rate significantly lower than the national average.

Source: Minnesota Department of Health. (2006). Wheel of public health interventions: A collection of "getting behind the wheel" stories, 2000–2006. Office of Public Health Practice, p. 19.

PHN Story #2

Most public health agencies face the reality of not having enough resources to meet the needs of clients. This can be a powerful impetus to working with other agencies, and the results achieved are often beyond those they would achieve on their own. Public health is working with a hospital in a rural area to provide lactation services to all new moms giving birth at the hospital. After establishing the goal of increasing breast-feeding rates, the local public health department approached maternity nurses at the hospital to partner with them in achieving this goal. The county agency had a PHN trained as a lactation consultant. Public health offered to provide hospital nurses with breast-feeding information and consultation knowing that the time immediately after birth is critical to successful initiation of breast-feeding. It also promoted consistent information being given to breast-feeding moms by the hospital and public health and provided a bridge between hospital and home for new moms. The program proved to be effective and gained support from physicians and hospital administrators. The moms were happy with the program and, therefore, it was a good marketing strategy for the hospital. It also provided a needed service to clients leading to increased breast-feeding rates. Currently the PHN who provides lactation consultation services has hospital privileges. She is scheduled 4 hours a week in the hospital and in that time she does rounds on new moms and is available for consultation with nurses. Because the service is located in the hospital, public health is receiving additional referrals for their universal home visiting program for new moms. The program is financially supported by both public health and the hospital.

Source: Minnesota Department of Health. (2006). Wheel of public health interventions: A collection of "getting behind the wheel" stories, 2000–2006. Office of Public Health Practice, p. 31.

PHN Story #3

A local newspaper reported that a statewide student health survey revealed their school district had one of the highest teen alcohol-use rates in the whole state. Numerous letters to the editor questioned why the community was not doing anything about the problem. Some viewed the report as an affront to the community's reputation (in the words of their city welcome sign) as a "great place to raise children." A demand was put out for community action.

A PHN from the public health agency partnered with other community groups and organizations to develop a plan to address alcohol use in the community. The plan included recommendations for enforcing existing laws (such as tightening sales of alcohol and enforcing "not a drop" laws with minors) and for developing acceptable (that is, "cool") alcohol-free activities for adolescents. The group's other major thrust was a decision to study assets and protective factors in adolescents to see if the community could find ways to develop assets in addition to preventing risk-taking behaviors. The representatives of each organization (including the PHN) were asked to take back this idea and get a commitment from their respective boards for the plan.

Source: Minnesota Department of Health. (2006). Wheel of public health interventions: A collection of "getting behind the wheel" stories, 2000–2006. Office of Public Health Practice, p. 31.

Reflections on Being a Public Health Nurse

We asked expert PHNs why they practice public health nursing and what they find rewarding in practice. Their comments capture the essence of what is important to PHNs and what inspires them to do their work. We hope that you connect with the meaning of what it means to be a PHN as you read and reflect on their words.

"Being a public health nurse is an honor and a privilege. You are constantly doing work important to the public 'common good.' You constantly give back each and every day. It is an amazing privilege to be allowed such an important place in others' lives." —Karen

"Being a public health nurse fits best with my philosophy—giving people the resources and supports they need to make good decisions that maximize their health, safety, and independence." —Chris

"Being a public health nurse includes looking beyond the obvious and looking for what is happening in the client situation that we do not yet know. Making genuine connections and building caring relationships undergirds public health. A public health nurse is both a nurse investigator and caregiver, blending holistic inquiry with thoughtful interventions that can make a real difference in people's everyday lives by impacting health and imparting hope." —Renee

"Public health nursing involves health care of an entire community. I personally thrive in a work environment where all aspects of nursing care might be required on any given day. A public health nurse needs to be flexible in her work day, since priorities can be continually changing." —BJ

"Public health nursing is rewarding when I help to improve the health of the community while assisting individuals to take action to optimize their own health." —Bruce

"I enjoy working with different cultures—learning about their traditions, beliefs, and how frequently there is a commonality to all people, regardless of what country they were born in or their economic status." —Mary

"I know that each family I visit will find their path a little easier and more focused because of me. As a public health nurse, I need to be flexible, nonjudgmental, caring, and empathetic, but also need to keep myself distanced enough to see the big picture and to help my clients look at options and goals for their health and their lives. I am a public health nurse because I want to make a difference." —Barb

"Being in the community is so rewarding—I work with people of all ages and backgrounds and establish partnerships to carry out the public health mission to reach those in need. Being a public health nurse means being a voice for prevention and early intervention, being a voice for making healthy choices, and being an advocate to help people to be healthy. For me, public health nursing is fulfilling, rewarding, challenging, and is my passion. It is a true calling and a blessing to be a public health nurse." —Bonnie

References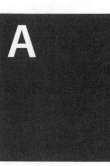

Introduction

Minnesota Department of Health (MDH), Division of Community Health Services, Public Health Nursing Section. (2001). *Public Health Interventions—Applications for Public Health Nursing Practice.* St. Paul, MN: Author. Retrieved June 29, 2010, from http://www.health.state.mn.us/divs/cfh/ophp/resources/docs/phinterventions_manual2001.pdf

Chapter 1

Abrams, S. (2004). From function to competency in public health nursing, 1931–2003. *Public Health Nursing, 21*(5), pp. 507–510.

American Nurses Association. (2007). *Public health nursing: Scope and standards of practice.* Silver Spring, MD: Nursesbooks.org

American Public Health Association, Public Health Nursing Section. (1996). Definition and role of public health nursing. Washington, D.C.: Author.

Clark, M. J. (2008). *Community health nursing.* Upper Saddle River, NJ: Pearson.

Core Public Health Functions Steering Committee. (1995). *Public health in America: Core functions and essential services of public health.* Adopted 1994. Retrieved June 12, 2010, from http://www.health.gov/phfunctions/public.htm

Dreher, M., Shapiro, D., & Asselin, M. (2006). *Healthy places, healthy people: A handbook for culturally competent community nursing practice.* Indianapolis, IN: Sigma Theta Tau International.

Friedman, M., Bowden, V., & Jones, E. (2003). *Family nursing: Research, theory, and practice* (5th ed.). Upper Saddle River, NJ: Prentice Hall.

Henry Street Consortium. (2003). Population-based public health nursing competencies. St. Paul, MN: Author. Retrieved 1/5/11 from http://www.health.state.mn.us/divs/cfh/ophp/consultation/phn/henrystreet/docs/core_competencies.pdf

Institute of Medicine. (1988). *The future of public health.* Washington, DC: National Academy Press.

Keller, L. O., Strohschein, S., & Schaffer, M. A. (in press). The cornerstones of public health nursing. *Public Health Nursing.*

Marmot, M. & Wilkinson, R. G. (1999). *Social determinants of health.* Oxford: Oxford University Press.

Minnesota Department of Health, Public Health Nursing Section. (2000). *Public health nursing practice for the 21st century: Competency development in population-based practice.* St. Paul, MN: Author. Retrieved June 12, 2010, from http://www.health.state.mn.us/divs/cfh/ophp/resources/docs/21stcentury-satellite-learning-guide.pdf

Minnesota Department of Health, Division of Community Health Services, Public Health Nursing Section. (2001). *Public health interventions: Applications for public health nursing practice.* St. Paul, MN: Author. Retrieved June 29, 2010, from http://www.health.state.mn.us/divs/cfh/ophp/resources/docs/phinterventions_manual2001.pdf

Minnesota Department of Health, Center for Public Health Nursing. (2003). Definition of population-based practice. Retrieved June 12, 2010, from http://www.health.state.mn.us/divs/cfh/ophp/resources/docs/population-based-practice_definition.pdf

Minnesota Department of Health, Center for Public Health Nursing. (2007). Cornerstones of Public Health Nursing. Adapted from Original by Center for Public Health Nursing, 2004. St. Paul: Author. Retrieved June 12, 2010,from http://www.health.state.mn.us/divs/cfh/ophp/resources/docs/cornerstones_definition_revised2007.pdf

Public Health Agency of Canada. (2002). Population health: What determines health? Retrieved March 4, 2010, from http://www.phac-aspc.gc.ca/ph-sp/determinants/index.html

Quad Council of Public Health Nursing Organizations. (2004). Public health nursing competencies. *Public Health Nursing, 21*(5), pp. 443–452.

Schaffer, M. A., Cross, S., Olson, L. O., Nelson, P., Schoon, P. M., & Henton, P. (2010). The Henry Street Consortium population-based competencies for educating public health nursing students. *Public Health Nursing, 28*(1), 78-90.

Stanhope, M. & Lancaster, J. (2008). *Public health nursing: Population-centered health care in the community* (7th ed.). St. Louis, MO: Mosby, Inc.

U.S. Department of Health and Human Services. (2000). *Healthy people 2010. A systematic approach to health improvement.* Retrieved June 12, 2010, from http://www.healthypeople.gov/Document/html/uih/uih_bw/uih_2.htm

U.S. Department of Health and Human Services. (2010). *Public health functions project. Public health in America statement.* Retrieved June 12, 2010, from http://www.health.gov/phfunctions

Zahner, S. J. & Block, D. E. (2006). The road to population health: Using Healthy People 2010 in nursing education. *Journal of Nursing Education, 45*(3), pp. 105–108.

Chapter 2

American Nurses Association. (2007). *Public health nursing: Scope and standards of practice.* Silver Spring, MD: Nursesbooks.org

Armstrong, K. L., Fraser, J. A., Dadds, M. R., & Morris J. (1999). A randomized, controlled trial of nurse home visiting to vulnerable families with newborns. *Journal of Paediatrics and Child Health, 35*(3), pp. 237–244.

Atkins, R. B., Williams, J. R., Silenas R., & Edwards, J. C. (2005). The role of PHNs in bioterrorism preparedness. *Disaster Management Response, 3*(4), pp. 98–105.

Brownson, R. C., Baker, E. A., Leet, T. L., & Gillespie, K. N. (Eds.) (2002). *Evidence-based public health.* New York, NY: Oxford University Press.

Corrarino, J. E. (2000). *Lessons learned: Successful strategies to implement a perinatal hepatitis B program.* Centers for Disease Control and Prevention Annual Hepatitis B Conference. San Diego, CA.

Corrarino, J. E., & Little, A. (2006). *Breathing easy: A public health nursing/community coalition success story.* American Public Health Association 128th Annual Meeting. Boston, MA.

Corrarino, J. E., Walsh, P. J., & Nadel, E. (2001). Does teaching scald burn prevention to families of young children make a difference? A pilot study. *Journal of Pediatric Nursing, 16*(4), pp. 256–62.

Corrarino, J. E., Williams, C., Campbell, W. S., 3rd, Amrhein, E., LoPiano, L., & Kalachik, D. (2000). Linking substance-abusing pregnant women to drug treatment services: A pilot program. *Journal of Obstetric, Gynecologic, and Neonatal Nurses, 29*(4), pp. 369–376.

Eckenrode, J., Ganzel, B., Henderson, C. R., Jr., Smith, E., Olds, D. L., Powers, J., Cole, R., Kitzman, H., & Sidora, K. (2000). Preventing child abuse and neglect with a program of nurse home visitation: The limiting effects of domestic violence. *Journal of the American Medical Association, 284*(11), pp. 1385–1391.

Fetrick, A., Christensen, M., & Mitchell, C. (2003). Does public health nurse home visitation make a difference in the health outcomes of pregnant clients and their offspring? *Public Health Nursing, 20*(3), pp. 184–189.

Fineout-Overholt, E., Melnyk, B. M., Stillwell, S., & Williamson, K. (2010). Critical appraisal of the evidence: Part I. *American Journal of Nursing, 110*(7), pp. 47–52.

Gupta, J. (2006). A model for interdisciplinary service-learning experience for social change. *Journal of Physical Therapy Education, 20*(3), pp. 55–60.

Institute of Medicine. (2004). *Academic health centers: Leading change in the 21st century.* National Academy of Sciences. National Academies Press. http://www.nap.edu/catalog/10734.html

Izzo, C. V., Eckenrode, J. J., Smith, E. G., Henderson, C. R., Cole, R., Kitzman, H., & Olds, D. L. (2005). Reducing the impact of uncontrollable stressful life events through a program of nurse home visitation for new parents. *Prevention Science, 6*(4), pp. 269–274.

Kearney, M. H., York, R., & Deatrick, J. A. (2000). Effects of home visits to vulnerable young families. *Journal of Nursing Scholarship, 32*(4), pp. 369–376.

Keller, L., Strohschein, S., Lia-Hoagberg, B., & Schaffer, M. (1998). Population-based public health nursing interventions: A model for practice. *Public Health Nursing, 15*(3), pp. 207–215.

Keller, L., Strohschein, S., Lia-Hoagberg, B., & Schaffer, M. (2004). Population-based public health interventions: Practice-based and evidence-supported. *Public Health Nursing, 21*(5), pp. 453–468.

Keller, L. & Strohschein, S. (2009). E$_2$ evidence exchange: Your public health nursing e-source. Public Health Nursing Faculty Conference, Otsego, MN, April 21, 2009.

MacNeil, J., Lobato, M., & Moore, M. (2005). An unanswered health disparity: Tuberculosis among correctional inmates, 1993 through 2003. *American Journal of Public Health, 95*(10), pp. 1800–1805.

Margolis, P. A., Lannon, C. M., Stevens, R., Harlan, C., Bordley, W. C., Carey, T., … Earp, J. L. (1996). Linking clinical and public health approaches to improve access to health care for socially disadvantaged mothers and children. A feasibility study. *Archives of Pediatric Adolescent Medicine, 150*(8), pp. 815–821.

Martin, K. S. (2005). *The Omaha System: A key to practice, documentation, and information management* (Reprinted 2nd ed.). Omaha, NE: Health Connections Press.

Melnyk, B. M. & Fineout-Overholt, E. (Eds.) (2005). *Evidence-based practice in nursing and healthcare: A guide to best practice* (1st ed.). Philadelphia: Lippincott Williams and Wilkins.

Milbank Memorial Fund. (1998). Partners in community health: Working together for a healthy New York. Milbank Memorial Fund.

Minnesota Department of Health, Center for Public Health Nursing. (2001). Public health interventions. St. Paul: Author. Retrieved June 12, 2010, from http://www.health.state.mn.us/divs/cfh/ophp/resources/docs/wheelbw.pdf

Minnesota Department of Health, Center for Public Health Nursing. (2003). The nursing process applied to population-based public health nursing practice. . St. Paul, MN: Author. Retrieved June 12, 2010, from http://www.health.state.mn.us/divs/cfh/ophp/resources/docs/nursing_process.pdf

Monsen, K. & Keller, L. O. (2002). A population-based approach to pediculosis management. *Public Health Nursing, 19*(3), pp. 201–208.

Newhouse, R. P., Dearholt, S. L., Poe, S. P., Pugh, L. C., & White, K. M. (2007). *Johns Hopkins evidence-based practice model and guidelines.* Indianapolis, IN: Sigma Theta Tau International.

Olds, D. L., Kitzman, H., Cole, R., Robinson, J., Sidora, K., Luckey, D. W., … Holmberg, J. (2004). Effects of nurse home-visiting on maternal life course and child development: Age 6 follow-up results of a randomized trial. *Pediatrics, 114*(6), pp. 1550–1559.

Olds, D., Kitzman, H., Hanks, C., Cole, R., Anson, E., Sidora-Arcoleo, K., … Bondy, J. (2007). Effects of nurse home visiting on maternal and child functioning: Age-9 follow-up of a randomized trial. *Pediatrics, 120*, pp. e832-e845, 2006-2111.

Olds, D. L., Robinson, J., O'Brien, R., Luckey, D. W., Pettitt, L. M., Henderson, C. R., Jr., … Talmi, A. (2002). Home visiting by paraprofessionals and by nurses: A randomized, controlled trial. *Pediatrics, 110*(3), pp. 486–496.

Olds, D. L., Robinson, J., Pettitt, L., Luckey, D. W., Holmberg, J., Ng R. K., … Henderson, C. R., Jr. (2004). Effects of home visits by paraprofessionals and by nurses: Age 4 follow-up results of a randomized trial. *Pediatrics, 114* (6), pp. 1560–1568.

Padget, S. M., Bekemeirer, B., & Berkowitz, B. (2004). Collaborative partnerships at the state level: Promoting systems changes in public health infrastructure. *Journal of Public Health Management Practice, 10*(3), pp. 251–257.

Quad Council of Public Health Nursing Organizations. (2007). The public health nursing shortage: A threat to the public's health. Endorsed by the Quad Council of Public Health Nursing Organizations, American Nurses Association, Congress on Nursing Practice & Economics, February 2007.

Stillwell, S. B., Fineout-Overholt, E., Melnyk, B. M., & Williamson, K. M. (2010). Evidence-based practice: Step by step. *American Journal of Nursing, 110*(5), pp. 41–47.

Tembreull, C. & Schaffer, M. (2005). The intervention of outreach: Best practices. *Public Health Nursing 22*(4), pp. 347–353.

Yousey, Y., Leake, J., Wdowik, M., & Janken, J. (2007). Education in a homeless shelter to improve the nutrition of young children. *Public Health Nursing, 24*(3), pp. 249–255.

Chapter 3

Abrams, S. E. (2008). The best of public health nursing, circa 1941. *Public Health Nursing, 25*(3), pp. 285–191.

Ailinger, R. L., Molloy, S. B., & Sacasa, E. R. (2009). Community health nursing student experience in Nicaragua. *Journal of Community Health Nursing, 26*, pp. 47-53.

Alkon, A., To, K., Mackie, J. F., Wolff, M., & Bernzweig, J. (2010). Health and safety needs in early care and education programs: What do directors, child health records, and national standards tell us? *Public Health Nursing, 27*(1), pp. 3–16.

Averill, J. (2003). Keys to the puzzle: Recognizing strengths in a rural community. *Public Health Nursing, 20*(6), pp. 449-455.

Centers for Disease Control and Prevention. (2010a). Definition of public health informatics. National Center for Public Health Informatics. Retrieved December 26, 2010, from http://www.cdc.gov/ncphi/about.html

Centers for Disease Control and Prevention. (2010b). CDC's Advisory Committee on Immunization Practices (ACIP) recommends universal annual influenza vaccination. CDC Online Newsroom, February 24, 2010. Retrieved December 30, 2010 from http://www.cdc.gov/media/pressrel/2010/r100224.htm

Clark, M. J. (2008). *Community health nursing.* Upper Saddle River, NJ: Pearson/Prentice Hall.

Cross, S. (2010). Public health teen parent program. *Unpublished, personal communication,* December 5, 2010.

Eide, P .J., Hahn, L., Bayne, T., Allen, C. B., & Swain, D. (2006). The population-focused analysis project for teaching community health. *Nursing Education Perspectives, 27*(1), pp. 22-27.

Eriksson, I. & Nilsson, K. (2008). Preconditions needed for establishing a trusting relationship during health counseling—An interview study. *Journal of Clinical Nursing, 17*(17), pp. 2352–2359.

Gardner, A. (2010). Therapeutic friendliness and the development of therapeutic leverage by mental health nurses in community rehabilitation settings. *Contemporary Nurse, 34*(2), pp. 140–148.

Jansson, A., Petersson, K., & Uden, G. (2001). Nurses' first encounters with parents of new-born children – public health nurses' views of a good meeting. *Journal of Clinical Nursing, 10*, pp. 140-151.

Keller, L. O., Strohschein, S., Lia-Hoagberg, B., & Schaffer, M. A. (2004). Population-based public health interventions. *Public Health Nursing, 21*(5), pp. 453–468.

Kleinfehn-Wald, N. (2010). Determining population needs in a rural/suburban county. *Unpublished, per-*

sonal communication, December 5, 2010.

Lanigan, C. (2010). In-home influenza immunizations. *Unpublished, personal communication,* December 1, 2010.

Mansfield, R. & Meyer, C. L. (2007). Making a difference with combined community assessment and change projects. *Journal of Nursing Education, 46*(3), pp. 132-134.

Martin, K. S. (2005). *The Omaha System: A key to practice, documentation, and information management* (Reprinted 2nd ed.). Omaha, NE: Health Connections Press.

Martin K. S., Monsen K. A., & Bowles K. H. (2011). The Omaha System and meaningful use: Applications for practice, education, and research. *CIN: Computers, Informatics, Nursing, 29*(1), pp. 52–58.

McCann, T. V. & Baker, H. (2001). Mutual relating: Developing interpersonal relationships in the community. *Journal of Advanced Nursing, 34*(4), pp. 530–537.

McNaughton, D. B. (2005). A naturalistic test of Peplau's theory in home visiting. *Public Health Nursing, 22*(5), pp. 429–438.

Meagher-Stewart, D., Edwards, N., Aston, M., & Young, L. (2009). Population health surveillance practice of public health nurses. *Public Health Nursing, 26*(6), pp. 553–560.

Minnesota Department of Health. (2001). Public health interventions—Application for public health nursing practice. St. Paul, MN: Author.

Minnesota Department of Health, Center for Public Health Nursing Practice. (2003). The nursing process applied to population-based public health nursing practice. Retrieved December 1, 2010, from http://www.health.state.mn.us/divs/cfh/ophp/resources/docs/nursing_process.pdf

Minnesota Department of Health, Office of Public Health Practice. (2006). A collection of "Getting Behind the Wheel Stories" 2000–2006. Retrieved December 20, 2010, from http://www.health.state.mn.us/divs/cfh/ophp/resources/docs/wheelbook2006.pdf

Monsen, K. A., Fitzsimmons, L. L., Lescenski, B. A., Lytton, A. B., Schwichtenberg, L. D., & Martin, K. S. (2006). A public health nursing informatics data-and-practice quality project. *CIN: Computers, Informatics, Nursing, 24*(3), pp. 152–158.

Monsen, K. A., Fulkerson, J. A., Lytton, A. B., Taft, L. L., Schwichtenberg, L. D., & Martin, K. S. (2010). Comparing maternal child health problems and outcomes across public health nursing agencies. *Maternal and Child Health Journal, 14*(3), pp. 412–421.

Omaha System. (2010). Omaha System web site. Retrieved December 6, 2010, from http://www.omaha-system.org

Otterness, N., Gehrke, P., & Sener, I. M. (2007). Partnerships between nursing education and faith communities: Benefits and challenges. *Journal of Nursing Education,* 46(1), pp. 39-44.

Racher, F. (2007). The evolution of ethics for community practice. *Journal of Community Health Nursing, 24*(1), pp. 65-76.

Reinberg, S. (2010). U.S. government sets new health goals for 2020. HealthDay. December 2, 2010. Retrieved December 4, 2010, from http://consumer.healthday.com/Article.asp?AID=646932

Schaffer, M. A., Jost, R., Peterson, B. J., & Lair, M. (2008). Pregnancy-free club: A strategy to prevent repeat adolescent pregnancy. *Public Health Nursing, 25*(4), pp. 304–311.

Schoon, P. (2010). Elementary school health assessment. *Unpublished, personal correspondence,* December 16, 2010.

Scroggins, L. M. (2008). The developmental processes for NANDA international nursing diagnoses. *International Journal of Nursing Terminologies and Classifications, 19*(2), pp. 57-64.

Truglio-Londrigan, M. & Lewenson, S. B. (2011). *Public health nursing: Practicing population-based care.* Sudbury, MA: Jones and Bartlett Publishers.

United States Department of Health and Human Services. (2000). *Healthy people 2010.* (2nd ed.). With *Understanding and improving health* and *Objectives for improving health.* (2 vols.). Washington, DC: U.S. Government Printing Office.

United States Department of Health and Human Services. (2010). Getting to Know Healthy People 2020. HealthyPeople.gov website. Retrieved December 28, 2010, from http://www.healthypeople.gov

Vance, E. A. & Fish, C. A. (2010). Omaha System case study. *Unpublished.* Personal correspondence from Karen S. Martin, Martin Associates, Omaha, NE. December 2, 2010.

Volbrecht, R. M. (2002). *Nursing ethics—Communities in dialogue.* Upper Saddle River, NJ: Pearson/ Prentice Hall.

Wilde, M. H., Albanese, E. P., Rennells, R., & Bullock, Q. (2004). Development of a student nurses' clinic for homeless men. *Public Health Nursing, 21*(4), pp. 354-360.

Chapter 4

Alfred, R. (2009). Sept. 8, 1854: Pump shutdown stops London cholera outbreak. Retrieved November 25, 2010, from http://www.wired.com/thisdayintech/2009/09/0908london-cholera-pump/

Aschengrau, A. & Seage, G. R. (2008). *Essentials of epidemiology in public health* (2nd ed.). Sudbury, Massachusetts: Jones and Bartlett Publishers.

Bigbee, J. L., Gehrke, P., & Otterness, N. (2009). Public health nurses in rural/frontier one-nurse offices. *Rural and Remote Health, 9*(4), pp. 1–12.

Centers for Disease Control and Prevention (CDC). (2010). Reported cases of Lyme disease—United States, 2009. Retrieved November 25, 2010, from http://www.cdc.gov/ncidod/dvbid/lyme/ld_Incidence.htm

Clark, M. J. (2003). *Community health nursing* (4th ed.). Upper Saddle River, NJ: Prentice Hall.

Earl, C. (2009). Medical history and epidemiology: Their contribution to the development of public health nursing. *Nursing Outlook, 57*(5), pp. 257–265.

Friis, R. H. & Sellers, T. A. (1999). *Epidemiology for public health practice* (2nd ed.). Gaithersburg, MD: Aspen.

Halfon, N. & Hochstein, M. (2002). Life course health development: An integrated framework for developing health, policy, and research. *Milbank Quarterly, 80*(3), pp. 433–479.

Klopf, L. (1998). Tuberculosis control in the New York State Department of Correctional Services: A case management approach. *American Journal of Infection Control, 26*(5), pp. 534–538.

Krieger, N. (1997). Epidemiology and the web of causation: Has anyone seen the spider? *Social Science and Medicine, 39*(7), pp. 887–903.

Krieger, N. (2001a). A glossary for social epidemiology. *Journal of Epidemiology and Community Health, 55*(10), pp. 693–700.

Krieger, N. (2001b). Theories for social epidemiology in the 21st century: An ecosocial perspective. *International Journal of Epidemiology, 30*(4), pp. 668–677.

Kuh, D., Ben-Shlomo, Y., Lynch, J., Hallqvist, J., & Power, C. (2003). Life course epidemiology. *Journal of Epidemiology and Community Health, 57*(10), pp. 778–783.

Le, C. T. (2001). *Health & numbers: A problem-based introduction to biostatistics* (2nd ed.). New York, NY: Wiley-Liss.

Lind, C. & Smith, D. (2008). Analyzing the state of community health nursing: Advancing from deficit to strengths-based practice using appreciative inquiry. *Advances in Nursing Science, 31*(1), pp. 28–41.

Lu, M. C. (2010). We can do better: Improving perinatal health in America. *Journal of Women's Health, 19*(3), pp. 569–574.

Merrill, R. M. & Timmreck, T. C. (2006). *Introduction to epidemiology* (4th ed.). Sudbury, MA: Jones and Bartlett Publishers.

Minnesota Department of Health (MDH). (2010). Reported cases of Lyme disease in Minnesota by year, 1986–2008. Retrieved November 25, 2010, from http://www.health.state.mn.us/divs/idepc/diseases/lyme/casesyear.html

Missouri Department of Health and Senior Services (MDHSS). (2010). Geographic Information Systems (GIS) and maps. Retrieved November 25, 2010, from http://www.dhss.mo.gov/GIS/

Pew Hispanic Center. (2006). Population pyramids by ethnicity, 2005. Cited in Hakimzadeh, S. (2006). 41.9 million and counting: A statistical view of Hispanics at mid-decade. Retrieved December 4, 2010, from http://pewresearch.org/pubs/251/419-million-and-counting

Reifsnider, E. (1995). The use of human ecology and epidemiology in nonorganic failure to thrive. *Public Health Nursing, 12*(4), pp. 262–268.

Richter, M. (2010). It does take two to tango! On the need for theory in research on the social determinants of health. *International Journal of Public Health, 55*, 457-458.

Stein, Z., Susser, M., Saenger, G., & Marolla, F. (1975). *Famine and human development: The Dutch hunger winter of 1944–45*. New York: Oxford University Press.

University of California, Los Angeles (UCLA). (2010). John Snow. Retrieved November 25, 2010, from http://www.ph.ucla.edu/epi/snow.html

Valanis, B. (1999). *Epidemiology in health care* (3rd ed.). Stamford, CT: Appleton & Lange.

Chapter 5

Ahern, M. M. & Hendryx, M. S. (2005). Social capital and risk for chronic illnesses. *Chronic Illness, 1*(3), pp. 183–90.

American Nurses Association. (2007). *Scope and standards of public health nursing practice.* Washington D.C: Author.

Aponte, J. & Nickitas, D. M. (2007). Community as client: Reaching an underserved urban community and meeting unmet primary healthcare needs. *Journal of Community Health Nursing, 24*(3), pp. 177–190.

Aronson, R. E., Wallis, A. B., O'Campo, P. J., & Schafer, P. (2007). Neighborhood mapping and evaluation: A methodology for participatory community health initiatives. *Maternal Child Health Journal, 11*(4), pp. 373–383.

Aston, M., Meagher-Stewart, D., Edwards, N., & Young, L. M. (2009). Public health nurses' primary health care practice: Strategies for fostering citizen participation. *Journal of Community Health Nursing, 26*, pp. 24–34.

Baker, I. R., Dennison, B. A., Boyer, P. S., Sellers, K. F., Russo, T. J., & Sherwood, N. A. (2007). An asset-based community initiative to reduce television viewing in New York state. *Preventive Medicine, 44*(5), pp. 437–441.

Bazarman, M. H. (Ed.) (2005). *Negotiating, decision making and conflict management.* Cheltenam, UK: Edward Elgar Publishing United.

Berger, P. L. & Neuhaus, R. J. (1977). *To empower people: The role of mediating structures in public policy.* Washington D.C.: American Enterprise Institute for Public Policy Research.

Brosnan, C. A., Upchurch, S. L., Meininger, J. C., Hester, L. E., Johnson, G., & Eissa, M. A. (2005). Student nurses participate in public health research and practice through a school-based screening program. *Public Health Nursing, 22*(3), pp. 260–266.

Burtman, B. (2010). The revolution will be mapped. *Miller-McCune.* Retrieved January 28, 2011 from http://www.miller-mccune.com/culture-society/the-revolution-will-be-mapped-7130/

Chaudry, R. V., Polivkia, B. J., & Kennedy, C. W. (2000). Public health nursing director's perceptions regarding interagency collaboration with community mental health agencies. *Public Health Nursing, 17*(2), pp. 75–84.

Clatworthy, W. (1999). Community care: Collaborative working. *Journal of Community Nursing, 13*(4), p. 4.

Community Tool Box. (2009). Identifying community assets and resources. University of Kansas: Work Group for Community Health and Development. Retrieved December 26, 2009, from http://ctb.ku.edu/en/tablecontents/sub_section_main_1043.htm

Crist, J. D. & Escandon-Dominguez, S. (2003). Identifying and recruiting Mexican American partners and sustaining community partnerships. *Journal of Transcultural Nursing, 14*(3), pp. 266–271.

Fawcett, S. B., Francisco, V. T., Paine-Andrews, A., & Schultz, J. A. (2000). A model memorandum of collaboration: A proposal. *Public Health Reports, 155*(2-3), pp. 174–90.

Findley, S. A., Irigoyen, M., See, D., Sanchez, M., Chen, S., Sternfels, P., & Caesar, A. (2003). Community-provider partnerships reduce immunization disparities: Field report from northern Manhattan. *American Journal of Public Health, 93*(7), pp. 1041–1044.

Foss, G. F., Bonaiuto, M. M., Johnson, Z. S., & Moreland, D. M. (2003). Using Polivka's model to create a service-learning partnership. *Journal of School Health, 73*(8), pp. 305–310.

Franklin, L., Exline, J., & Stringer, K. (2002). Using coalition and community-based partnerships to improve immunization rates in Mississippi: A case study. *Texas Journal of Rural Health, 20*(3), pp. 31–37.

Gamm, L. D. (1998). Advancing community health through community health partnerships. *Journal of Healthcare Management, 43*(1), pp. 51–67.

Hendryx, M. S., Ahern, M. M., Lourich, N. P., & McCurdy, A. H. (2002). Access to health care and community social capital. *Health Services Research, 37*(1), pp. 87–103.

Henneman, E. A., Lee, J. L., & Cohen, J. I. (1995). Collaboration: A concept analysis. *Journal of Advanced Nursing, 21*(1), pp. 103–109.

Institute for Clinical and Translational Science. (2009). The 9 principles of the community-based participatory research model. University of Iowa. Retrieved February 6, 2010, from http://icts.uiowa.edu/content/9-principles-community-based-participatory-research-model

Israel, B. A., Eng, E., Schulz, A. J., & Parker, E. A. (Eds.) (2005). *Methods for community-based participatory research for health.* San Francisco, CA: Jossey-Bass.

Kang, R. (1995). Building community capacity for health promotion: A challenge for public health nurses. *Public Health Nursing, 12*(5), pp. 312–318.

Keller, L. O., Strohschein, S., Lia-Hoagberg, B., & Schaffer, M. A. (2004). Population-based public health interventions: Practice-based and evidence supported. Part 1. *Public Health Nursing, 21*(5), pp. 453–468.

Kenny, G. (2002). Children's nursing and interprofessional collaboration: Challenges and opportunities. *Journal of Clinical Nursing, 11*(3), pp. 306-313.

Kreulen, G. J., Bednarz, P. K., Wehrwein, T., & Davis, J. (2008). Clinical education partnership: A model for school district and college of nursing collaboration. *The Journal of School Nursing, 24*(6), pp. 360–369.

Lindsey, E., Sheilds, L., & Stajduhar, K. (1999). Creating effective nursing partnerships: Relating community development to participatory action research. *Journal of Advanced Nursing, 29*(1), pp. 1238–1245.

Looman, W. S. & Lindeke, L. L. (2005). Health and social context: Social capital's utility as a construct for nursing and health promotion. *Journal of Pediatric Health Care, 19*(2), pp. 90–94.

McNeill, L. H., Kreuter, M. W., & Subramanian, S. V. (2006). Social environment and physical activity: A review of concepts and evidence. *Social Science & Medicine, 63*(4),pp. 1011-22 .

Michael, Y. L., Farquhar, S. A., Wiggins, N., & Green, M. K. (2008). Findings from a community-based participatory prevention research intervention designed to increase social capital in Latino and African-American communities. *Journal of Immigrant & Minority Health, 10*(3), pp. 281–289.

Potter, P. A. & Perry, A. (2009). *Fundamentals of nursing.* St. Louis, MO: Mosby Elsevier.

Savage, C. L., Xu, Y., Lee, R., Rose, B. L., Kappesser, M., & Anthony, J. S. (2006). A case study in the use of community-based participatory research in public health nursing. *Public Health Nursing, 23*(5), pp. 472–478.

Schaffer, M. A. (2009). A virtue ethics guide to best practices for community-based participatory research. *Progress in Community Health Partnerships: Research, Education, and Action, 3*(1), pp. 83–90. Retrieved December 27, 2009, from http://www.press.jhu.edu/journals/progress_in_community_health_partnerships/

Seifer, S. D. & Connors, K. (Eds). (2007). Faculty toolkit for service-learning in higher education. Community-Campus Partnership for Health, Learn and Serve America's National Service-Learning Clearinghouse. Retrieved December 26, 2009, from http://www.servicelearning.org/filemanager/download/HE_toolkit_with_worksheets.pdf

Skybo, T. & Polivka, B. (2006). Health promotion model for childhood violence prevention. *Journal of Clinical Nursing, 16*, pp. 38-45.

Timmerman, G. M. (2007). Addressing barriers to health promotion in underserved women. *Family & Community Health, Supplement, 30*(15), pp. S34–S42.

Tuckman, B. W. (1965). Development sequences in small groups. *Psychology Bulletin, 63*(6), pp. 384–399.

Williams-Barnard, C., Sweatt, A., Harkness, G., & DiNapoli, P. (2004). The clinical home community: A model for community-based education. *International Nursing Review, 51*(2), pp. 104–112.

Chapter 6

2009-2010 H1N1 Flu Pandemic: Dakota county's response. (April 16, 2010). Working draft.

American Lung Association. (2010). About OAS. Retrieved December 28, 2010 from http://www.lungusa.org/lung-disease/asthma/in-schools/open-airways/about-oas.html

American Nurses Association. (2007). *Public health nursing: Scope and standards of practice.* Silver Spring, MD: Author.

Carter, K. F., Kaiser, K. L., O'Hare, P. A., & Callister, L. C. (2006). Use of PHN competencies and ACHNE essentials to develop teaching-learning strategies for generalist C/PHN curricula. *Public Health Nursing, 23*(2), pp. 146–160.

Encyclopedia of Everyday Law: Child Abuse/Child Safety/Child Discipline. (2010). Retrieved December 28, 2010 from http://www.enotes.com/everyday-law-encyclopedia/child-abuse-child-safety-discipline#history

Horlich, G., Shaw, F. E., Gorji, M., & Fishbein, D. B. (2008). Delivering new vaccines to adolescents: The role of school-entry laws. *Pediatrics, 121*, pp. S79–S84.

Keller, L. O. & Litt, E. A. (2008). *Report on public health nurse to population ratio.* Association of State and Territorial Directors of Nursing (ASTDN).

Land, M. & Barclay, L. (2008). Nurses' contribution to child protection. *Neonatal, Paediatric and Child Health Nursing, 11*(10), pp. 18–24

Lanigan, C. (2010). Director of QI and Analysis for Family Health, Minneapolis Visiting Nurse Agency. *Unpublished, personal communication,* October 18, 2010.

Minnesota Department of Health. (2003a). *Communicable disease reporting and HIPAA. Immunization sharing and HIPAA.* Retrieved December 28, 2010 from http://www.health.state.mn.us/divs/idepc/dtopics/reportable/rule/hipaacomm.html.

Minnesota Department of Health. (2003b). *Immunization sharing and HIPAA.* Retrieved December 28, 2010 from http://www.health.state.mn.us/divs/idepc/immunize/hippadata.html

Minnesota Department of Health. (2005a). Isolation and quarantine procedures. Retrieved December 28, 2010 from http://www.health.state.mn.us/divs/opa/isolation05.pdf

Minnesota Department of Health. (2005b). *Communicable disease rule, Chapter 4605.* Retrieved December 28, 2010 from http://www.health.state.mn.us/divs/idepc/dtopics/reportable/rule/rule.html

Minnesota Department of Health. (2008). *Minnesota responds medical reserve corps volunteer protections.* Minnesota Department of Health fact sheet. Retrieved December 28, 2010 from http://www.health.state.mn.us/divs/opa/mrcfs08.pdf

Minnesota Department of Health (2009b). *Community health assessment and action planning (CHAAP): 2005–2009, Introduction & handbook.* Office of Public Health Practice. Retrieved December 28, 2010 from http://www.health.state.mn.us/divs/cfh/ophp/system/planning/chaap/index.html

Minnesota Department of Health. (2009a). *Department of health local public health act overview.* Retrieved December 28, 2010 from http://www.health.state.mn.us/divs/cfh/ophp/resources/docs/factsheetlphactivities-2009.pdf

Minnesota Department of Health State Community Health Services Advisory Committee (1992). *Controlling public health nuisances: A guide for community health boards.* Retrieved December 28, 2010 from http://www.health.state.mn.us/divs/eh/local/CHBoardGuide1992.pdf

Minnesota Rulemaking Manual. (2009). *Chapter 3 - Rule Development.* Retrieved December 28, 2010 from http://www.health.state.mn.us/rules/manual/03rl-dev.doc

Minnesota Statutes. (2005). *Section 144.419. Isolation and quarantine of persons.* Retrieved December 28, 2010 from http://www.revisor.leg.state.mn.us/data/revisor/statutes/2005/144/419.html

Minnesota Statutes 145A.03–145A.10. (2009). Minnesota Office of the Revisor of Statutes. Retrieved December 28, 2010 from https://www.revisor.mn.gov/statutes/?year=2009&id=145A

National Alliance on Mental Illness. (2006). *Understanding the civil commitment process.* Retrieved December 28, 2010 from http://nami.beardog.net/AdvHTML_Upload/CivilCommitment.pdf

National Association of County and City Health Officials (NACCHO). (2008a). *Fast facts: 2008 national profile of local health departments.* Retrieved December 28, 2010 from http://www.naccho.org/topics/infrastructure/profile/resources/2008report/index.cfm

National Association of County and City Health Officials (NACCHO). (2008b). *Medical reserve corps.* Retrieved December 28, 2010 from http://www.naccho.org/topics/emergency/MRC/index.cfm

National Association of County and City Health Officials (NACCHO). (2010). *Public health law.* Retrieved December 28, 2010 from http://www.naccho.org/topics/infrastructure/PHLaw/index.cfm

Pozgar, G. D. (2005). *Legal and ethical issues for health professionals.* Sudbury, MA: Jones and Bartlett Publishers.

Schwartz, M. B. & Brownell, K. D. (2007). Actions necessary to prevent childhood obesity: Creating the climate for change. *Journal of Law, Medicine & Ethics, 31*(1), pp. 78–89.

Stanhope, M. & Lancaster, J. (2008). *Public health nursing: Population-centered health care in the community.* St. Louis, MO: Mosby Elsevier.

Chapter 7

Aiken, T. (2004). *Legal, ethical, and political issues in nursing.* Philadelphia: Davis.

American Nurses Association. (1992). Registered nurse utilization of unlicensed assistive personnel. *American Nurses Association Position Statement.*

American Nurses Association. (2007). *Public health nursing: Scope and standards of practice.* Silver Spring, MD: Nursesbooks.org

Beauchamp, T. & Childress, J. (1979). *Principles of biomedical ethics.* New York: Oxford University Press.

California Board of Registered Nursing. (2006). *California nursing practice act with regulations and related statutes.* Charlottesville, VA: Matthew Bender & Company, Inc.

Clancy, A. & Svensson, T. (2007). 'Faced' with responsibility: Levinasian ethics and the challenges of responsibility in Norwegian public health nursing. *Nursing Philosophy, 8*(3), pp. 158–166.

Easley, C. E. & Allen, C. E. (2007). A critical intersection: Human rights, public health nursing, and nursing ethics. *Advances in Nursing Science, 30*(4), pp. 367–382.

Evanson, T. A. (2006). Intimate partner violence and rural public health nursing practice: Challenges and opportunities. *Online Journal of Rural Nursing and Health Care, 6*(1), pp. 7–20.

Gallop, R. (1998). Postdischarge social contact: A potential area for boundary violation. *Journal of the American Psychiatric Nurses Association, 4*(4), pp. 105–110.

Griffith, R. (2007). Understanding confidentiality and disclosure of patient information. *British Journal of Community Nursing, 12*(11), pp. 530–534.

Jacobson, G. A. (2002). Maintaining professional boundaries: Preparing nursing students for the challenge. *Journal of Nursing Education, 41*(6), pp. 279–281.

Keller, L. O. & Litt, E. A. (2008). *Report on public health nurse to population ratio.* Association of State and Territorial Directors of Nursing (ASTDN).

McGarry, J. (2003). The essence of 'community' within community nursing: A district nursing perspective. *Health and Social Care in the Community, 11*(5), pp. 423–430.

Meagher-Stewart, D., Underwood, D., & Schoenfeld, B. et al. (2009). Building Canadian public health nursing capacity: Implications for action. Nursing Health Services Research Unit. Number 15. Retrieved March 30, 2010, from http://www.nhsru.com/documents/Series%2015%20McMaster_Building-CanadianPublicHealth.pdf

National Council of State Boards of Nursing and American Nurses Association. (2006). Joint statement on delegation. Retrieved December 29, 2010 from https://www.ncsbn.org/Joint_statement.pdf

Oberle, K. & Tenove, S. (2000). Ethical issues in public health nursing. *Nursing Ethics, 7*(5), pp. 425–438.

Purtilo, R. (2005). *Ethical dimensions in the health professions* (4th ed.). Philadelphia: Elsevier Saunders.

Racher, F. E. (2007). The evolution of ethics for community practice. *Journal of Community Health Nursing, 24*(1), pp. 65–76.

Schneiderman, J. U. (2003). *Exploration of the role of nurses in caring for children in foster care.* (Doctoral Dissertation). University of Southern California. Los Angeles, CA.

Schneiderman, J. U. (2006). Innovative pediatric nursing role: Public health nurses in child welfare. *Pediatric Nursing, 32*(4), pp. 317–321.

Scoville Walker, S. (2004). Ethical quandaries in community health nursing. In E. Anderson & J. McFarlane (Eds.) *Community as partner: Theory and practice in nursing* (4th ed.).(pp. 83–113). Philadelphia: Lippincott, Williams & Wilkins.

Volbrecht, R. M. (2002). *Nursing ethics: Communities in dialogue.* Upper Saddle River, NJ: Prentice Hall.

Williams, J. K. & Cooksey, M. M. (2004). Navigating the difficulties of delegation: Learn to improve teamwork in the unit by delegating duties appropriately. *Nursing, 34*(9), p. 32.

Chapter 8

Anderson, D. G., Richmond, C., & Stanhope, M. (2004). Enhanced undergraduate public health nursing experience: A collaborative experience with the Kentucky department for public health. *Family & Community Health, 27*(4), pp. 291–297.

Bennett, G. G. & Glasgow, R. E. (2009). The delivery of public health interventions via the internet: Actualizing their potential. *Annual Review of Public Health, 30,* pp. 273–293.

Black, A. (2008). Health literacy and cardiovascular disease: Fostering client skills. *American Journal of Health Education, 39*(1), pp. 55–57.

Calle, E. E., Miracle-McMahill, H. L, Moss, R. E., & Heath, C. W., Jr. (1994). Personal contact from friends to increase mammography usage. *American Journal of Preventive Medicine, 10*(6), pp. 361–366.

Carey, R. (1989). How values affect the mutual goal setting process with multiproblem families. *Journal of Community Health Nursing, 6*(1), pp. 7–14.

Chaffee, M. (2000). Health communications: Nursing education for increased visibility and effectiveness. *Journal of Professional Nursing, 16*(1), pp. 31–38.

Clark, M. J. (2008). *Community health nursing: Advocacy for population health.* Upper Saddle River, NJ: Pearson Education, Inc.

DeBuono, B. A. (2002). *Pfizer health literacy initiative.* New York: Pfizer Graphic.

DiClemente, C. & Proshaska, J. (1998). Toward a comprehensive transtheoretical model of change. In W. R. Miller & N. Heather (Eds.) *Treating addictive behaviors* (pp. 3–24). New York: Plenum Press.

Ervin, N. E. & Cowell, J. M. (2004). Integrating research into teaching public health nursing. *Public Health Nursing, 21*(2), pp. 183–190.

Evans, D. E. & McCormack, L. (2008). Applying social marketing in health care: Communicating evidence to change consumer behavior. *Medical Decision Making, 28,* pp. 781–792.

Goodrow, B., Scherzer, G., & Florence, J. (2004). An application of multidisclipinary education to a campus-community partnership to reduce motor vehicle accidents. *Education for Health, 17*(2), pp. 152–162.

Green, A. (2006). A person-centered approach to palliative care nursing. *Journal of Hospice and Palliative Nursing, 8*(5), pp. 294–301.

Holmes, B. J. (2008). Communicating about emerging infectious disease: The importance of research. *Health, Risk & Society, 10*(4), pp. 349–360.

Institute of Medicine. (2004). *Health literacy: A prescription to end confusion.* Washington D. C.: National Academy Press.

Jakeway, C. C., Cantrell, E. E., Cason, J. B., & Talley, B. S. (2006). Developing population health competencies among public health nurses in Georgia. *Public Health Nursing, 23*(2), pp. 161–167.

Keller, L. O., Strohschein, S., Lia-Hoagberg, B., & Schaffer, M. A. (2004). Population-based public health interventions: Practice-based and evidence-supported (Part I). *Public Health Nursing, 21*(5), pp. 453–468.

Kolb, D. A. (1984) *Experiential learning experience as a source of learning and development.* New Jersey: Prentice Hall.

Kolb, D. A. (2005). *The Kolb learning style inventory. Version 3.1.* David A. Kolb, Experience Based Learning Systems, Inc.

Kreps, G. L. & Sparks, L. (2008). Meeting the health literacy needs of immigrant populations. *Patient Education and Counseling, 71*(3), pp. 328–332.

Levy-Storms, L. (2005). Strategies for diffusing public health innovations through older adults' health communication networks. *Generations, 29*(2), pp. 70-75.

Maltby, H. (2006). Use of health fairs to develop public health nursing competencies. *Public Health Nursing, 23*(2), pp. 183–189.

McGrath, J. (1995). The gatekeeping process: The right combinations to unlock the gates. In E. Maibach & R. L. Parrott (Eds.) *Designing Health Messages—Approaches from Communication Theory and Public Health Practice* (pp. 199–216). Thousand Oaks, CA: Sage.

Miller, W. R. (2004). Motivational interviewing in service to health promotion. *American Journal of Health Promotion, 18*, pp. A1–A10.

Netiquette Home Page. (2006). Retrieved December 30, 2010 from http://www.albion.com/netiquette/

Onega, L. L. & Devers, E. (2008). Health education and group process. In M. Stanhope & J. Lancaster *Public health nursing: Population-centered health care in the community* (pp. 289–338). St. Louis, MO: Mosby Elsevier.

Public Health Nursing Section. (2001). *Public Health Interventions—Application for Public Health Nursing Practice.* St. Paul: Minnesota Department of Health.

Shinitzky, H. E. & Kub, J. (2001). The art of motivating behavior change: The use of motivational interviewing to promote health. *Public Health Nursing, 18*(3), pp. 178–185.

Sowan, N. A., Moffatt, S. G., & Canales, M. K. (2004). Creating a mentoring partnership model: A university-department of health experience. *Family & Community Health, 27*(4), pp. 326-337.

St. Catherine University. (2008). Teaching Plan. *Unpublished, personal communication* from Patricia M. Schoon, September 15, 2010.

Substance Abuse & Mental Health Service Administration Network. (1994). *You can prepare easy to read materials.* Technical Assistance Bulletin, National Clearinghouse for Alcohol and Drug Information. Retrieved December 30, 2010 from http://www.actforyouth.net/documents/YDM%20pdf6.4C%20handout.pdf

Toofany, S. (2006). Patient empowerment: Myth or reality? *Nursing Management, 13*(6), pp. 18–22.

Tveiten, S. & Severinsson, E. (2006). Communication—A core concept in client supervision by public health nurses. *Journal of Nursing Management, 14*(3), pp. 235–243.

Weiss, B. D. (2007). *Health literacy and patient safety: Help patients understand.* Chicago, IL: American Medical Association Foundation and American Medical Association.

Westdahl, C. & Page-Goertz, S. (2006). Promotion of breastfeeding—Beyond the benefits. *International Journal of Childbirth Education, 22*(4), pp. 8–16.

Whitman, N. I. (1998). Assessment of the learner. In M. D. Boyd, C. J. Gleit, B. A. Grahm, & N. I. Whitman, *Health Teaching in Nursing Practice: A Professional Model* (pp. 157-180). Stamford, CT: Appleton & Lange.

Wright, A. L, Naylor, A., Wester, R., Bauer, M., & Sutcliffe, E. (1997). Using cultural knowledge in health promotion: Breastfeeding among the Navajo. *Health Education & Behavior, 24*(5), pp. 625–639.

Zahner, S. J. & Gredig, Q. B. (2005). Improving public health nursing education: Recommendations of local public health nurses. *Public Health Nursing, 22*(5), pp. 445–450.

Zerwekh, J. V. (1991). A family caregiving model for public health nursing. *Nursing Outlook, 39*(5), pp. 213–217.

Chapter 9

Aronowitz, T. (2005). The role of "envisioning the future" in the development of resilience among at-risk youth. *Public Health Nursing, 22*(3), pp. 200–208.

Aston, M., Meagher-Stewart, D., Sheppard-Lemoine, D., Vukic, A., & Chircop, A. (2006). Family health nursing and empowering relationships. *Pediatric Nursing, 32*(1), pp. 61–67.

Austin, W., Bergum, V., & Dossitor, J. (2003). Relational ethics: An action ethic as a foundation for health care. In Tschudin, V. (Ed.) *Approaches to Ethics: Nursing Beyond Boundaries.* Woburn, MA: Buttersworth-Heinenmann.

Chafey, K. (1996). "Caring" is not enough: Ethical paradigms for community-based care. *Nursing and Health Care Perspectives on Community, 17*(1), pp. 10–15.

Chismar, D. (1988). Empathy and sympathy: The important difference. *The Journal of Value Inquiry, 22*(4), pp. 257–266.

Crisp, B. & Lister, P. (2004). Child protection and public health: nurses' responsibilities. *Journal of Advanced Nursing, 47*(6), pp. 656-663.

Fawcett, J. (2000). *Analysis and evaluation of contemporary nursing knowledge: Nursing models and theories.* Philadelphia: F.A. Davis Company.

Fazzone, P. A., Barloon, L. F., McConnell, S. J., & Chitty, J. A. (2000). Personal safety, violence, and home health. *Public Health Nursing, 17*(1), pp. 43–52.

Fredriksson, L., & Eriksson, K. (2006). The ethics of the caring conversation. *Nursing Ethics, 13*(1), pp. 138-148.

Gantert, T., McWilliam, C., Ward-Griffin, C., & Allen, N. (2009). Working it out together: Family caregivers' perceptions of relationship-building with in-home service providers. *Canadian Journal of Nursing Research, 41*(3), pp. 44-63.

Gellner, P., Landers, S., O'Rourke, D., & Schlegel, M. (1994). Community health nursing in the 1990s—Risky business? *Holistic Nursing Practice, 8*(2), pp. 15–21.

Heaman, M., Chalmers, K., Woodgate, R., & Brown, J. (2007). Relationship work in an early childhood home visiting program. *Journal of Pediatric Nursing, 22*(4), pp. 319–330.

Jack, S. M., DiCenso, A., & Lohfeld, L. (2005). A theory of maternal engagement with public health nurses and family visitors. *Journal of Advanced Nursing, 49*(2), pp. 182–190.

Jackson, C. (2010). Using loving relationships to transform health care: A practical approach. *Holistic Nursing Practice, 24*(4), pp. 181–186.

Kendra, M. A., Weiker, A., Simon, S., Grant, A., & Shullick, D. (1996). Safety concerns affecting delivery of home health care. *Public Health Nursing, 13*(2), pp. 83–89.

Ladd, R. E., Pasquerella, L., & Smith, S. (2000). What to do when the end is near: Ethical issues in home health care nursing. *Public Health Nursing, 17*(2), pp. 103–110.

Marcellus, L. (2005). The ethics of relation: Public health nurses and child protection clients. *Journal of Advanced Nursing, 51*(4), pp. 414–420.

McNaughton, D. B. (2005). A naturalistic test of Peplau's theory in home visiting. *Public Health Nursing, 22*(5), pp. 429–438.

Morse, J. M., Bottorff, J., Neander, W., & Solberg, S. (1991). Comparative analysis of conceptualizations and theories of caring. *IMAGE: Journal of Nursing Scholarship, 23*(2), pp. 119–126.

Morse, J. M., Solberg, S. M., Neander, W. L., Bottorff, J. L., & Johnson, J. L. (1990). Concepts of caring and caring as a concept. *Advances in Nursing Science, 13*(1), pp. 1–14.

Mulcahy, H., & McCarthy, G. (2008). Participatory nurse/client relationships: Perceptions of public health nurses and mothers of vulnerable families. *Applied Nursing Research, 21*(3), pp. 169–172.

Nagano, H. (2000). Empathic understanding: Constructing an evaluation scale from the microcounseling approach. *Nursing and Health Sciences, 2*(1), pp. 17–27.

Olthuis, G., Dekkers, W., Leget, C., & Vogelaar, P. (2006). The caring relationship in hospice care: An analysis based on the ethics of the caring relationship. *Nursing Ethics, 13*(1), pp. 29–40.

Ridgeway, S. (2010). Lillian Wald, founded public health nursing. *Working Nurse.* Retrieved September 27, 2010, from http://www.workingnurse.com/articles/Lillian-Wald-Founded-Public-Health-Nursing

Schaffer, M. A., Jost, R., Pederson, B. J., & Lair, M. (2008). Pregnancy-free club: A strategy to prevent repeat adolescent pregnancy. *Public Health Nursing, 25*(4), pp. 304–311.

Schulte, J. (2000). Finding ways to create connections among communities: Partial results of an ethnography of urban public health nurses. *Public Health Nursing, 17*(1), pp. 3-10.

Schulte, J. M., Nolt, B. J., Williams, R. L., Spinks, C. L., & Hellsten, J. J. (1998). Violence and threats of violence experienced by public health field workers. *Journal of the American Medical Association, 280*(5), pp. 439–442.

SmithBattle, L. (2003). Displacing the "rule book" in caring for teen mothers. *Public Health Nursing, 20* (5), pp. 369-376.

SmithBattle, L., Drake, M.A., & Diekemper, M. (1997). The responsive use of self in community health nursing practice. *Advances in Nursing Science, 20*(2), pp. 75–89.

SmithBattle, L., Diekemper, M., & Leander, S. (2004a). Getting your feet wet: Becoming a public health nurse, part 1. *Public Health Nursing, 21*(1), pp. 3–11.

SmithBattle, L., Diekemper, M., & Leander, S. (2004b). Moving upstream: Becoming a public health nurse, part 2. *Public Health Nursing, 21*(2), pp. 95–102.

Smith-Campbell, B. (1999). A case study on expanding the concept of caring from individuals to communities. *Public Health Nursing, 16*(6), pp. 405–411.

Sundelof, E. A., Hansebo, G., & Ekman, S. (2004). Friendship and caring communion: The meaning of caring relationship in district nursing. *International Journal for Human Caring, 8*(3), pp. 13–20.

Warelow, P., Edward, K. L., & Vinek, J. (2008). Care: What nurses say and what nurses do. *Holistic Nursing Practice, 22*(3), pp. 146–153.

Chapter 10

American Nurses Association (ANA). (2001). *Code of ethics for nurses with interpretive statements.* Washington, DC: Nursesbooks.org.

American Nurses Association (ANA). (2007). *Public Health Nursing—Scope and Standards of Practice.* Silver Springs, MD: Nursesbooks.org.

American Nurses Association (ANA). (2010a). *Guide to the code of ethics for nurses—Interpretation and application.* Silver Springs, MD: Nursebooks.org

American Nurses Association (ANA). (2010b). Nurses human rights. ANA position statements on ethics and human rights. Silver Springs, MD: Nursing World. Retrieved November 14, 2010, from http://www.nursingworld.org/MainMenuCategories/EthicsStandards/Ethics-Position-Statements.aspx

Baum, N., Gollust, S., Goold, S., & Jacobson, P. (2007). Looking ahead: Addressing ethical challenges in public health practice. *Journal of Law, Medicine, and Ethics, 35*(4), pp. 657–667.

Boutain, D. (2008). Social justice as a framework for undergraduate community health clinical in the United States. *International Journal of Nursing Education Scholarship, 5*(1), pp. 1-12.

Braveman, P. & Gruskin, S. (2003). Defining equity in health. *Journal of Epidemiology and Community Health, 57*, pp. 254–258.

Bu, X. & Jezewski, M. A., (2006). Developing a mid-range theory of patient advocacy through competency analysis. *Journal of Advanced Nursing, 57*(1), pp. 101–110.

Budetti, P. (2008). Market justice and US healthcare. *Journal of the American Medical Association, 299*(1), pp. 92–94.

Center for Vulnerable Populations Research. (2008). CVPR Newsletter, 5(1). Los Angeles, CA: University of California, Los Angeles, School of Nursing. Retrieved November 28, 2010, from http://www.nursing.ucla.edu/orgs/cvpr/who-are-vulnerable.html

Center for Vulnerable Populations Research. (2010). Who are the vulnerable? Los Angeles, CA: University of California, Los Angeles, School of Nursing. Retrieved November 28, 2010, from http://www.nursing.ucla.edu/orgs/cvpr/who-are-vulnerable.html

Cohen, B. & Reutter, L. (2007). Development of the role of public health nurses in addressing child and family poverty: A framework for action. *Journal of Advanced Nursing, 60*(1), pp. 96–107.

Congressional Budget Office. (2008). Growing disparities in life expectancy. *Economic and Budget Issue Brief*. Retrieved November 24, 2010, from http://www.cbo.gov/ftpdocs/91xx/doc9104/04-17-LifeExpectancy_Brief.pdf

Curtin, L. (1979). The nurse as advocate: A philosophical foundation for nursing. *Advances in Nursing Science, 1*(3), pp. 1–10.

Denehy, J. (2007). National Association of School Nurses: Speaking up for children. *Journal of School Nursing, 23*(3): pp. 125–27.

Easley, C. E. & Allen, C. E. (2007). A critical intersection—Human rights, public health nursing, and nursing ethics. *Advances in Nursing Science, 30*(4), pp. 367–382.

Ensign, J. (2001). The health of shelter-based foster youth. *Public Health Nursing, 18*(1), pp. 19–23.

Falk-Rafael, A. (2005a). Speaking truth to power: Nursing's legacy and moral imperative. *Advances in Nursing Science, 28*(3), pp. 212–223.

Falk-Rafael, A. (2005b). Advancing nursing theory through theory-guided practice –the emergence of a critical caring perspective. *Advances in Nursing Science, 28*(1), pp. 38–49.

Gadow, S. (1999). Relational narrative: The postmodern turn in nursing ethics. *Scholarly Inquiry for Nursing Practice: An International Journal, 13*(1), pp. 57–70.

Galer-Unti, R. (2010). Advocacy 2.0: Advocating in the digital age. *Health Promotion Practice, 11*(6), pp. 784–787.

Gostin, L. O. & Powers, M. (2006). What does social justice require for the public's health? Public health ethics and policy imperatives. *Health Affairs, 25*(4), pp. 1053–1060.

Gruskin, S., Cottingham, J., Hilber, A. M., Kismodi, E., Lincetto, O., & Roseman, M. J. (2008). Using human rights to improve maternal and neonatal health: History, connections and a proposed practical solution. *Bulletin of the World Health Organization, 86*(8), pp. 589–593.

Health Resources and Service Administration. (2009). Life Expectancy Table retrieved November 28, 2010, from http://mchb.hrsa.gov/whusa09/hstat/hi/pages/207le.html

Horton, S. & Johnson, R. J. (2010). Improving access to health care for uninsured elderly patients. *Public Health Nursing, 27*(4), pp. 362–370.

Hughes, J. (2010). Putting the pieces together: How public health nurses in rural and remote Canadian communities respond to intimate partner violence. *Online Journal of Rural Nursing and Health Care, 10*(1), pp. 34–47.

International Council of Nurses. (2006). The ICN position statement on nurses and human rights. Geneva, Switzerland: Author. Retrieved November 30, 2010, from http://www.icn.ch/images/stories/documents/publications/position_statements/E10_Nurses_Human_Rights.pdf

Jenkins, C., McNary, S., Carlson, B. A., King, M. G., Hossler, C. L., Magwood, G., … Imani, M. (2004). Reducing disparities for African Americans with diabetes: Progress made by the REACH 2010 Charleston and Georgetown diabetes coalition. *Public Health Reports, 119*, pp. 322–330.

Jones, P., Waters, C., Oka, R., & McGhee, E. (2010). Increasing community capacity to reduce tobacco-related health disparities in African American communities. *Public Health Nursing, 27*(6), pp. 552–560.

Kalnins, I. (2008). Enda Dell Weinel, champion of public health nursing—excerpts from an oral history. *Public Health Nursing, 25*(2), pp. 194–199.

Keller, L. O. (2010). Table: Comparison of value structure. *Unpublished,* personal correspondence.

Kleinfehn-Wald, N. (2010). Social justice and human rights issues identified by practicing public health nurses. Unpublished research.

Lavery, S. H., Smith, M. L., Esparza, A. A., Hrushow, A., Moore, M., & Reed, D. F. (2005). The community action model: A community-driven model designed to address disparities in health. *American Journal of Public Health, 95*(4), pp. 611–616.

MacDonald, H. (2006). Relational ethics and advocacy in nursing: Literature review. *Journal of Advanced Nursing, 57*(2), pp. 119–126.

Mallik, M. (1997). Advocacy in nursing—A review of the literature. *Journal of Advanced Nursing, 25*(1), pp. 130–138.

Minnesota Department of Health (MDH). (2001). *Public health interventions—Application for public health nursing practice.* St. Paul, MN: Author.

Office of Minority Health and Health Disparities. (2010). About Minority Health. Retrieved December 7, 2010, from http://www.cdc.gov/omhd/AMH/AMH.htm

Pacquiao, D. (2008). Nursing care of vulnerable populations using a framework of cultural competence, social justice and human rights. *Contemporary Nurse, 28*(1–2), pp. 189–197.

Racher, F. E. (2007). The evolution of ethics for community practice. *Journal of Community Health Nursing, 24*(1), pp. 65–76.

Satcher, D. & Higginbotham, E. J. (2008). The public health approach to eliminating disparities in health. *American Journal of Public Health, 98*, pp. 400–403.

Smith, D., Jacobson, L., & Yiu, L. (2008). Primary health care. In L. Stamler & L. Yiu (Eds.), *Community Health Nursing: A Canadian Perspective* (2nd ed.) (pp. 111 – 124). Toronto, ON: Pearson Prentice Hall.

Strass, P. & Billay, E. (2008). *A public health nursing initiative to promote antenatal health. Canadian Nurse, 104*(2), pp. 29–33.

United Nations. (1948). The universal declaration of human rights. Geneva, Switzerland: Author. Retrieved November 15, 2010, from http://www.un.org/Overview/rights.html

Unnatural Causes. (2010). Unnatural Causes. Retrieved November 15, 2010, from http://www.unnatural-causes.org

U. S. Department of Health and Human Services. Understanding the Affordable Care Act. Healthcare.gov. Retrieved November 20, 2010, from www.healthcare.gov

Vanderburg, S., Wright, L., Boston, S., & Zimmerman, G. (2010). Maternal child home visiting program improves nursing practice for screening of woman abuse. *Public Health Nursing, 27*(4), pp. 347–352.

Volbrecht, R. M. (2002). *Nursing ethics—Communities in dialogue.* Upper Saddle River, NJ: Pearson Prentice Hall.

Chapter 11

Aston, M., Meagher-Stewart, D., Sheppard-Lemoine, D., Vukic, A., & Chircop, A. (2006). Family health nursing and empowering relationships. *Pediatric Nursing, 32*(1), pp. 61–67.

Cioffi, J. (2003). Communicating with culturally and linguistically diverse patients in an acute care setting: Nurses' experiences. *International Journal of Nursing Studies, 40*(3), pp. 299-306.

Dillon, R. (1992). Respect and care: Toward a moral integration. *Canadian Journal of Philosophy, 22*(1), pp. 105-132.

Flores, G. (2005). The impact of medical interpreter services on the quality of health care: A systematic review. *Medical Care Research Review, 62*(3), pp. 255–299.

Garrett, P. (2009). Healthcare interpreter policy: Policy determinants and current issues in the Australian context. *Interpreting & Translation, 1*(2), pp. 44–54.

Goldsborough, J. D. (1970). On becoming nonjudgmental. *The American Journal of Nursing, 70*(11), pp. 2340–2343.

Leininger, M. (1978). Transcultural nursing theories and research approaches. In Leininger, M. (Ed.) *Transcultural Nursing.*(pp. 31 – 51). New York, NY: Wiley and Sons.

Mack, M., Uken, R., & Powers, J. (2006). People improving the community's health: Community health workers as agents of change. *Journal of Health Care for the Poor and Underserved, 17*(1), pp. 16–25.

Nagano, H. (2000). Empathic understanding: Constructing an evaluation scale from the microcounseling approach. *Nursing & Health Sciences, 2*(1), pp. 17–27.

Segal, J., Smith, M. A. & Jaffe, J. Nonverbal communication skills: The power of nonverbal communication and body language. *HELPGUIDE.org.* Retrieved December 23, 2009, from http://www.helpguide.org/mental/eq6_nonverbal_communication.htm

O'Brien, M. J., Squires, A. P., Bixby, R. A., & Larson S. C. (2009). Role development of community health workers: An examination of selection and training processes in the intervention literature. *American Journal of Preventive Medicine, 37*(6), pp. s262–s269.

Pasco, A. C. Y., Morse, J. M., & Olson, J. K. (2004). The cross-cultural relationships between nurses and Filipino Canadian patients. *Journal of Nursing Scholarship, 36*(3), pp. 239–246.

Payne, R. K., DeVol, P. E., & Smith, T. D. (2001). *Bridges out of poverty: Strategies for professionals and communitie*s. Texas: aha! Process, Inc.

Pesznecker, B. L. (1984). The poor: A population at risk. *Public Health Nursing, 1*(4), pp. 237–249.

Porr, C. (2005). Shifting from preconceptions to pure wonderment. *Nursing Philosophy, 6*(3), pp. 189–195.

Ramarajan, L., Barsade, S. G., & Burack, O. R. (2008). The influence of organizational respect on emotional exhaustion in the human services. *The Journal of Positive Psychology, 3*(1), pp. 3–18.

Volbrecht, R. M. (2001). *Nursing Ethics: Communities in dialogu*e. New Jersey: Prentice Hall, Inc.

Wright, L. M., & Leahey, M. (2005). *Nurses and families: A guide to family assessment and intervention* (4th ed.) Philadelphia: F.A. Davis Company.

Chapter 12

Crisp, B. R. & Green Lister, P. (2004). Child protection and public health: Nurses' responsibilities. *Journal of Advanced Nursing, 47*(6), pp. 656–663.

DeMay, D. A. (2003). The experience of being a client in an Alaska public health nursing home visitation program. *Public Health Nursing, 20*(3), pp. 228–236.

Flynn, M. A., Hall, K., Noack, A., Clovechok, S., Enns, E., Pivnick, J., …Pryce, C. (2005). Promotion of healthy weights at preschool public health vaccination clinics in Calgary: An obesity surveillance program. *Canadian Journal of Public Health, 96*(6), pp. 421–426.

Friedman, M. M., Bowden, V. R., & Jones, E. G. (2003). *Family nursing: Research, theory and practice* (5th ed.). Upper Saddle River, NJ: Prentice Hall.

Hayes, J. C., Davis, J. A., & Miranda, M. L. (2006). Incorporating a built environment module into an accelerated second-degree community health nursing course. *Public Health Nursing 23*(5), pp. 442–452.

Hayter, M. (2005). Reaching marginalized young people through sexual health nursing outreach clinics: Evaluating service use and the views of service users. *Public Health Nursing, 22*(4), pp. 339–346.

Kemp, L., Anderson, T., Travaglia, J., & Harris, E. (2005). Sustained nursing home visiting in early childhood: Exploring Australian nursing competencies. *Public Health Nursing, 22*(3), pp. 254–259.

Kemper, A. R., Fant, K. E., & Clark, S. J. (2005). Informing parents about newborn screening. *Public Health Nursing, 22*(4), pp. 332–338.

Labun, E. (1988). Spiritual care: An element in nursing care planning. *Journal of Advanced Nursing, 13*(3), pp. 314–320.

McKeown, F. (2007). The experiences of older people on discharge from hospital following assessment by the public health nurse. *Journal of Clinical Nursing, 16*(3), pp. 469–476.

McSherry, W., Cash, K., & Ross, L. (2004). Meaning of spirituality: Implications for nursing practice. *Journal of Clinical Nursing, 13*(8), pp. 934–941.

Minnesota Department of Health (MDH). (2007). Community Health Assessment and Action Planning Handbook (CHAAP) 2005–2009. Office of Public Health Practice, Division of Community and Family Health. St. Paul, Minnesota.

Minnesota Department of Health (MDH). (2009). Early identification of young children with special health care needs. *Minnesota Department of Health Fact Sheet: Title V (MCH) Block Grant Children and Adolescents with Special Health Care Needs*. St. Paul, Minnesota.

Mondy, C., Cardenas, D., & Avila, M. (2003). The role of an advanced practice public health nurse in bioterrorism preparedness. *Public Health Nursing, 20*(6), pp. 422–431.

Olds, D. L., Kitzman, H., Hanks, C., Cole, R., Anson, E., Sidora-Arcoleo, K., … Bondy, J. (2007). Effects of nurse home visiting on maternal and child functioning: Age-9 follow-up of a randomized trial. *Pediatrics, 120*(4), pp. 832–845.

Ricketts, S. A., Murray, E. K., & Schwalberg, R. (2005). Reducing low birthweight by resolving risks: Results from Colorado's Prenatal Plus Program. *American Journal of Public Health, 98*(11), pp. 1952–1957.

Schim, S., Doorenbos, A., Benkert, R., & Miller, J. (2007). Culturally congruent care: Putting the puzzle together. *Journal of Transcultural Nursing, 18*(2), pp. 103–110.

Schneiderman, J. U. (2006). Innovative pediatric nursing role: Public health nurses in child welfare. *Pediatric Nursing, 32*(4), pp. 317–321.

Sittner, B., Hudson, D., & Defrain, J. (2007). Using the concept of family strengths to enhance nursing care. *MCN: The American Journal of Maternal/Child Health Nursing, 32*(6), pp. 353–357.

Somervell, A. M., Saylor, C., & Mao, C. L. (2005). Public health nurse interventions for women in a dependency drug court. *Public Health Nursing, 22*(1), pp. 59–64.

Strass, P., & Billay, E. (2008). A public health nursing initiative to promote antenatal health. *Canadian Nurse, 104*(2), pp. 29–33.

World Health Organization (WHO). Environmental Health. Retrieved September 14, 2010, from http://www.who.int/topics/environmental_health/en/

Chapter 13

American Nurses Association. (2007). *Public health nursing: Scope and standards of practice.* Silver Springs, MD: Nursesbooks.org.

American Public Health Association. (2010). Top ten rules of advocacy. Retrieved November 15, 2010, from www.apha.org

Avolio, B. J., Walumbwa, F. O., & Weber, T. J. (2009). Leadership: Current theories, research, and future directions. *Annual Review of Psychology, 60*, pp. 421–449.

Blackburn, C. (1992). *Improving health and welfare work with families in poverty: A handbook.* Buckingham, UK: Open University Press.

Brueshoff, B. (2010). Leadership for entry-level public health nurses. *Unpublished, personal correspondence,* December 1, 2010.

Cashman, K. (2008). *Leadership from the inside out: Becoming a leader for life* (2nd ed.). San Francisco, CA: Berrett-Koehler Publishers, Inc.

Cohen, B. E. & Reutter, L. (2007). Development of the role of public health nurses in addressing child and family poverty: A framework for action. *Journal of Advanced Nursing, 60*(1), pp. 96–107.

Dakota County Public Health. (2004). Dakota County Clinical Menu modified from Henry Street Consortium Clinical Menu (2004). West St. Paul, MN: Author.

Deschaine, J. & Schaffer, M. (2003). Strengthening the role of public health nurse leaders in policy development. *Policy, Politics, & Nursing Practice, 4*(4), pp. 266–274.

Falk-Rafael, A. (2005). Speaking truth to power: Nursing's legacy and moral imperative. *Advances in Nursing Science, 28*(3), pp. 212–223.

Henry Street Consortium. (2004). The Henry Street Consortium Clinical Menu. St. Paul, MN: Author. Retrieved December 14, 2010, from http://www.health.state.mn.us/divs/cfh/ophp/consultation/phn/henrystreet/

Hill, K. S. (2008). Leading change: The creativity of a public health nurse leader. *Journal of Nursing Administration, 38*(11), pp. 459–460.

Kalb, K. B., Cherry, N. M., Kauzloric, J., Brender, A., Green, K., Miyagawa, L., et al. (2006). A competency-based approach to public health nursing performance appraisal. *Public Health Nursing, 29*(3), pp. 115–138.

Mason, D. J., Backer, B. A., & Georges, C. A. (1991). Toward a feminist model for the political empowerment of nurses. *Image Journal of Nursing Scholarship, 23*(2), pp. 72–77.

Meagher-Stewart, D., Underwood, J., MacDonald, M., Schoenfeld, B., Blythe, J., Knibbs, K., … Crea, M. (2010). Organizational attributes that assure optimal utilization of public health nurses. *Public Health Nursing, 27*(5), pp. 433–441.

Minnesota Department of Health. (2001). Public Health Interventions – Applications for Public Health Nursing Practice. St.Paul, MN: Author

Morrison, R. S., Jones, L., & Fuller, B. (1997). The relation between leadership style and empowerment on job satisfaction of nurses. *Journal of Nursing Administration, 27*(5), pp. 27–34.

Nissen, L. B., Merrigan, D. M., & Kraft, M. K. (2005). Moving mountains together: Strategic community leadership and systems change. *Child Welfare, 84*(2), pp. 123–140.

Quad Council. (2004). Public health nursing competencies—Quad Council of Public Health Nursing Organizations. *Public Health Nursing, 21*(5), pp. 443–452.

Racher, F. (2007). The evolution of ethics for community practice. *Journal of Community Health Nursing, 24*(1), pp. 65–76.

Robinson, F. P. (2009). Servant teaching: The power and promise for nursing education. *International Journal of Nursing Education Scholarship*, 6(1), Article 5, Electronic Press.

Russell, R. F. & Stone, A. G. (2002). A review of servant leadership attributes: Developing a practical model. *Leadership and Organizational Development Journal, 23*(3), pp. 145–157.

Schoon, P.M. (2010). Student Leadership Examples at Three Levels of Practice. *Unpublished. Personal correspondence, January 25, 2011.*

Stanley, D. (2006). Recognizing and defining clinical nurse leaders. *British Journal of Nursing, 15*(2), pp. 108–111.

Stanley, D. (2008). Congruent leadership: Values in action. *Journal of Nursing Management, 16*(5), pp. 519–524.

Swearingen, S. & Liberman, A. (2004). Nursing leadership—Serving those who serve others. *The Health Care Manager,* 23(2), pp. 100–109.

Underwood, J. M., Mowat, D. L., Meagher-Stewart, D. M., Deber, R. B., Baumann, A. O., MacDonald, M. B., … Munroe, V. J. (2009). Building community and public health nursing capacity: A synthesis report of the national community health nursing study. *Canadian Journal of Public Health, 100*(5), pp. I-1–I-11.

U. S. Health and Human Services. (2020). Healthy People 2020—The road ahead. Retrieved December 14, 2010 from http://www.healthypeople.gov/hp2020

Volbrecht, R. M. (2002). *Nursing ethics—Communities in dialogue.* Upper Saddle River, NJ: Pearson Prentice Hall.

Zilembo, M. & Monterosso, L. (2008). Nursing students' perceptions of desirable leadership qualities in nurse preceptors: A descriptive survey. *Contemporary Nurse, 27*(2), pp. 194–206.

Chapter 14

Anonymous. (2010). Competency Portfolio: Student Story #1. *Unpublished.*

Anonymous. (2010). Competency Portfolio: Student Story #2. *Unpublished.*

Anonymous. (2010). Competency Portfolio: Student Story #3. *Unpublished.*

Minnesota Department of Health. (2006). *Wheel of Public Health Interventions: A collection of "getting behind the wheel" stories, 2000-2006.* Office of Public Health Practice.

Chapter 3

National Public Health Goals and Strategies

1. Healthy People 2020: http://www.healthypeople.gov

2. Task Force on Community Preventive Services: http://www.thecommunityguide.org/index.html

Public Health Nursing Informatics

1. Omaha System Case Studies: http://www.omahasystem.org

Public Health Nursing Practice and Process

1. The Nursing Process Applied to Population-Based Public Health Nursing Practice—Minnesota Department of Health: http://www.health.state.mn.us/divs/cfh/ophp/resources/docs/nursing_process.pdf

2. Wisconsin's Public Health Nursing Practice Model—Linking Education and Practice for Excellence in Public Health Nursing Project (LEAP Project): http://videos.med.wisc.edu/videoInfo.php?videoid=3385

3. Public Health Nursing Process and Documentation—County of Los Angeles, California:http://www.publichealth.lacounty.gov/phn/docs/Documentation12_02_08.pdf

Public Health Nursing Stories

1. Case Study on Indoor Air Quality in Family with Young Children: http://www.medscape.com/viewarticle/718616_5

2. National Association of School Nurses Radio: http://www.nasn.org/Default.aspx?tabid=597

3. Nurse-Family Partnership Stories: http://www.nursefamilypartnership.org/nurses/stories-from-nurses

4. Nurses Share Their Stories: http://www.missouristate.edu/nursing/38989.htm

5. Public Health Nursing Stories: http://www.health.state.mn.us/divs/cfh/connect/index.cfm?article=phstories.categorysearch&qCategoryId=200029

Chapter 4

1. Centers for Disease Control and Prevention (CDC): http://www.cdc.gov

2. National Center for Health Statistics: http://www.cdc.gov/nchs/

3. Resources for Creating Public Health Maps: http://www.cdc.gov/epiinfo/maps.htm

4. CDC Wonder: http://wonder.cdc.gov/

5. U.S. Environmental Protection Agency (EPA): http://www.epa.gov/

6. Census Bureau Home Page: http://www.census.gov/

7. National Institute of Nursing Research (NINR): http://www.ninr.nih.gov/

8. Indian Health Service (HIS): http://www.ihs.gov/

9. Agency for Healthcare Research and Quality Home Page (AHRQ): http://www.ahrq.gov/

10. U.S. Health Resources and Services Administration (HRSA): http://www.hrsa.gov/index.html

11. Pan American Health Organization (PAHO): http://new.paho.org/

12. About John Snow: http://www.ph.ucla.edu/epi/snow.html

13. Epidemiology Data Center: http://www.edc.gsph.pitt.edu/

14. Fed Stats: http://www.fedstats.gov/

15. Population Reference Bureau: http://www.prb.org/

16. Epidemiology and Disease Control Program—Maryland Department of Health: http://edcp.org/

17. Brooks, G. (2001). *Year of wonders: A novel of the plague.* London, England: Penguin Books.

18. Balshem, M. (1993). *Cancer in the community: Class and medical authority.* Washington D.C.: Smithsonian Institution Press.

19. Maternal and Child Health Bureau. Life course resources: http://mchb.hrsa.gov/lifecourseresources.htm

Chapter 5

1. Community-Campus Partnerships for Health (CCPH). A nonprofit organization that promotes health (broadly defined) through partnerships between communities and higher educational institutions. CCPH has many resources for partnership development. http://www.ccph.info/

2. Public Health Interventions—Applications for Public Health Nursing Practice. St. Paul: Minnesota Department of Health. (2001). (Collaboration is located on pp. 177–210.) http://www.health.state.mn.us/divs/cfh/ophp/resources/docs/phinterventions_manual2001.pdf

3. Community Tool Box. Identifying community assets and resources. (2009). University of Kansas: Work Group for Community Health and Development. http://ctb.ku.edu/en/tablecontents/ sub_section_main_1043.htm

4. Linking Education and Practice for Excellence in Public Health Nursing (LEAP). The purpose is to improve competency for public health nursing practice in a changing public health system by educating public health nurses, student nurses, and nursing faculty in the knowledge and skills required for providing population-based, culturally competent public health nursing services. http://www.son.wisc.edu/LEAP/

5. Community Engagement through Service Learning Manual. Narsavage, G. & Lindell, D. (2001). *Community engagement through service learning manual.* Fort Collins, CO: Case Western Reserve University & Frances Payne Bolton School of Nursing. http://depts.washington.edu/ccph/ pdf_files/CETSLmanual4.pdf

6. Engaging the Community in Decision Making. Lasker, R. D. & Guidry, J. A. (2009). *Engaging the community in decision making: Case studies in tracking participation, voice and influence.* Jefferson, NC: McFarland & Company, Inc. www.mcfarlandpub.com

Chapter 6

General Health Information

1. Online Source for Health Information. Centers for Disease Control and Prevention. (2010). Health and safety topics. http://www.cdc.gov/

Coordinated School Health Focus Areas

2. Minnesota Department of Health. (2010). Resources for 5 focus areas: HIV/AIDS/STD, nutrition, physical activity, teen pregnancy, and tobacco. http://www.health.state.mn.us/schools/csh/ focusareas/index.html

Immunization

3. Information and Resources for Individuals, Families, and Professional about Influenza. www.flu.gov

4. Resources about Immunization for Nurses. American Nurses Association. (2010). ANA immunize. www.anaimmunize.org

Obesity Prevention

5. Recommended Obesity Prevention Strategies. Centers for Disease Control and Prevention. (2010). Division of Nutrition, Physical Activity and Obesity. http://www.cdc.gov/nccdphp/dnpao/

6. Recommendations, Statistics, and Strategies for Obesity Prevention. Centers for Disease Control and Prevention. (2010). Overweight and obesity. http://www.cdc.gov/obesity/

7. Systematic Reviews on Obesity Prevention. Guide to Community Preventive Services. (2010). Obesity prevention and control. http://www.thecommunityguide.org/obesity/index.html

Chapter 7

Confidentiality

1. The Health Insurance Portability and Accountability Act of 1996 (HIPAA) Privacy and Security Rules. Retrieved December 29, 2010 from http://www.hhs.gov/ocr/privacy/

Delegation

2. Joint Statement on Delegation. National Council of State Boards of Nursing and American Nurses Association. (2006). Retrieved December 29, 2010 from https://www.ncsbn.org/Joint_statement. pdf

Ethics Resources

3. American Nurses Association. The Center for Ethics and Human Rights. Code of Ethics, Genetics and Genomics, ANA Positions on Ethics and Human Rights. Retrieved January 29, 2011 from http://nursingworld.org/MainMenuCategories/EthicsStandards/Ethics-Position-Statements.aspx

4. American Nurses Association. Code of Ethics for Nurses. (2001). Retrieved January 29, 2011 from http://www.nursingworld.org/MainMenuCategories/EthicsStandards/CodeofEthicsforNurses.aspx

5. Nursing Ethics (journal). Retrieved December 29, 2010 from http://nej.sagepub.com/

6. North Carolina Institute for Public Health. Offers a short course on ethics—offers questions about ethics in public health. Retrieved December 29, 2010 from http://oce.sph.unc.edu/phethics/

7. Fowler, M. D. M. (Ed.) (2008). *Guide to the Code of Ethics for Nurses: Interpretation and Application.* Silver Springs, MD: American Nurses Association.

Professional Boundaries

8. Professional Boundaries: A Nurse's Guide to the Importance of Professional Boundaries. National Council of State Boards of Nursing. Retrieved December 29, 2010 from https://www.ncsbn.org/Professional_Boundaries_2007_Web.pdf

Chapter 8

Health Promotion Education

1. Professional E-mail Communication

   • Netiquette guidelines for ethical and respectful online communication. http://www.albion.com/netiquette

   • Friedman, D. (2005). Tips for More Effective Email Communication. *Connections Magazine.* Retrieved January 29, 2011 from http://www.connectionsmagazine.com/articles/5/072.html

Health Literacy

2. Improving Communication from the Federal Government to the Public. www.plainlanguage.gov

3. Pfizer Clear Health Communication Initiative: Public Health Professionals. http://www.pfizer-healthliteracy.com/public-health-professionals/default.html

4. Simply Put: A Guide for Creating Easy-To-Understand Materials (2009). Centers for Disease Control and Prevention. http://www.cdc.gov/healthmarketing/pdf/Simply_Put_082010.pdf

Adolescent and School Health

5. Center for Disease Control—tools, curriculum, statistics. http://www.cdc.gov/HealthyYouth/index.htm

Flu Vaccine: Centers for Disease Control Public and Prevention Service Message

6. You Tube Video: Why Flu Matters: Personal Stories from Families Affected by Influenza (for parents). http://www.youtube.com/user/cdcflu

Handwashing: Hand Hygiene Print Materials

7. Signs, posters, brochures, manuals, curricula, and other hand hygiene materials that you can print and use. Available from Ramsey County Health Department, Minnesota. http://www.health.state.mn.us/handhygiene/materials.html

Oral Health

8. Guidelines, assessment tools, anticipatory guidance, posters, and public education materials. http://www.mchoralhealth.org/Toolbox/professionals.html

9. Minnesota Department of Health Child and Teen Checkups—Five modules. http://www.health.state.mn.us/divs/fh/mch/webcourse/dental/index.cfm

Physical Activity: Blue Cross Blue Shield of Minnesota "Do" Campaign

10. Do is based on a simple idea: By moving your body each day, you can improve your overall health and reduce your risk of heart disease, stroke, diabetes, and other illnesses. The *do* physical activity campaign was developed by Blue Cross and Blue Shield of Minnesota, based on guidelines set by the Centers for Disease Control and Prevention and the American Heart Association. http://www.do-groove.com/

Tobacco Prevention and Control: North Carolina Division of Public Health

11. Provides information on preventing the initiation of smoking and other tobacco use, eliminating exposure to secondhand smoke, helping tobacco users quit, and addressing tobacco-related health disparities. http://www.tobaccopreventionandcontrol.ncdhhs.gov/

Chapter 9

Relationship-Building

1. Henry Street Settlement: http://www.henrystreet.org/site/PageServer?pagename=abt_lwald

2. Jewish Women's Archives: http://jwa.org/historymakers/wald

3. Visiting Nurse Service of New York: http://www.vnsny.org/community/our-history/lillian-wald/

4. Working Nurse: http://www.workingnurse.com/articles/Lillian-Wald-Founded-Public-Health-Nursing

Caring Relationships

5. Anderson, M., & Braun. J. (1995). *Caring for the Elderly Client*. Philadelphia: F. A. Davis Company

6. MacKay, R., Hughes, J., & Carver, E. (Eds.) (1989). *Empathy in the Helping Relationship*. New York: Springer.

Chapter 10

1. Highlights in Minority Health at the Office of Minority Health and Health Disparities: http://www.cdc.gov/omhd/Highlights/Highlight.htm. Look for examples of important health disparities by population.

2. National Partnership for Action to End Health Disparities: http://minorityhealth.hhs.gov/npa/templates/browse.aspx?lvl=1&lvlid=13. Read about the business case for eliminating health disparities.

3. The Office on Women's Health—Quick Health Data Online: http://www.healthstatus2010.com/owh/disparities/ChartBookData_search.asp

Advocacy

4. American Nurses Association—Practice standards, position papers and publications: http://www.nursingworld.org

5. American Public Health Association—Position papers: http://www.apha.org

6. International Council for Nursing—Practice standards, position papers: http://www.icn.ch/

7, Human Rights Watch: http://www.hrw.org/

8, Public Health Advocacy—National Association of County and City Health Officials: http://www.naccho.org/advocacy/

9. United Nations: http://unfoundation.org

Health Disparities

10. Centers for Disease Control and Prevention: http://www.cdc.gov

11. CDC—Health Disparities: http://www.cdc.gov/omhd/Topic/healthdisparities.html

12. Health Care Reform: http://www.healthcare.gov/

13. Healthy People 2020: http://www.healthypeople.gov/hp2020/

14. Institute of Medicine Reports: http://www.iom.edu/Reports.aspx

15. Kaiser Foundation—Health Policy explained: http://www.KaiserEDU.org

16. Robert Wood Johnson Foundation—Health Policy, Vulnerable Populations and Health Disparities: http://www.rwjf.org/

17. Surgeon General's Reports: http://www.surgeongeneral.gov/library/

18. World Health Organization, Commission on the Social Determinants of Health: http://www.who.int/en/

Chapter 11

1. Lipson, J. G., & Dibble, S. L. (Eds). (2005). *Culture & Clinical Care*. San Francisco, CA: UCSF Nursing Press.

2. *Bridges out of Poverty* (Note that this presents examples at the individual level primarily.) A curriculum and a DVD series provide communities with strategies to address poverty. YouTube link for the DVD series: http://www.youtube.com/watch?v=G_8F7XQSX4Y

3. O'Connor, A. (2001). *Poverty Knowledge: Social Science, Social Policy, and the Poor in Twentieth-Century U.S. History* (Politics and Society in Twentieth Century America). Princeton, NJ: Princeton University Press.

4. Pipher, M. (2002). *The Middle of Everywhere*. San Diego, CA: Harcourt, Inc. (Helping refugees enter the American community)

5. *Unnatural Causes* DVD series: http://www.unnaturalcauses.org

Chapter 12

1. Center for Disease Control and Prevention (CDC): http://www.cdc.gov

2. Child Development Screening Instruments: Ages and Stages and the ESI-R: http://www.health.state.mn.us/divs/fh/mch/devscrn/glance.html

3. Environmental Pollution Agency (EPA) – Indoor Air Quality for Schools: http://www.epa.gov/iaq/schools/toolkit.html

4. EPA – Healthy School Environments: http://www.epa.gov/schools/

5. Home Safety Council: http://www.homesafetycouncil.org

6. Health Care Without Harm: http://www.noharm.org

7. Immunization Action Coalition: http://www.immunize.org

8. Kids Health: http://kidshealth.org

9. NCAST programs include screening tools used in PHN practice to assess relationship and bonding between mother/parent and infant/child: http://www.ncast.org/index.cfm?category=2

10. Pediatric Home Assessment Tool for asthma: http://www.healthyhomestraining.org/Nurse/PEHA.htm

11. American Association of Poison Control Centers: http://www.aapcc.org/dnn/default.aspx

Chapter 13

1. Alliance of Young Nurse Leaders and Advocates: http://www.aynla.org/.

2. United Nations Millennium Development Goals: http://mdgs.un.org/unsd/mdg/Default.aspx

3. Regina Clark—7 C's of Leadership on YouTube: http://www.youtube.com/watch?v=dACu_uc-ghuA

4. 25 Most Famous Nurses in History: http://onlinebsn.org/2009/25-most-famous-nurses-in-history/

5. The Five Most Influential Nurses in History: http://noedb.org/library/features/the-five-most-influential-nurses-in-history

6. Nursing Empowerment: http://www.youtube.com/watch?v=lzjbe7ZOCKk&feature=related

7. Katrina—Nature at its worse. Nursing at its best.: http://www.youtube.com/watch?v=JPSbDq2NjDg&feature=channel

8. Colin Powell's 13 Rules of Leadership: http://www.youtube.com/watch?v=C-vve55FDaU&feature=related

9. Robert Wood Johnson Foundation—Leadership resources—Webinars: http://www.rwjfleaders.org/resources

Leadership Books

10. Dickenson-Hazard, N. (2008). *Ready, set, go lead!* Indianapolis: Sigma Theta Tau International.

11. Hansen-Turton, T., Sherman, S., & Ferguson, V. (2009). *Conversations with leaders: frank talk from nurses (and others) on the frontlines of leadership.* Indianapolis: Nursing Knowledge International.

12. Houser, B. P., &Player, K. (2010). *Pivotal moments in nursing: leaders who changed the path of a profession, Vol. 1.* Sigma Theta Tau International, Center for Nursing Press.

13. Houser, B. P., Player, K. (2007). *Pivotal Moments in Nursing: Leaders Who Changed the Path of a Profession, Vol. II.* Indianapolis: Sigma Theta Tau International.

14. George, B. (2003). *Authentic Leadership: Rediscovering the Secrets to Creating Lasting Value.* Jossey-Bass/Wiley.

15. Pausch, R., with Zaslow, J. (2008). *The Last Lecture.* Hyperion Books.

16. Maxwell, J. C. (2005). *The 21 Irrefutable Laws of Leadership: Follow Them and People Will Follow You.* Thomas Nelson Books.

ENTRY-LEVEL POPULATION-BASED PUBLIC HEALTH NURSING COMPETENCIES

For The New Graduate Or Novice Public Health Nurse

PHN KNOWLEDGE AND SKILLS

CORNERSTONE

Public Health Nursing Practice focuses on entire populations and reflects community priorities and needs

1. **Applies the public health nursing process to communities, systems, individuals and families**
   A. Identifies the population(s) for which the PHN is accountable
   B. Assesses the health status of communities, systems, individuals and families
      1) Identifies and understands the use of key health determinants
      2) Identifies relevant and appropriate data and information sources for the populations to which the PHN is accountable
         a. Familiar with data used in the health department
         b. Familiar with data in the programs in which the PHN works
      3) Works in partnership with communities, systems, individuals or families to attach meaning to collected quantitative and qualitative data
      4) Works in partnership with communities, systems, individuals and families to establish priorities
   C. In partnership with communities, systems, individuals and families, develops a plan based on priorities (including nursing care plans for individuals/families)
      1) Selects desired outcomes that are measurable, meaningful, and manageable
      2) Selects public health interventions that
         a. Are evidence-based
         b. Have the greatest potential for improving the health of the population
         c. Respect the culture and ethnic beliefs of the community
         d. Are consistent with professional standards, the Nurse Practice Act, existing laws, ordinances, and policies
      3) Selects level(s) of intervention (community, systems, individuals and families)
      4) Selects level(s) of prevention (primary, secondary, tertiary)
   D. Implements the plan with communities, systems, individuals and families
      1) Works in partnership with communities, systems, individuals and families to implement public health interventions
      2) Utilizes best practices when implementing the public health nursing intervention
   E. Evaluates
      1) Measures outcomes of public health nursing interventions
      2) Documents public health nursing process by completing forms, records, and charts for communities, systems, individuals and families

CORNERSTONE

Public Health Nursing Practice promotes health through strategies driven by epidemiological evidence

2. **Utilizes basic epidemiological (the incidence, distribution, and control of disease in a population) principles in public health nursing practice**
   A. Understands the relationship between community assessment and health department programs, especially the populations and programs with which the PHN works
   B. Understands the relationships between risk/protective factors and health issues
   C. Obtains and interprets information regarding risks and benefits to the community
   D. Applies epidemiological triangle (host, agent, environment) when assessing and intervening with communities, systems, individuals and families

CORNERSTONE

Public health nursing practice collaborates with community resources to achieve those strategies… but can and will work alone if necessary

3. **Utilizes collaboration to achieve public health goals**
   A. Demonstrates effective participation on interdisciplinary teams (contributes, are prepared, bring things back)
   B. Develops relationships and builds partnerships with communities, systems, individuals and families
   C. Utilizes community assets to empower communities, systems, individuals and families

4. **Works within the responsibility and authority of the governmental public health system**
   A. Describes the relationship among the federal, state, and local levels of public health system
   B. Identifies the individual's and organization's responsibilities within the context of the Essential Public Health Services and Core Functions
   C. Recognizes that public health has statutory authority such as public health nuisance, quarantine, and commitment
   D. Differentiates the public health model from medical model
   E. Understands the independent public health nursing role as described in the Scope and Standards of Public Health Nursing
   F. Describes the role of government in the delivery of community health services
   G. Aware of components of health care system
      1) Funding streams such as Medicare, Medicaid, PMAP, categorical grants
      2) Programs utilized by local health departments, such as WIC, home visiting
      3) Community resources
   H. Understands legal issues such as data privacy and mandated reporting

CORNERSTONE

The authority for the independent practice of public health nursing emanates from the Nurse Practice Act.

5. Practices within the auspices of the Nurse Practice Act
A. Understands the scope of nursing practice (independent nursing functions and delegated medical functions)
B. Establishes appropriate professional boundaries
C. Maintains confidentiality
D. Demonstrates ethical, legal and professional accountability
E. Delegates and supervises other personnel
F. Understands the role of a public health nurse as described under public health nursing registration

ALL CORNERSTONES

6. Effectively communicates with communities, systems, individuals, families and colleagues
A. Interacts respectfully, sensitively and effectively with everyone
B. Presents accurate demographic, statistical, programmatic, and scientific information
C. Selects appropriate communication methods, such as audiovisual, technological, multi-media tools
D. Organizes written materials that are clear, concise, accurate, and complete
E. Utilizes sound teaching/learning principles that consider specific characteristics of the community, system, individual or family
F. Communicates electronically utilizing basic word processing, Internet, email, Netiquette, attachments, and Web-based systems

PHN CHARACTERISTICS & VALUES

CORNERSTONE

Public Health Nursing Practice establishes caring relationships with the communities, systems, individuals and families that comprise the populations PHNs serve

7. **Establishes and maintains caring relationships with communities, systems, individuals, and families**
   A. Demonstrates trust, respect, empathy
   B. Follows through with commitments
   C. Maintains appropriate boundaries
   D. Demonstrates tact and diplomacy
   E. Seeks assistance when needed in managing relationships

CORNERSTONE

Public Health Nursing Practice is grounded in social justice, compassion, and sensitivity to diversity, and respect for the worth of all people, especially the vulnerable

8. **Shows evidence of commitment to social justice, the greater good, and the public health principles**
   A. Differentiates between social justice and market justice
   B. Applies principles of social justice to promote and maintain the health and well-being of populations
   C. Advocates for the populations for which the PHN is accountable

9. **Demonstrates nonjudgmental/unconditional acceptance of people different from self**
   A. Listens to others in an unbiased manner
   B. Respects points of view of others
   C. Promotes the expression of diverse opinions and perspectives *(encourages involvement of diverse populations)*
   D. Identifies the role of cultural, social, spiritual, religious, and behavioral factors when selecting or designing public health interventions
   E. Interacts respectfully, sensitively and effectively with persons from diverse cultural, socioeconomic, educational, racial, ethnic, gender, sexual orientation, religious backgrounds, health status, age, and lifestyle preferences

CORNERSTONE

Public Health Nursing Practice encompasses the mental, physical, emotional, social, spiritual, and environmental aspects of health

10. Incorporates mental, physical, emotional, social, spiritual, and environmental aspects of health into assessment, planning, implementation, and evaluation

   A. Assesses mental, physical, emotional, social, spiritual, and environmental health of communities, systems, individuals and families

   B. Develops intervention plans that consider the mental, physical, emotional, social, spiritual, and environmental health of communities, systems, individuals and families

   C. Implements interventions that improve the mental, physical, emotional, social, spiritual, and environmental health of communities, systems, individuals and families

   D. Evaluates the impact of public health nursing interventions on the mental, physical, emotional, social, spiritual, and environmental health of communities, systems, individuals and families

ALL CORNERSTONES

11. Demonstrates leadership in public health nursing with communities, systems, individuals and families

   A. Seeks learning opportunities

   B. Works independently; autonomous in practice

   C. Willing to work in an unstructured environment, tolerates ambiguity

   D. Seeks consultation and support   (reality check, end of rope phenomenon)

   E. Takes initiative; is a self-starter

   F. Adapts to change

   G. Is willing and able to respond to population needs

   H. Demonstrates flexibility

   I. Contributes to team efforts

   J. Prioritizes and organizes workload, time, materials and resources

March 2003
Developed by the Henry Street Consortium
*Linking Public Health Nursing Practice and
Education To Promote Population Health*
http://www.health.state.mn.us/divs/chs/phn/partnerships.html

APPENDIX

Personal characteristics that contribute to effective practice
1. Passion
2. Creativity
3. Courage
4. Confidence
5. Adaptability
6. Humor
7. Persistence
8. Independent
9. Positive attitude
10. Life long learner
11. Risk taker
12. Hard worker
13. Leader
14. Resourceful
15. Flexibility
16. Caring
17. Compassion
18. Self-care

Basic public health nursing knowledge base:
1. Human Growth & Development across the lifespan: prenatal, infancy, preschool, school-age, adolescent, adult, elderly
2. Family development
3. Antepartum/Postpartum
4. Parenting
5. Health promotion: infant, pre-school, school-age, adolescent, women, men, elderly
6. Chronic disease prevention and management
7. Injury prevention
8. Violence prevention
9. Chemical health issues and/or behaviors
10. Mental Health
11. Death and dying; grief and loss
12. Human sexuality
13. Family planning
14. Nutrition
15. Disaster and bioterrorism response
16. Disease prevention and control, including universal precautions
17. Immunizations across the lifespan
18. Environmental Health and Safety
19. Technical Nursing Skills
20. Medication administration/management
21. Health determinants
22. Social and market justice

Comparison of Henry Street Entry-Level PHN Competencies to Other Public Health Practice Frameworks

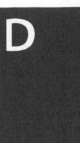

D

Entry-Level Population-Based PHN Competencies Henry Street Consortium, 2003 *11 Competencies*	Core Competencies for Public Health Professionals Council on Linkages, 2001; QUAD Council [ANA, APHA, ACHNE, ASTDN] Competencies, 2003 *18 Domains*	Scope and Standards of Public Health Nursing American Nurses Association, 2007 *6 Standards of Care; 8 Standards of Professional Performance*	Essential Public Health Services Core Public Health Functions Steering Committee, 1994 *10 Core Functions*
#1 Applies the public health nursing process to communities, systems, individuals, and families	• Analytic/Assessment Skills • Policy Development and Program Planning Skills • Cultural Competency Skills • Community Dimensions of Practice Skills	*Standards of Care* Assessment; Diagnosis; Outcome Identification; Planning; Assurance; Evaluation	• Monitor Health • Diagnose and Investigate • Inform, Educate, and Empower • Link to/Provide Care • Evaluate • System Management and Research
#2 Utilizes basic epidemiological principles (the incidence, distribution, and control of disease in a population) in public health nursing practice	• Analytic/Assessment Skills • Community Dimensions of Practice Skills • Basic Public Health Sciences Skills	*Standards of Care* Assessment; Diagnosis; Outcome Identification; Planning; Assurance; Evaluation	• Diagnose and Investigate

Entry-Level Population-Based PHN Competencies Henry Street Consortium, 2003 *11 Competencies*	Core Competencies for Public Health Professionals Council on Linkages, 2001; QUAD Council [ANA, APHA, ACHNE, ASTDN] Competencies, 2003 *18 Domains*	Scope and Standards of Public Health Nursing American Nurses Association, 2007 *6 Standards of Care; 8 Standards of Professional Performance*	Essential Public Health Services Core Public Health Functions Steering Committee, 1994 *10 Core Functions*
#3 Utilizes collaboration to achieve public health goals	• Communication Skills • Leadership and Systems Thinking Skills	Collaboration Collegiality	• Mobilize Community Partnerships • Link to/Provide Care
#4 Works within the responsibility and authority of the governmental public health system	• Policy Development and Program Planning Skills • Cultural Competency Skills • Community Dimensions of Practice Skills • Financial Planning and Management Skills • Leadership and Systems Thinking Skills	Quality of Care Performance Appraisal Resource Utilization	• Develop Policies • Enforce Laws
#5 Practices public health nursing within the auspices of the Nurse Practice Act	• Analytic/Assessment Skills • Policy Development and Program Planning Skills • Community Dimensions of Practice Skills	*Standards of Care* Assessment; Diagnosis; Outcome Identification; Planning; Assurance; Evaluation	• Assure Competent Workforce
#6 Effectively communicates with communities, systems, individuals, families and colleagues	• Communication Skills • Cultural Competency Skills • Financial Planning and Management Skills	Education	• Link to/Provide Care

Entry-Level Population-Based PHN Competencies Henry Street Consortium, 2003 *11 Competencies*	Core Competencies for Public Health Professionals Council on Linkages, 2001; QUAD Council [ANA, APHA, ACHNE, ASTDN] Competencies, 2003 *18 Domains*	Scope and Standards of Public Health Nursing American Nurses Association, 2007 *6 Standards of Care; 8 Standards of Professional Performance*	Essential Public Health Services Core Public Health Functions Steering Committee, 1994 *10 Core Functions*
#7 Establishes and maintains caring relationships with communities, systems, individuals, and families	• Communication Skills • Cultural Competency Skill • Leadership and Systems Thinking Skills	Quality of care Education Ethics	• Inform, Educate, and Empower • Mobilize Community Partnerships • Link to/Provide Care
#8 Shows evidence of commitment to social justice, the greater good, and the public health principles	• Analytic/Assessment Skills • Communication Skills • Leadership and Systems Thinking Skills	Quality of Care Ethics	• Inform, Educate, and Empower • Mobilize Community Partnerships • Develop Policies
#9 Demonstrates nonjudgmental and unconditional acceptance of people different from self	• Communication Skills • Cultural Competency Skills • Leadership and Systems Thinking Skills	Ethics	• Inform, Educate, and Empower • Mobilize Community Partnerships
#10 Incorporates mental, physical, emotional, social, spiritual, and environmental aspects of health into assessment, planning, implementation, and evaluation	• Analytic/Assessment Skills • Cultural Competency Skills	*Standards of Care* Assessment; Diagnosis; Outcome Identification; Planning; Assurance; Evaluation	• Inform, Educate, and Empower • Link to/Provide Care

Entry-Level Population-Based PHN Competencies Henry Street Consortium, 2003 *11 Competencies*	Core Competencies for Public Health Professionals Council on Linkages, 2001; QUAD Council [ANA, APHA, ACHNE, ASTDN] Competencies, 2003 *18 Domains*	Scope and Standards of Public Health Nursing American Nurses Association, 2007 *6 Standards of Care; 8 Standards of Professional Performance*	Essential Public Health Services Core Public Health Functions Steering Committee, 1994 *10 Core Functions*
#11 Demonstrates leadership	• Policy Development and Program Planning Skills • Communication Skills • Community Dimensions of Practice Skills • Financial Planning and Management Skills • Leadership and Systems Thinking Skills	Quality of Care Performance Appraisal Education Collegiality Ethics Collaboration Resource Utilization	• Mobilize Community Partnerships • Develop Policies • Assure Competent Workforce

Index

L